Congenital and Structural Heart Disease

Editors

DAMIEN KENNY

ZIYAD M. HIJAZI

INTERVENTIONAL CARDIOLOGY CLINICS

www.interventional.theclinics.com

Consulting Editors
SAMIN K. SHARMA
IGOR F. PALACIOS

January 2013 • Volume 2 • Number 1

ELSEVIER

1600 John F. Kennedy Boulevard • Suite 1800 • Philadelphia, Pennsylvania 19103-2899

http://www.theclinics.com

INTERVENTIONAL CARDIOLOGY CLINICS Volume 2, Number 1
January 2013 ISSN 2211-7458, ISBN-13: 978-1-4557-7108-0

Editor: Barbara Cohen-Kligerman
Developmental Editor: Teia Stone

Interventional Cardiology Clinics (ISSN 2211-7458) is published quarterly by Elsevier Inc., 360 Park Avenue South, New York, NY 10010-1710. Months of issue are January, April, July, and October. Subscription prices are USD 188 per year for US individuals, USD 126 per year for US students, USD 281 per year for Canadian individuals, USD 144 per year for Canadian students, USD 281 per year for international individuals, and USD 144 per year for international students. To receive student/resident rate, orders must be accompanied by name of affiliated institution, date of term, and the *signature* of program/residency coordinator on institution letterhead. Orders will be billed at individual rate until proof of status is received. Foreign air speed delivery is included in all *Clinics* subscription prices. All prices are subject to change without notice. **POSTMASTER:** Send address changes to *Interventional Cardiology Clinics*, Elsevier Health Sciences Division, Subscription Customer Service, 3251 Riverport Lane, Maryland Heights, MO 63043. **Customer Service: Telephone: 1-800-654-2452** (U.S. and Canada); **1-314-447-8871** (outside U.S. and Canada). **Fax: 1-314-447-8029. E-mail: journalscustomerservice-usa@elsevier.com** (for print support); **journalsonlinesupport-usa@elsevier.com** (for online support).

Reprints. For copies of 100 or more of articles in this publication, please contact the Commercial Reprints Department, Elsevier Inc., 360 Park Avenue South, New York, NY 10010-1710. Tel.: 212-633-3812; Fax: 212-462-1935; E-mail: reprints@elsevier.com.

Printed and bound by CPI Group (UK) Ltd, Croydon, CR0 4YY

Transferred to digital print 2012

Contributors

CONSULTING EDITORS

SAMIN K. SHARMA, MD, FSCAI, FACC
Director of Clinical Cardiology; Director of
Cardiac Catheterization Laboratory, Mount
Sinai Medical Center, New York, New York

IGOR F. PALACIOS, MD, FSCAI
Director of Interventional Cardiology,
Cardiology Division, Heart Center,
Massachusetts General Hospital; Associate
Professor of Medicine, Harvard Medical
School, Boston, Massachusetts

EDITORS

DAMIEN KENNY, MB, MD, MRCPCH
Assistant Professor of Pediatrics and Director
of Heart Failure; Associate Director of the
Cardiac Catheterization Hybrid Suite, Rush
Center for Congenital and Structural Heart
Disease, Rush University Medical Center,
Chicago, Illinois

**ZIYAD M. HIJAZI, MD, MPH, FSCAI,
FACC, FAAP**
Professor of Pediatrics and Internal Medicine;
University Chair, Director and Section Chief,
Pediatric Cardiology, Rush Center for
Congenital & Structural Heart Disease, Rush
University Medical Center, Chicago, Illinois

AUTHORS

MAZENI ALWI, MBBS, MRCP
Department of Paediatric Cardiology, Institut
Jantung Negara (National Heart Institute),
Kuala Lumpur, Malaysia

LEE N. BENSON, MD, FRCPC, FACC, FSCAI
Division of Cardiology, Department of
Pediatrics, The Labatt Family Heart Center,
The Hospital for Sick Children, University of
Toronto School of Medicine, Toronto, Ontario,
Canada

ELCHANAN BRUCKHEIMER, MBBS
Director, Pediatric Cardiac Catheterization,
Schneider Children's Medical Center Israel,
Petach Tikva, Israel

GIANFRANCO BUTERA, MD, PhD
Pediatric Cardiology and GUCH Unit,
Policlinico San Donato IRCCS, San Donato
Milanese, Italy

MARIO CARMINATI, MD
Pediatric Cardiology and GUCH Unit,
Policlinico San Donato IRCCS, San Donato
Milanese, Italy

FRANCESCO CASILLI, MD
Emodinamica e Radiologia Cardiovascolare,
Policlinico San Donato, San Donato Milanese,
Italy

**JOHN P. CHEATHAM, MD, FAAP, FACC,
FSCAI**
Director, Cardiac Catheterization and
Interventional Therapy; Professor, Pediatrics
and Internal Medicine, Cardiology Division, The
Heart Center, Nationwide Children's Hospital,
The Ohio State University, Columbus, Ohio

MASSIMO CHESSA, MD, PhD
Pediatric Cardiology and GUCH Unit,
Policlinico San Donato IRCCS, San Donato
Milanese, Italy

TED FELDMAN, MD, FESC, FACC, FSCAI
NorthShore University HealthSystem,
Evanston, Illinois

MARK HAMILTON, MRCP, FRCR
Department of Radiology, Bristol Heart
Institute, Bristol, United Kingdom

**ZIYAD M. HIJAZI, MD, MPH, FSCAI,
FACC, FAAP**
Professor of Pediatrics and Internal Medicine;
University Chair, Director and Section Chief,
Pediatric Cardiology, Rush Center for
Congenital and Structural Heart Disease,
Rush University Medical Center, Chicago,
Illinois

RALF J. HOLZER, MD, MSc, FSCAI
Assistant Director, Cardiac Catheterization
and Interventional Therapy; Associate
Professor of Pediatrics, Division of
Cardiology, The Heart Center, Nationwide
Children's Hospital, The Ohio State University,
Columbus, Ohio

ERIC M. HORLICK, MD, CM, FRCPC
Division of Cardiology, Department of
Medicine, Toronto General Hospital, University
Health Network, University of Toronto School
of Medicine, Toronto, Ontario, Canada

FRANK F. ING, MD
Director, Cardiac Catheterization Laboratory;
Associate Chief, Pediatric Cardiology,
Children's Hospital Los Angeles; Clinical
Professor of Pediatrics, University of Southern
California, Los Angeles, California

IGNACIO INGLESSIS, MD
Director of Adult Congenital Interventions,
Interventional Cardiology, Massachusetts
General Hospital; Assistant Professor of
Medicine, Harvard Medical School, Boston,
Massachusetts

SAIBAL KAR, MD, FACC, FSCAI
Associate Professor of Medicine and Director,
Interventional Cardiac Research, Heart
Institute, Cedars Sinai Medical Center,
UCLA, Los Angeles, California

DAMIEN KENNY, MB, MD, MRCPCH
Assistant Professor of Pediatrics and Director
of Heart Failure; Associate Director of the
Cardiac Catheterization Hybrid Suite, Rush
Center for Congenital and Structural Heart
Disease, Rush University Medical Center,
Chicago, Illinois

ASRA KHAN, MD
Assistant Professor of Pediatrics, Baylor
College of Medicine, Houston, Texas

AMEYA KULKARNI, MD
Clinical Research Fellow, Interventional
Cardiology, Massachusetts General Hospital,
Harvard Medical School, Boston,
Massachusetts

**ROBIN P. MARTIN, MB ChB, FRCP,
FRCPCH**
Bristol Heart Institute, Bristol, United Kingdom

MARHISHAM CHE MOOD, MD
Department of Paediatric Cardiology, Institut
Jantung Negara (National Heart Institute),
Kuala Lumpur, Malaysia

GARETH J. MORGAN, MPhil, MRCPCH
Bristol Heart Institute, Bristol, United Kingdom

CHRISTIAN NAGY, MD
Division of Cardiology, Department of
Medicine, Toronto General Hospital, University
Health Network, University of Toronto School
of Medicine, Toronto, Ontario, Canada

MAMOO NAKAMURA, MD
Heart Institute, Cedars Sinai Medical Center,
Los Angeles, California

EUSTAQUIO ONORATO, MD, FSCAI
Unità di Cardiologia Invasiva, Clinica
Montevergine, Avellino, Italy; Cardiovascular
Department, Humanitas Gavazzeni,
Bergamo, Italy

MARK D. OSTEN, MD
Division of Cardiology, Department of
Medicine, Toronto General Hospital, University
Health Network, University of Toronto School
of Medicine, Toronto, Ontario, Canada

CARLOS AUGUSTO CARDOSO PEDRA, MD, PhD
Director, Catheterization Laboratory for Congenital Heart Disease, Instituto Dante Pazzanese de Cardiología; Co-director, Catheterization Laboratory for Congenital Heart Disease, Hospital do Coração, Sao Paulo, Brazil

SIMONE FONTES PEDRA, MD, PhD
Director, Echocardiography Laboratory for Congenital Heart Disease, Instituto Dante Pazzanese de Cardiología; Director, Cardiac Fetal Unit, Hospital do Coração da Associação Sanatório Sírio, Sao Paulo, Brazil

ALEJANDRO ROMÁN PEIRONE, MD, FSCAI
Director, Pediatric Cardiology Section, Hospital Privado de Córdoba, Córdoba, Argentina

C. FABIO PERALTA, MD, PhD
Director, Fetal Medicine Program, Hospital do Coração da Associação Sanatório Sírio, Sao Paulo, Brazil

ALICE PERLOWSKI, MD
University of Chicago Hospital, Chicago, Illinois

LUCIANE PIAZZA, MD
Pediatric Cardiology and GUCH Unit, Policlinico San Donato IRCCS, San Donato Milanese, Italy

ANTONIO SARACINO, MD
Pediatric Cardiology and GUCH Unit, Policlinico San Donato IRCCS, San Donato Milanese, Italy

HARSIMRAN S. SINGH, MD, MSc
Division of Cardiology, Department of Medicine, New York Presbyterian Hospital, Weill Cornell Medical College, New York, New York; Division of Cardiology, Department of Medicine, Toronto General Hospital, University Health Network, University of Toronto School of Medicine, Toronto, Ontario, Canada

MARK S. TURNER, PhD, FRCP
Bristol Heart Institute, Bristol, United Kingdom

ANDREA W. WAN, MD, FRCPC
Division of Cardiology, Department of Pediatrics, The Labatt Family Heart Center, The Hospital for Sick Children, University of Toronto School of Medicine, Toronto, Ontario, Canada

Contents

> Fetal interventions for congenital heart disease have become important treatment modalities in the past 10 to 15 years. The basic hypothesis has been that a prenatal intervention may remodel cardiac morphology and function to such an extent that it may favorably alter the in utero natural history, resulting in improved prenatal and postnatal outcomes, including an increased likelihood of achieving biventricular circulation. This review discusses the current indications, techniques, and outcomes of fetal cardiac interventions and provides a glimpse into the future with regard to technical improvements and newer treatment modalities, such as maternal oxygenation and in utero pacemaker implantation.

> Percutaneous neonatal cardiac interventions are effective in management strategies. Aortic valve dilation has become a first line therapy with excellent outcomes and low morbidity equivalent to surgery. Percutaneous intervention for coarctation of the aorta can safely postpone surgical intervention in small unwell neonates, allowing stabilization and growth. Stent implantation can provide a stable and predictable relief of obstruction; however, care should be taken to implant stents so that they can be removed subsequently. As experience increases, the role of percutaneous techniques in the management of high-risk neonates with coarctation of the aorta will become better defined and improve the outcomes.

> Hybrid therapies have increased and offer a valuable alternative to standard catheter or surgical therapies in selected patient. These hybrid therapies often combine the best of both techniques, in particular for ventricular septal defect closure and intraoperative pulmonary artery stent placement. For patients with hypoplastic left heart syndrome, the hybrid approach is an important alternative therapeutic strategy, providing similar results to conventional Norwood-type palliation. Further studies are needed and are underway to evaluate the neurodevelopmental outcome in these patients.

> Ostium secundum–type atrial septal defect closure has evolved from a surgical procedure requiring cardiopulmonary bypass to a percutaneous, catheter-based procedure usually requiring only an overnight hospital stay. The overall safety and

effectiveness has compared favorably with surgical repair. Although rare, complications have been described, including erosion, device embolization, or malfunction and arrhythmias. The overall long-term clinical outcomes have been excellent: good quality of life, functional class improvement, and ventricular remodeling have been the rule after the procedure. It is mandatory to recommend indefinite follow-up of patients undergoing this procedure for potential long-term complications.

Patent foramen ovale (PFO) is considered a risk factor for serious clinical syndromes, the most important of which is cryptogenic stroke in the setting of paradoxic embolism. The safety and feasibility of transcatheter PFO closure have been addressed in several studies; this procedure is performed worldwide with excellent results. Variations in the atrial septal configuration and PFO are frequent and have an impact on the technical aspects and success in transcatheter PFO closure. To minimize the rate of complications of percutaneous closure of PFO, patients must be carefully selected on the basis of morphology and location of the interatrial defect.

Isolated perimembranous ventricular septal defect (VSD) is the most common congenital heart defect (after bicuspid aortic valve). Surgery is considered the gold standard for the treatment of these VSDs. However, it is associated with morbidity and mortality. Less invasive techniques have been developed, and percutaneous closure of perimembranous VSDs is now considered a possible alternative to the standard surgical approach. The main problem associated with transcatheter closure of VSD is the occurrence of complete atrioventricular block and need for pacemaker implantation. Improvements in technology and design will help to reduce the occurrence of this problem in the near future.

Stenting of patent ductus arteriosus (PDA) is an attractive alternative to the surgical aortopulmonary shunt in the palliation of cyanotic congenital heart disease. However, the diverse morphology of PDA in this setting limits its role, as stenting an overly tortuous duct may not be feasible, and in a significant number of patients, ductus-related pulmonary artery stenosis contraindicates this procedure. The major acute complications are stent migration, thrombosis, and cardiac failure. Early failure of palliation caused by in-stent stenosis is another limitation of this procedure.

The narrowing of the lumen in coarctation of the aorta can be relieved with a high degree of immediate success by transcatheter methods. All methods are associated with immediate and longer-term complications, including dissection, aneurysm formation, and recoarctation. The introduction of the use of covered stents in aortic coarctation is encouraging because the material cover provides additional protection to the acutely disrupted aortic wall and can provide long-term protection of the dilated segment and the downstream area of poststenotic dilation. This review discusses the currently available options for stenting aortic coarctation.

Pulmonary artery (PA) stenosis represents a heterogeneous defect with a wide morphology and etiology. Interventions to treat PA stenosis should be based on the location, severity, and cause of stenosis as well as the size of the patient at presentation. Specialized dilation balloons, stents, and delivery techniques have been developed to treat a variety of PA stenoses in small infants through adulthood. Early and intermediate results of angioplasty and stenting are superior to surgical results, while long-term data on angioplasty and stenting are becoming available for these proven safe and effective techniques.

We describe 3 distinct ACHD lesions amenable to percutaneous repair: (1) venous baffle obstruction in transposition of the great arteries, (2) coronary artery fistulas, and (3) ruptured sinus of Valsalva aneurysms. For each entity, we chronicle the typical clinical scenario and indications for intervention to supplement the technical approach and potential pitfalls with treatment.

Percutaneous transcatheter device closure for post-myocardial infarction ventricular septal defect is a feasible alternative to open surgical patch repair. Patient selection, imaging, timing of intervention, technique, and results are discussed.

Although established, transcatheter pulmonary valve replacement is in its infancy compared with surgical pulmonary valve replacement. Extended clinical experience and follow-up have identified new challenges; however, careful evaluation of data through clinical trials has facilitated effective evolution of responses to these challenges. The limited patient population has resulted in less interest in new valve design, but having been the older sibling to transcatheter aortic valve replacement, transcatheter pulmonary valve replacement is likely to benefit in the future from design modifications to the more popular and commercially viable transcatheter aortic valve revolution. Improving valve longevity and applying the technology to native outflow tracts remain the short-to-medium term goals.

Pulmonary vein stenosis (PVS) is a known complication of pulmonary vein isolation in the treatment of atrial fibrillation. Patients with PVS can present with a great variety of symptoms. Clinicians should have a low threshold to evaluate for this potentially morbid and treatable condition. PVS can be treated by stenting affected pulmonary veins via transseptal access to the left atrium and use of bare metal biliary stents.

Percutaneous interventions for mitral valve disease represent both the oldest and the newest of catheter interventions. Balloon mitral valvuloplasty was among the first effective catheter therapies for valvular heart disease. The technique and device approach was initially reported by Inoue in 1982 and, remarkably, is virtually unchanged between then and now. Conversely, novel catheter therapies to repair mitral regurgitation are now in their infancy, with only the earliest human experience. This article details the spectrum of these therapies.

The left atrial appendage is a primary source of thrombi in patients with nonvalvular atrial fibrillation. Transcatheter left atrial appendage occlusion/exclusion is a novel technology with the potential as an alternative approach for lifelong anticoagulation to prevent potential catastrophic embolic stroke. This article discusses important evaluation, procedural steps, and the clinical data for left atrial appendage closure.

INTERVENTIONAL CARDIOLOGY CLINICS

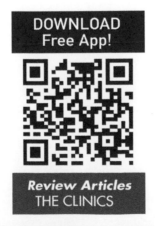

DOWNLOAD Free App!

Review Articles
THE CLINICS

NOW AVAILABLE FOR YOUR iPhone and iPad

Preface
Congenital and Structural Heart Disease

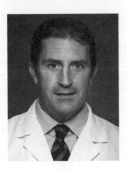 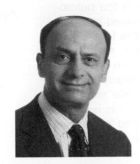

Damien Kenny, MB, MD, MRCPCH   Ziyad M. Hijazi, MD, MPH, FSCAI, FACC, FAAP
Editors

With increasing demand for less invasive strategies to deal with growing numbers of patients with congenital and structural heart disease, transcatheter interventional approaches have grown exponentially to meet patient expectations.

With the development of low-profile balloons and stents, interventions on small infants with stenotic valves (balloon valvuloplasty) and/or inadequate pulmonary or systemic blood flow (ductal stenting) are now commonly practiced. Indeed, some of these interventions are carried out in fetal life in an attempt to arrest the progressive structural changes that may lead to hypoplastic right or left heart.

In patients of all ages transcatheter approaches may be limited by access issues, with the delivery of occlusion devices or stents requiring relatively large delivery sheaths that are not maneuverable around the curves of the heart. Thus, surgeons and interventionalists are now working together through "hybrid" procedures, including perventricular ventricular septal defect (VSD) closure to optimize outcomes with minimal trauma to the heart.

Some challenges remain, including a viable device for transcatheter closure of perimembranous VSDs. Other approaches are evolving, including transcatheter pulmonary valve replacement, and battlegrounds lie in ensuring the optimal approach for the patient is supported by accurate data and consideration of economics rather than on the opinion of the surgeon or interventionalist. Some conditions continue to haunt us, including transcatheter closure of postinfarct VSDs, with suboptimal outcomes despite various strategies.

Transcatheter interventions for other structural heart lesions are also covered in this issue of *Interventional Cardiology Clinics*, including

Intervent Cardiol Clin 2 (2013) xiii–xiv
http://dx.doi.org/10.1016/j.iccl.2012.10.001
2211-7458/13/$ – see front matter

percutaneous mitral valve interventions, advances with transcatheter occlusion of the left atrial appendage, and pulmonary vein stenting for acquired pulmonary vein stenosis. Novel and up-to-date approaches to more established congenital heart lesions such as atrial and ventricular septal defects, as well as stenting of the pulmonary arteries and aorta, are also covered in detail.

We are very fortunate to have the input from world-renowned experts in their respective fields and many of our contributors are true innovators developing and driving many of the approaches you will read about. We sincerely hope you will learn from and enjoy this issue of *Interventional Cardiology Clinics* and hope that it will add to your clinical practice in a meaningful way.

Damien Kenny, MB, MD, MRCPCH
Rush Center for Congenital and
Structural Heart Disease
Rush University Medical Center
1653 W. Congress Parkway
Chicago, IL 60612, USA

Ziyad M. Hijazi, MD, MPH, FSCAI, FACC, FAAP
Pediatric Cardiology
Rush Center for Congenital &
Structural Heart Disease
Rush University Medical Center
Suite 770 Jones, 1653 W. Congress Parkway
Chicago, IL 60612, USA

E-mail addresses:
Damien_Kenny@rush.edu (D. Kenny)
Ziyad_Hijazi@rush.edu (Z.M. Hijazi)

Future Directions of Fetal Interventions in Congenital Heart Disease

Simone Fontes Pedra, MD, PhD[a], C. Fabio Peralta, MD, PhD[b],
Carlos Augusto Cardoso Pedra, MD, PhD[a,c,*]

KEYWORDS

- Fetal Medicine • Interventions • Congenital heart disease • Echocardiography

KEY POINTS

- Fetal interventions for congenital heart disease have become an important treatment modality with well-established indications, such as aortic stenosis and evolving hypoplastic left heart syndrome (HLHS), HLHS with intact or highly restrictive interatrial septum, and pulmonary atresia or critical pulmonary stenosis with intact ventricular septum and evolving hypoplastic right heart syndrome.
- Fetal interventions should be performed by a well-trained multidisciplinary team at a referral center with a large number of patients and an institutional commitment to support a fully developed fetal cardiac program.
- The technique has been standardized with catheters being inserted through needles that are advanced across the maternal abdomen and the fetal heart in anesthetized patients.
- These procedures may alter the natural history of such diseases, resulting in improved postnatal outcomes measured by better clinical stability, survival, and achievement of a biventricular circulation.
- Expansion of indications, better imaging and catheter technologies, and introduction of new forms of therapy are expected in the near future.

 Videos of fetal position; fetal anesthesia; pulmonary valvuloplasty; aortic valvuloplasty; and pericardial drainage accompany this article at http://www.interventional.theclinics.com/

INTRODUCTION: NATURE OF THE PROBLEM

Fetal aortic valvuloplasty was first reported by Maxwell and colleagues in 1990 in the United Kingdom.[1] Initial worldwide experience with this procedure showed disappointing results.[2] With better patient selection and evolving catheter and imaging technologies, however, fetal interventions have become an important therapeutic modality in the past 10 to 15 years for some forms of congenital heart disease (CHD).[3–16] These include aortic stenosis (AS) and evolving hypoplastic left heart syndrome (HLHS), HLHS with intact or highly restrictive interatrial septum (IAS), and pulmonary atresia (PA) or critical pulmonary stenosis (CPS) with intact ventricular septum (IVS) and evolving hypoplastic right heart syndrome (HRHS). The basic hypothesis behind these procedures has been that a prenatal intervention may remodel cardiac morphology and function to such an extent that they may favorably alter the in utero natural history,

[a] Echocardiograhy Laboratory for Congenital Heart Disease, Instituto Dante Pazzanese de Cardiologia, Av Dante Pazzanese 500, 14o andar, Sao Paulo 04012-180, Brazil; [b] Fetal Medicine Program, Hospital do Coração da Associação Sanatório Sírio, Rua Desembargador Eliseu Guilherme 147, CEP: 04003-905, São Paulo, Brazil; [c] Catheterization Laboratory for Congenital Heart Disease, Hospital do Coração, Sao Paulo, Brazil
* Corresponding author. Catheterization Laboratory for Congenital Heart Disease, Instituto Dante Pazzanese de Cardiologia, Av Dante Pazzanese 500, 14o andar, Sao Paulo 04012-180, Brazil.
E-mail address: cacpedra@uol.com.br

Intervent Cardiol Clin 2 (2013) 1–10
http://dx.doi.org/10.1016/j.iccl.2012.09.005

resulting in improved prenatal and postnatal outcomes, including an increased likelihood of achieving a biventricular (BV) circulation. Although there are many case reports and case series encountered in the literature of successful fetal cardiac interventions,[3–16] some may consider these procedures still experimental because they are routinely performed in only a few selected centers in the world. Although this is true, data in the literature support our belief that they are reproducible, safe, and effective in different hands, with well-established and acceptable outcomes.

The aim of this review was to discuss the indications and technical aspects of these procedures and pregnancy and postnatal outcomes. Also, a snapshot of our own experience at a referral cardiology institution in Brazil will be presented whenever possible.

RELEVANT ANATOMY AND PREPROCEDURE PLANNING

The indications for fetal interventions for CHD are as follows:

1. Critical AS and evolving HLHS.[3–9]
   a. AS should be the dominant lesion with no additional major cardiac or extracardiac malformations. The diagnosis is based on echocardiographic visualization of a thickened, immobile aortic valve with turbulent or decreased color Doppler flow. The Doppler-derived gradient can be misleading because of frequently associated left ventricular (LV) dysfunction and endocardial fibroelastosis (EFE).
   b. The LV diastolic length should be above the lower limit of normal (z-score > –2) at the time of diagnosis. Occasionally, aortic valvuloplasty is considered in smaller LVs (LV diastolic length z-score below –2), not only with the hope to avert LV hypoplasia but also to ameliorate LV function and promote antegrade flow across the aortic valve to theoretically improve cerebral and myocardial perfusion in prenatal and postnatal periods, respectively.
   c. All fetuses should demonstrate reversed blood flow in the transverse aortic arch (TAA), left-to-right flow across the IAS, monophasic mitral valve (MV) inflow, and severe LV dysfunction in midgestation.
   d. Fetal aortic valvuloplasty should be generally performed before 30 weeks' gestational age.
2. HLHS and intact or highly restrictive IAS.[10,11]
   a. All patients should have an unequivocal prenatal echocardiographic diagnosis of established HLHS with either an intact IAS or a tiny ($\leq$1 mm) patent foramen ovale (PFO) and prominent reverse flow in the pulmonary veins.
   b. Fetal atrial septoplasty should be performed between 26 and 32 weeks' gestation. Earlier interventions may be ineffective due to spontaneous closure of the newly created atrial septal defect (ASD).
3. PA/IVS or CPS/IVS with impending HRHS.[12–15]
   a. Fetuses are considered for pulmonary valvuloplasty when they have a prenatal echocardiographic diagnosis of PA/IVS or CPS/IVS with the following features[1]: membranous pulmonary atresia, with identifiable pulmonary valve (PV) leaflets or membrane, no or minimal systolic opening, and no or minimal color Doppler ultrasound flow across the PV[2]; an intact ventricular septum[3]; left-to-right shunting across a patent ductus arteriosus (PDA); and[4] right heart hypoplasia, with a tricuspid valve (TV) annulus z-score $\leq$2 and an identifiable but qualitatively small right ventricle (RV). No increase in the size of the RV over a period of 4 to 6 weeks may also be considered in the decision-making process.
   b. Cases with fetal diagnosis of major coronary-to-RV fistulas should be excluded.
   c. Pulmonary valvuloplasty should be performed between 28 and 29 weeks' gestation.
4. Critical AS, massive mitral regurgitation (MR), giant left atrium (LA), and fetal hydrops.[17,18]
   a. These form a unique and challenging subgroup of patients who have been described as such only recently. They usually have dilated LV and reversed flow in the TAA.
   b. Aortic valvuloplasty and atrial septoplasty can be attempted between 30 and 34 weeks' gestation as a "salvage" procedure to diminish the risk of fetal demise owing to conspicuous hydrops associated with pulmonary veins and RV compression.

Fetal cardiac interventions should be performed in centers with obstetrics backup.[16] Although special units have been designed and used for these procedures, they are usually conducted in the operating room (OR) by a multidisciplinary team.

The multidisciplinary team includes a fetal medicine specialist, a fetal/pediatric cardiologist, and an interventionalist. In our experience, the fetal cardiologist is responsible for patient selection and preprocedural and postprocedural echocardiographic assessment. The fetal medicine specialist conducts fetal positioning and anesthesia, and simultaneously controls the puncture needle and the ultrasound probe. The interventionalists (usually 2) handle the catheters and wires while the fetal medicine specialist holds onto the needle to keep its position during the procedure.

PREPARATION AND PATIENT POSITIONING

Although maternal general anesthesia has been used for fetal interventions,[3–16] we have performed them under maternal conscious sedation and regional spinal blockade conducted by an anesthesiologist.

Uterine contractions prophylaxis is recommended with maternal use of nifedipine (20 mg, 3 times a day, starting 12 hours before the procedure, with 2 additional doses after it is finished). Significant polihydramnios can be drained using a 15-cm-long 20-gauge Chiba needle (Cook Inc, Bloomington, IN) before starting the procedure.

Optimal fetal position for needle entry and proper alignment with the target structure should be achieved by manual external version, if needed (Video 1). Avoiding maternal general anesthesia keeps the fetus awake to "fight" with the ultrasound probe during external version performed by the fetal medicine specialist. This may be important to attain an optimal fetal position and minimize the need for laparotomy and uterus exposure, which is eschewed in our experience.

After optimal fetal position is attained, the fetus is anesthetized using a mixture of fentanyl (5–10 μg/kg), pancuronium (10 μg/kg), and atropine (20 μg/kg) given intramuscularly or in the umbilical cord (Video 2).

DESCRIPTION OF THE PROCEDURE

Cardiac access is obtained using techniques similar to those previously described and standardized by the Boston group.[3–8,10,11,15,16]

Under continuous 2-dimensional ultrasound guidance, a 15-cm-long 17-gauge to 19-gauge Chiba needle (with a stylet) is advanced through the maternal abdomen, uterine wall, and fetal chest wall and into the target cardiac chamber (LV, RV, or right atrium [RA]) (Videos 3 and 4). The imaging plane should be carefully adjusted to yield a picture in which both the entire needle length and the target cardiac chamber are included in the field of view.

Intracardiac epinephrine (1–10 μg/kg) may be given to avoid fetal bradycardia, especially for valvuloplasties. A premarked system (a rapid-exchange 6-mm-long to 10-mm-long coronary balloon premounted over a cutoff 0.014-inch floppy tip guide wire) is advanced to the desired location (Fig. 1). The LV or the RV is entered at the apex, with the

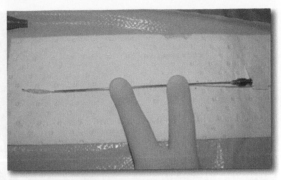

Fig. 1. Premarked system used to perform the fetal cardiac procedures. The wire is secured with a tape with its tip advancing 1 to 2 cm beyond the tip of the catheter balloon. The catheter balloon shaft is marked with a tape that abuts the hub of the needle when the system is advanced through it.

needle course parallel to the outflow track directed at the stenotic/atretic semilunar valves (see Videos 3 and 4). In this way, the valves should be crossed almost blindly, with minimal wire and catheter manipulation. Occasionally, a transplacentary and/or subcostal transhepatic needle course is required to reach the desired location depending on the placenta and fetal positions.

Balloons are inflated with pressure gauges to allow precise estimates of inflation diameters (10%–30% larger than the valve annulus if possible). Two to 4 inflations are performed depending on the fetal clinical status (Videos 4 and 5).

For atrial septoplasties, a 17-gauge Chiba needle with a greater internal lumen diameter may be used to accommodate the profile of larger dilating balloons (the largest possible, usually 4 mm, expandable to 4.5–4.7 mm). Although we have not attempted to implant stents in the IAS, this may be achieved by using special catheters specifically designed by the Boston group for fetal interventions.[11] The 17-gauge Chiba needle is advanced through the thin-walled RA in a perpendicular course toward the IAS. The same needle is used to perforate the IAS to gain access to the LA. Once the tip of the needle is seen in the body of the dilated LA, the premarked system is advanced until the tape mark on the catheter balloon shaft reaches the proximal hub of the Chiba needle. At this point, the whole system is brought back as a unit until the balloon straddles the IAS. The balloon is inflated with enough pressure to achieve the maximum balloon diameter under the bursting pressure limit (Fig. 2). A second puncture within the IAS may be performed using similar techniques if the newly created ASD is judged to be too small to relieve left atrial hypertension.

After the valves or the IAS are dilated, the whole system (needle + balloon + wire) is withdrawn as

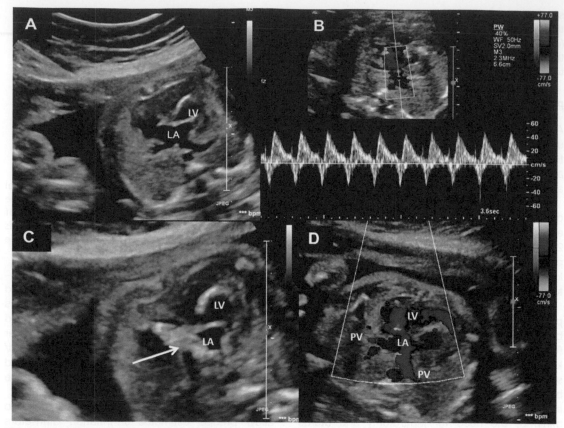

Fig. 2. Fetal atrial septostomy in a patient with hypoplastic left heart syndrome and restrictive atrial septal defect. Echocardiographic views. (*A*) The left atrium and the pulmonary veins are dilated. (*B*) Doppler pattern in the pulmonary vein showing bidirectional flow owing to a prominent A wave. (*C*) Balloon (*arrow*) inflated across the interatrial septum after transeptal puncture. (*D*) Immediate result after fetal atrial septostomy showing reduction in left atrial size and an unobstructed flow across the interatrial septum on color flow mapping (*red color*). LA, left atrium; LV, left ventricle; PV, pulmonary vein.

a unit through the fetal cardiac wall and out of the fetal and maternal bodies (Video 6). To avoid shearing off the balloon from the catheter shaft, no attempt to bring the balloon back into the needle lumen should be made.

After the intervention, small-volume-unit doses of epinephrine (1–10 μg/kg) and atropine should be available for immediate fetal intracardiac injection to treat hemodynamic instability owing to significant and persistent fetal bradycardia.[19] Also a new 20-gauge Chiba needle should be readily available for pericardial drainage in case of tamponade (Video 7).

IMMEDIATE POSTPROCEDURAL CARE, REHABILITATION, AND RECOVERY

A technically successful aortic or pulmonary valvuloplasty is defined as unequivocal evidence of antegrade flow and/or new aortic/pulmonary regurgitation (AR or PR) as assessed by color Doppler echocardiography (**Figs. 3 and 4**). In this regard, postprocedural AR improves significantly or disappears until birth for an unknown reason. It is well tolerated during fetal life owing to the low systemic vascular resistance determined by the placental circulation and high end-diastolic LV pressure secondary to severe LV dysfunction.

A technically successful atrial septoplasty is defined as the unequivocal presence of a newly created ASD at the conclusion of the intervention with significant improvement in the left to right shunt, associated with reduction in LA size and improvement in the pulmonary vein Doppler pattern on the following day. The ASD size is determined by measuring the width of the color jet (vena contracta) (see **Fig. 2**).

After the procedure, mothers are hospitalized overnight. Fetuses are assessed by ultrasound before planned maternal discharge. Patients can be followed at either the performing center or the referring institution. Echocardiography should be

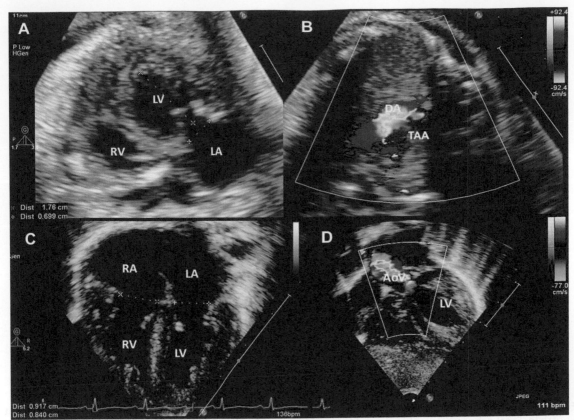

Fig. 3. Outcomes after fetal aortic valvuloplasty for critical aortic stenosis and evolving hypoplastic left heart syndrome. Fetal and neonatal echocardiographic views. (*A*) Measurements of the mitral valve annulus and left ventricular length in a 2-chamber view in fetal life. The left ventricle has a globular shape owing to severe systolic dysfunction. (*B*) Flow reversal in the fetal aortic arch as determined by color flow mapping (*red color*). (*C*) Four-chamber view in neonatal period showing adequate size left ventricle and mitral valve. (*D*) Subcostal long-axis view in the neonatal period showing flow acceleration across the aortic valve. The left ventricular function was normal, generating a 70 mm Hg gradient across the valve. A biventricular circulation was achieved after percutaneous transcarotid aortic valvuloplasty. AoV, aortic valve; DA, ductus arteriosus; LA, left atrium; LV, left ventricle; RA, right atrium; RV, right ventricle; TAA, transverse aortic arch.

performed at intervals determined by the primary fetal cardiologist.

It is recommended that these mothers should give birth at the referral institution with a fully developed neonatal cardiology program. Although these fetuses may be delivered transvaginally, we believe that a C-section poses less stress on such fragile patients. They should be immediately transferred to the neonatal intensive care unit and started on a prostaglandin drip.

Postnatal management varies with the underlying anatomy and the institution providing care, but generally includes percutaneous aortic valvuloplasty, Norwood or Norwood/Sano operation, bilateral pulmonary artery banding and ductal stenting through a median sternotomy (the so-called "hybrid approach"), atrial septostomy using a variety of techniques, surgical aortic valvuloplasty, surgical mitral valvuloplasty or replacement, and percutaneous pulmonary valvuloplasty ± ductal stenting.

CLINICAL RESULTS IN THE LITERATURE

The technical success and clinical outcomes after fetal cardiac interventions seem to be reproducible in different hands providing that such interventions are performed by a well-trained multidisciplinary team at a referral center with a large number of patients and an institutional commitment to support a fully developed fetal cardiac program.[3–16] Our preliminary experience on 19 interventions in 18 patients (unpublished submitted data) showed a high rate of technical success (18 of 19). One fetus underwent aortic valvuloplasty and ASD creation at the same setting.

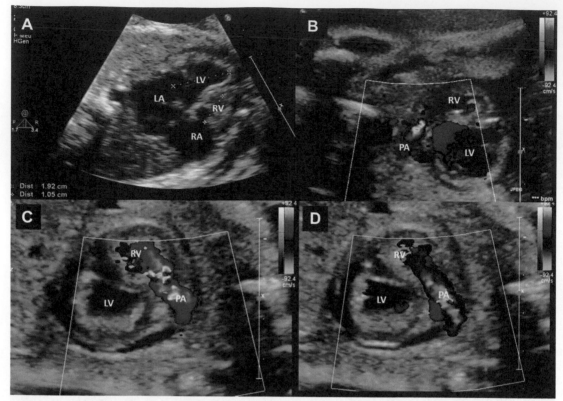

Fig. 4. Outcomes after fetal pulmonary valvuloplasty for critical pulmonary valve stenosis and a hypoplastic right ventricle. Fetal echocardiographic views. (*A*) Four-chamber view in fetal life. The right ventricle is hypertrophied and does not reach the apex of the heart. Right and left ventricular lengths are measured. The tricuspid valve is smaller than the mitral valve. (*B*) Flow acceleration is seen across the pulmonary valve in this fetus with critical pulmonary valve stenosis and flow reversal in the ductus. (*C*) Pulmonary insufficiency in the fetus after successful balloon valvuloplasty as determined by color flow mapping (*red color*). (*D*) Unobstructed forward flow across the pulmonary valve in the fetus after successful balloon valvuloplasty as determined by color flow mapping (*blue color*). LA, left atrium; LV, left ventricle; PA, pulmonary artery; RA, right atrium; RV, right ventricle.

Ethical issues can be significant when offering a fetal intervention, which is one of those rare procedures with the potential to cause damage or death to 2 individuals with a single operation. Because the objective assessment of maternal and fetal risks in such interventions is somewhat limited by the available knowledge, its perception becomes more dependent on each individual's value system. What is a tolerable risk for some parents may differ from others with a different culture, socioeconomic class, religious background, or personal family situation. Proper parental counseling with more than one individual and institutional surveillance are crucial to ensure that parents are aware of the current state of knowledge and possible alternatives to fetal catheter intervention. This highlights the importance of establishing a complete fetal cardiac program with its own peculiarities from diagnostic to prenatal and postnatal cardiologic and neonatal treatment capabilities, and parental support.

It seems that optimal patient selection is crucial to achieve better outcomes in fetuses with critical AS and evolving HLHS.[7,8] As such, only a subset of patients will eventually achieve a BV circulation (see **Fig. 3**). This can be best predicted by a multivariable threshold scoring system, which includes an LV long-axis z-score greater than 0, an LV short-axis z-score greater than 0, an aortic annulus z-score greater than 3.5, an MV annulus z-score greater than 2, a high-pressure LV defined by the presence of MR or AS with a maximum systolic gradient of 20 mm Hg or higher and milder degrees of EFE.

One may argue that even fetuses who have smaller LVs may benefit from the procedure because of improved coronary flow and preservation of myocardial function, which may have a positive impact on neonatal outcomes.[20] In addition, promoting forward flow across the aortic valve in utero may theoretically help to minimize the neurodevelopmental abnormalities secondary to retrograde TAA perfusion observed in fetuses with established HLHS. An improvement in cerebral hemodynamics has not been seen after successful aortic valvuloplasty as yet.[21] It is important to note that the preceding arguments remain purely speculative and further studies are necessary to test these hypotheses.

Additionally, much has been debated on the assumption that patients undergoing BV repair after fetal palliation have better outcomes and overall quality of life than patients undergoing a UV pathway with its attendant complications. Based on recently published information on postnatal LV diastolic dysfunction in patients with BV circulation after fetal aortic valvuloplasty,[22] a word of caution is recommended, especially considering that some of these neonates will still have to undergo endocardial resection to remove EFE.[23–25] Even acknowledging these follow-up issues, we still believe that pursuing a BV circulation is justifiable in our environment given our suboptimal results in neonates with established HLHS, no matter what kind of strategy is used.

In our own experience with fetal aortic valvuloplasty (unpublished submitted data), technical success was attained in 7 of 8 patients. In 2 patients, a BV circulation was achieved already in the neonatal period after successful percutaneous aortic valvuloplasties (see **Fig. 3**). Two patients were born with borderline LVs and were initially managed with palliative procedures but succumbed to late complications. Because no improvement of the LV size was observed over time in one patient, the family opted for neonatal palliative care. Interestingly, 2 patients with borderline ventricles in fetal life achieved an eventual BV circulation after an initial neonatal hybrid approach followed by operations for LV overhaul before 1 year of age.

The occasional fetus with critical AS associated with severe MR and conspicuous hydrops is challenging to manage.[17,18] A recent published series showed that this condition is commonly associated with either fetal loss or prematurity and carries a somber prognosis no matter what is performed in the prenatal or postnatal periods.[17] Perhaps in utero ASD creation or enlargement should have been given the same importance as aortic valve dilation. Establishing a reliable decompressing pathway for the giant LA seems to be crucial to alleviate pulmonary vein and RV compression, systemic venous congestion, and increase cardiac output.[17] In our limited experience, 2 of 3 patients with this condition died in the early neonatal period of prematurity and hydrops despite successful fetal aortic valve dilation. The remaining patient died at the age of 5 months after complications arising from percutaneous and surgical aortic valvuloplasties and mitral valve replacement.

In utero pulmonary valvuloplasty for PA/IVS or CPS/IVS is more challenging from the technical standpoint because of the heavy trabeculated RV and a smaller RV cavity, which may be associated with a significant failure rate, especially at the beginning of the learning curve.[15] Despite that, it seems that fetuses who undergo a successful intervention show a significant growth of the right ventricular structures from midgestation to late gestation when compared with control fetuses who did not undergo prenatal intervention and had univentricular outcomes after birth.[15] In our limited experience with 3 fetuses, technical failure was observed in one. The remaining 2 patients had CPS/IVS and showed significant growth of the RV structures, achieving an eventual BV circulation after initial neonatal palliation with pulmonary valvuloplasty and ductal stenting (see **Fig. 4**).

Although it has been demonstrated that in utero ASDs can be successfully created in fetuses with established HLHS and intact or highly restrictive IAS,[10,11] the neonatal outcomes for these patients remain disappointing. Although such patients are born with higher saturations and a more stable clinical course,[11] surgical mortality after the Norwood operation remains higher than in patients who were not intervened in utero. It is unclear whether the procedure performed in late gestation is efficacious in terms of preventing the development of secondary pulmonary vascular and parenchymal changes. Our experience consists of 4 technically successful cases. One fetus died the following day of unclear reasons. In 2 patients, the IAS was highly restrictive at birth and resultant systemic hypoxia prompted urgent atrial septostomy. Both died of several complications after a hybrid approach and prolonged hospitalization. In the other patient, in whom a 3.5-mm ASD was created at 32 weeks' gestation, in spite of an initial favorable clinical course and remarkable neonatal clinical stability, she eventually died of pulmonary arterial hypertension due to pulmonary vein arterialization at the age of 6 months after a Glenn/Norwood operation.

POTENTIAL COMPLICATIONS AND MANAGEMENT

Significant morbidity to the mothers is rarely encountered in the literature; however a "simple" needle puncture of the uterus does have the potential to cause problems, such as bleeding, infection, or premature labor. Because these risks are theoretically increased if a laparotomy is required under general anesthesia, our group decided not to use this approach at the outset of our program. We believe that proper fetal access can be attained using alternative techniques, such as those described previously.

Premature labor may be incited by the intervention. It seems that adequate uterine relaxation and contractions prevention help to avoid this complication.

Fetal hemodynamic instability owing to fetal bradycardia and significant hemopericardium are common complications.[19] Several mechanisms have been postulated to explain fetal hemodynamic instability including a cholinergically mediated bradycardic response triggered by a ventricular reflex and potentiated by sympathetic withdrawal, and reduced cardiac output resulting from ventricular distortion during ventricular puncture. Given the high frequency of such complications, prophylactic atropine administration during fetal anesthesia, intracardiac therapeutic injection of epinephrine and atropine, and prompt pericardial drainage should be considered part of the standard of care in such interventions (see Video 7). Although significant bradycardia is almost exclusive of procedures that involve ventricular access, it occasionally may be seen in atrial septoplasties, especially in prolonged procedures.

Fetal loss of uncertain etiology may also be observed. Although it is more commonly reported to be associated with hemodynamic instability and hemopericardium, other contributing factors, such as fetal and maternal anesthetic issues and mechanical stimuli may also play a role.[19]

FUTURE DIRECTIONS

Once the multidisciplinary team is well acquainted with the techniques, the indications might be expanded. Fetuses with Ebstein malformation of the tricuspid valve and restrictive ASD are at risk of intrautero demise owing to massive dilatation of the RA and cardiac silhouette, low cardiac output, and pulmonary hypoplasia. It has been speculated that early fetal atrial septostomy may help to avert these deleterious effects. Device closure of the RV in selected patients sounds too far-fetched nowadays but may become a reality in the near future.

Although fetal interventions can be performed using standard coronary balloons and Chiba needles, there is room for technical improvement. Shear of the balloon can happen if the catheter is pulled back into these sharp needles. Nontraumatic cannulas specifically designed for fetal interventions may help to minimize this problem and allow for the use of larger balloons or even stents, which may be required to achieve adequate relief of the LA hypertension in patients with HLHS and intact IAS. Catheters with shorter shafts may also

expedite the procedure. An alternative vascular/cardiac route, such as a transhepatic access to gain the inferior vena cava may be an option for some cases of atrial septostomy and pacemaker implantation in the future (Dietmar Schranz, 2012, personal communication).

Although the quality of pictures is satisfactory in most of cases, this may not be the truth when the procedure is geared toward 20 to 23 weeks of gestational age and smaller fetuses. Miniaturized catheters for pressure measurement[26] and fetal transesophageal echocardiography[27] have also been described in case reports as adjunctive tools to better monitor the intervention. Given the technical demands of the procedure and the need for speed, however, it is unlikely that these modalities can be used routinely without introducing additional risks.

The impact of maternal hyperoxygenation on the fetal left cardiac structures has also been studied.[28] Because of pulmonary vasodilation, pulmonary blood flow is increased. The resultant increased pulmonary venous flow works as a stimulus for LV growth in selected fetuses with small LV associated with coarctation of the aorta and other left-sided lesions. It is unclear whether this strategy works for well-established anatomic obstructions, such as critical AS and evolving HLHS. Other potential applications are CHD with hypoplastic pulmonary arteries, such as Tetralogy of Fallot and others.

Fetal pacing for congenital heart block is still an open area for research. Experimental devices have been tested in vitro and in vivo with encouraging results.[29] Proper timing of pacemaker insertion and optimal cardiac/vascular access remain open questions.

Finally, intracardiac inoculation of stem cells in the fetus might be a therapeutic alternative in the future for myocardial diseases, and, perhaps, ventricular hypoplasias.

SUMMARY

We believe that the current data available in the literature justify expanding the availability of fetal catheter intervention as a treatment option to centers with the infrastructure and commitment to do these procedures. Nevertheless, they should still be restricted to referral centers that can amass a critical volume of experience to ensure clinical competence.

Maternal risks are low and there are data indicating that some fetuses do benefit from these interventions, especially balloon aortic valvuloplasty. In this regard, prenatal intervention on the aortic valve should be regarded only as a part of a process of overhaul of left heart structures, which will need to continue postnatally, no matter of the type of eventual circulation. Perhaps, the success of a fetal intervention should be judged not only by achievement of a BV circulation but also by the medium-term and long-term functional outcome of either a BV or a UV circulation reflecting the optimization of the pulmonary and myocardial development that may result from successful and timely fetal intervention.

Clearly, more fetuses need to be studied both with and without fetal intervention, preferentially in a multicenter registry or a prospective randomized trial. This will allow a more accurate comparison of outcomes following any intervention with the natural history, which will, in turn, result in better clinical practice.

SUPPLEMENTARY DATA

Supplementary data related to this article can be found online at http://dx.doi.org/10.1016/j.iccl.2012.09.005.

REFERENCES

1. Maxwell D, Allan L, Tynan MJ. Balloon dilation of the aortic valve in the fetus: a report of two cases. Br Heart J 1991;65:256–8.
2. Kohl T, Sharland G, Allan LD, et al. World experience of percutaneous ultrasound-guided balloon valvuloplasty in human fetuses with severe aortic valve obstruction. Am J Cardiol 2000;85:1230–3.
3. Tworetzky W, Wilkins-Haug L, Jennings RW, et al. Balloon dilation of severe aortic stenosis in the fetus: potential for prevention of hypoplastic left heart syndrome: candidate selection, technique, and results of successful intervention. Circulation 2004;110:2125–31.
4. Marshall AC, Tworetzky W, Bergersen L, et al. Aortic valvuloplasty in the fetus: technical characteristics of successful balloon dilation. J Pediatr 2005;147(4):535–9.
5. Wilkins-Haug LE, Tworetzky W, Benson CB, et al. Factors affecting technical success of fetal aortic valve dilation. Ultrasound Obstet Gynecol 2006;28(1):47–52.
6. Mäkikallio K, McElhinney DB, Levine JC, et al. Fetal aortic valve stenosis and the evolution of hypoplastic left heart syndrome: patient selection for fetal intervention. Circulation 2006;113:1401–5.
7. McElhinney DB, Marshall AC, Wilkins-Haug LE, et al. Predictors of technical success and postnatal biventricular outcome after in utero aortic valvuloplasty for aortic stenosis with evolving hypoplastic left heart syndrome. Circulation 2009;120(15):1482–90.
8. McElhinney DB, Vogel M, Benson CB, et al. Assessment of left ventricular endocardial fibroelastosis in fetuses with aortic stenosis and evolving hypoplastic left heart syndrome. Am J Cardiol 2010;106:1792–7.
9. Arzt W, Werttaschnigg D, Veit I, et al. Intrauterine aortic valvuloplasty in fetuses with critical aortic stenosis: experience and results of 24 procedures. Ultrasound Obstet Gynecol 2011;37:689–95.
10. Marshall AC, van der Velde ME, Tworetzky W, et al. Creation of an atrial septal defect in utero for fetuses with hypoplastic left heart syndrome and intact or highly restrictive atrial septum. Circulation 2004;110(3):253–8.
11. Marshall AC, Levine J, Morash D, et al. Results of in utero atrial septoplasty in fetuses with hypoplastic left heart syndrome. Prenat Diagn 2008;28(11):1023–8.
12. Tulzer G, Arzt W, Franklin RC, et al. Fetal pulmonary valvuloplasty for critical pulmonary stenosis or atresia with intact septum. Lancet 2002;360(9345):1567–8.
13. Arzt W, Tulzer G, Aigner M, et al. Invasive intrauterine treatment of pulmonary atresia/intact ventricular septum with heart failure. Ultrasound Obstet Gynecol 2003;21(2):186–8.
14. Galindo A, Gutierrez-Larraya F, Velasco JM, et al. Pulmonary balloon valvuloplasty in a fetus with critical pulmonary stenosis/atresia with intact ventricular septum and heart failure. Fetal Diagn Ther 2006;21(1):100–4.
15. Tworetzky W, McElhinney DB, Marx GR, et al. In utero valvuloplasty for pulmonary atresia with hypoplastic right ventricle: techniques and outcomes. Pediatrics 2009;124:e510–8.
16. Wilkins-Haug LE, Benson CB, Tworetzky W, et al. In-utero intervention for hypoplastic left heart syndrome—a perinatologist's perspective. Ultrasound Obstet Gynecol 2005;26(5):481–6.
17. Vogel M, McElhinney DB, Wilkins-Haug LE, et al. Aortic stenosis and severe mitral regurgitation in the fetus resulting in giant left atrium and hydrops. Pathophysiology, outcomes, and preliminary experience with pre-natal cardiac intervention. J Am Coll Cardiol 2011;57:348–55.
18. Rogers LS, Peterson AL, Gaynor JW, et al. Mitral valve dysplasia syndrome: a unique form of left-sided heart disease. J Thorac Cardiovasc Surg 2011;142(6):1381–7.
19. Mizrahi-Arnaud A, Tworetzky W, Bulich LA, et al. Pathophysiology, management, and outcomes of fetal hemodynamic instability during prenatal cardiac intervention. Pediatr Res 2007;62(3):325–30.
20. Selamet Tierney ES, Wald RM, McElhinney DB, et al. Changes in left heart hemodynamics after technically successful in-utero aortic valvuloplasty. Ultrasound Obstet Gynecol 2007;30(5):715–20.
21. McElhinney DB, Benson CB, Broen DW, et al. Cerebral blood flow characteristics and biometry in fetuses undergoing prenatal interventions for aortic

stenosis with evolving left heart syndrome. Ultrasound Med Biol 2010;36(1):29–37.

22. Friedman KG, Margossian R, Graham DA, et al. Postnatal left ventricular diastolic function after fetal aortic valvuloplasty. Am J Cardiol 2011;108:556–60.

23. Tworetzky W, del Nido PJ, Powell AJ, et al. Usefulness of magnetic resonance imaging of left ventricular endocardial fibroelastosis in infants after fetal intervention for aortic valve stenosis. Am J Cardiol 2005;96:1568–70.

24. Hasan BS, Keane JF, Tworetzky W, et al. Postnatal angiographic appearance of left ventricular myocardium in fetal patients with aortic stenosis having in-utero aortic valvuloplasty. Am J Cardiol 2009;104: 1271–5.

25. Emani SM, Bacha EA, McElhinney DB, et al. Primary left ventricular rehabilitation is effective in maintaining two-ventricle physiology in the borderline left heart. J Thorac Cardiovasc Surg 2009;138:1276–82.

26. Goldstein BH, Fifer CG, Armstrong AK, et al. Use of a pressure guidewire in fetal cardiac intervention for critical aortic stenosis. Pediatrics 2011;128(3):e716–9.

27. Kohl T, Breuer J, Heep A, et al. Fetal transesophageal echocardiography during balloon valvuloplasty for severe aortic valve stenosis at 28+6 weeks of gestation. J Thorac Cardiovasc Surg 2007;134:256–7.

28. Kohl T. Chronic intermittent materno-fetal hyperoxygenation in late gestation may improve on hypoplastic cardiovascular structures associated with cardiac malformations in human fetuses. Pediatr Cardiol 2010;31:250–63.

29. Assad RS, Zielinsky P, Kalil R, et al. New lead for in utero pacing for fetal congenital heart block. J Thorac Cardiovasc Surg 2003;126(1):300–2.

Neonatal Interventions for Left-Sided Obstructive Lesions
Alternatives to Surgery

Andrea Wan, MD, FRCPC, Lee Benson, MD, FRCPC, FSCAI*

KEYWORDS

- Neonate • Aortic stenosis • Coarctation of the aorta • Catheter management

KEY POINTS

- Percutaneous balloon aortic valve dilation is a first-line treatment for neonates with aortic valve stenosis and effectively postpones the need for surgery.
- Premature, low-weight, and critically unwell neonates with coarctation of the aorta have significantly increased morbidity and mortality with primary surgical repair.
- Percutaneous coarctation balloon dilation or stent implantation in high-risk neonates may postpone the need for surgery and improve outcomes.

Obstructive lesions of the left heart presenting in the neonatal period can occur at multiple levels, from mitral valve stenosis, hypoplasia of the left ventricle, obstruction of the outflow tract (subvalvar, valvar, or supravalvar) through to hypoplasia or coarctation of the aortic arch. In the current era, treatment strategies have evolved to include percutaneous techniques in acute and longer term management. This article focuses specifically on percutaneous balloon aortic valve dilation for neonatal aortic valve stenosis and palliative interventions for neonates with coarctation of the aorta.

NEONATAL AORTIC STENOSIS
The Nature of the Problem

Left ventricular outflow tract obstruction in the neonate can occur at any level in the outflow: Subvalvar, valvar, or supravalvar. Valvar aortic stenosis is the most common form, occurring in 3% to 6% of children with congenital heart lesions and having an incidence of 2.5 to 5 per 10,000 live births.[1] Neonates with aortic valvar stenosis can have a variable clinical presentation. Indeed, those

neonates with preserved ventricular function despite severe stenosis may have few symptoms, whereas others with poor function may present with cardiovascular collapse. Neonates with duct-dependent systemic perfusion are defined as having "critical" aortic valve stenosis.

Natural history studies have shown a poor prognosis for untreated aortic stenosis in neonates[2,3] with mortality in excess of 90%. Even in a more recent series, 5.9% of neonates with critical aortic valve stenosis (and variable degrees of left heart hypoplasia) died before any intervention could be performed.[3]

Relevant Anatomy

The pathologic lesion is not solely because of fusion of the commissures, but often associated with thickened, so-called dysplastic leaflets with unequal cuspal dimensions and variable degrees of annular hypoplasia. Although the valve itself is most frequently bicuspid in structure, it can also be uni-, tri-, or quadricuspid (**Fig. 1**). Although such stenosis can occur in isolation, associated

Division of Cardiology, The Department of Pediatrics, The Labatt Family Heart Center, The Hospital for Sick Children, School of Medicine, The University of Toronto, 555 University Avenue, Toronto M5G1X8, Canada
* Corresponding author.
E-mail address: lee.benson@sickkids.ca

Intervent Cardiol Clin 2 (2013) 11–22
http://dx.doi.org/10.1016/j.iccl.2012.09.001
2211-7458/13/$ – see front matter © 2013 Elsevier Inc. All rights reserved.

interventional.theclinics.com

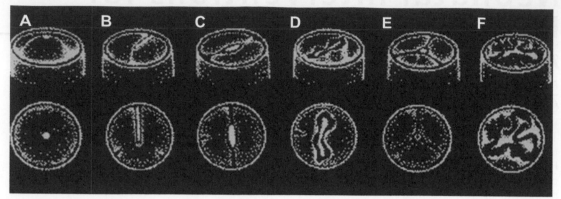

Fig. 1. Different morphologies of congenitally stenotic aortic valves. (*From* Freedom RM, Mawson JB, Yoo SJ, et al. Congenital heart disease - textbook of angiocardiography. Futura Publishing Company, Inc; 1997; with permission.)

lesions including arch coarctation and variable degrees of left heart hypoplasia with or without endocardial fibroelastosis are not infrequent. In neonates with aortic stenosis in the setting of left heart hypoplasia, assessment of suitability for a bi-ventricular management strategy can be complex and the reader is referred to in-depth reviews beyond the scope of this article.[3,4]

AORTIC VALVE BALLOON DILATION

Balloon aortic valve dilation was first reported in 1984 by Lababidi,[5] who published a case series of 23 children aged 2 to 17 years. Successful application of this percutaneous technique was quickly applied in infants[6] and neonates[7] and has since become first-line treatment for neonates.

Indications

Indications for balloon dilation in those newborns with isolated valvar stenosis were recently published by the American Heart Association[8] and are summarized in **Box 1**. The severity of the lesion is graded as trivial (<25 mm Hg), mild (25–49 mm Hg), moderate (50–79 mm Hg), severe (≥80 mm Hg), and "critical" in those with a ductal dependent systemic circulation, based on a scheme used in the Joint Study on the Natural History Study of Congenital Heart Defects.[9] In the recent American Heart Association guidelines, the hemodynamic thresholds were based on catheter-derived peak to peak gradients (with the patient sedated), which are lower than echocardiographic Doppler-derived peak instantaneous gradients.[10–12] Echocardiographic Doppler-derived gradients are low in the setting of reduced left ventricular function; thus, the guidelines recommend to proceed with intervention in those neonates with depressed function. Peak-to-peak transvalvar gradients can

---

Box 1
American Heart Association indications for aortic valve dilation in isolated valvar aortic stenosis (AS)[8] (relevant to neonates)

Class 1

1. Aortic valvuloplasty is indicated regardless of valve gradient in the newborn with isolated critical valvar AS who is ductal dependent or in children with isolated valvar AS who have depressed left ventricular systolic function (level of evidence: B).

2. Aortic valvuloplasty is indicated in children with isolated valvar AS who have a resting peak systolic valve gradient (by catheter) of ≥50 mm Hg[a] (level of evidence: B).

3. Aortic valvuloplasty is indicated in children with isolated valvar AS who have a resting peak systolic valve gradient (by catheter) of ≥40 mm Hg[a] if there are symptoms of angina or syncope or ischemic ST-T wave changes on electrocardiography (level of evidence: C).

Class IIb

1. Aortic valvuloplasty may be considered for asymptomatic patients with a catheter-obtained peak systolic gradient of <50 mm Hg when the patient is heavily sedated or anesthetized if a nonsedated Doppler study finds the mean valve gradient to be >50 mmHg (level of evidence: C).

[a] These refer to pressure gradients measured with a patient sedated during cardiac catheterization. Catheter gradients obtained with a patient under general anesthesia are likely to be somewhat lower.
   From Feltes TF, Bacha E, Beekman RH, 3rd, et al. Indications for cardiac catheterization and intervention in pediatric cardiac disease: a scientific statement from the American Heart Association. Circulation 2011;123:2607–52; with permission.

be estimated from echocardiographic Doppler-derived pressures using the formula: Peak-to-peak systolic gradient = 6.02 + 1.49 × (mean gradient) − 0.44 × (pulse pressure).[11,12]

Procedural Approach

Balloon dilation can be successfully accomplished through several different approaches (**Table 1**). The standard approach is retrograde via the femoral artery,[5] using a 4- or 5-Fr sheath. However, owing to the risk of femoral arterial complications (primarily thrombosis) in the small neonate, alternative approaches have evolved.[22] At present, there is no consensus as to which approach is optimal.

Procedural Technique

The procedure is typically performed under general anesthesia. Critically ill patients may benefit from the expertise of a pediatric cardiac anesthetist if available. Cardiovascular surgical assistance with cut down access if a carotid approach is used may also be helpful, and preparation for mechanical support with extracorporeal membrane oxygenation should be considered before commencing the procedure, depending on the child's status. Neonates with severe or critical aortic stenosis are at greater risk for

developing arrhythmias and may not tolerate catheter or wire manipulation; therefore, all equipment should be prepared in advance.

The vascular access site should be selected based on patient size and stability, as well as operator experience and available resources. When arterial access is used, a 4-Fr introducer sheath is typically used and should be sufficient to accommodate a low-profile balloon of adequate diameter (see below). For the antegrade approach, a 4- or 5-Fr sheath can be placed in the femoral vein. An additional arterial line may be placed for monitoring if desired, and an additional venous sheath can be used for rapid right ventricular pacing in cases where ventricular function is not compromised.

Balloon Size

Balloon diameter to valve annulus ratios of approximately 90% are generally recommended.[23,24] A study performed in lambs[25] showed that balloon to annulus ratios of less than 1.1 did not cause significant damage to the left ventricular outflow tract, whereas ratios of more than 1.2 can cause tears or hematomas of the aortic and mitral valves, as well as the interventricular septum. Data from the Valvuloplasty and Angioplasty of Congenital Anomalies registry[26] showed the optimal balloon

Table 1
Vascular access sites for balloon aortic valve dilation in the neonate

Approach	Advantages	Disadvantages
Femoral artery[13–15]	Standard approach, familiar technique	Risk of vascular complication Can be difficult to cross the valve retrograde
Femoral vein[15,16]	Avoids cannulation of femoral artery Potentially more stable balloon position, less likely to perforate cusp	Risk of left ventricular perforation, mitral valve damage (rare). Useful if there is very poor ventricular function
Carotid artery[17–19]	Avoids cannulation of femoral artery Direct approach to cross aortic valve	Requires surgical cut down and repair of artery Possible risk of carotid artery compromise/neurologic sequelae
Umbilical artery[20]	Avoids cannulation of femoral artery	Unlikely to be feasible in older neonates Umbilical-iliac system can be tortuous Infection risk
Axillary/subscapular artery[21]	Avoids cannulation of femoral artery Compromise of axillary/subscapular artery unlikely to cause functional problems with arm	Requires surgical cut down and repair of artery Not feasible if aberrant right subclavian artery May be difficult to maneuver from innominate artery to ascending aorta

to annulus ratio to be 0.9 to 1.0. Undersized balloons resulted in significant residual stenosis and oversized balloons increased the risk of significant aortic insufficiency.

Balloon Stability

A stable balloon position is critical to ensure the operator that the valve was maximally dilated. However, in the presence of normal left ventricular function, systolic contraction ejects the inflated balloon into the aorta, thus missing the target lesion. Additionally, a stable balloon position minimizes potential trauma to the valve (ie, avulsion of the leaflets from the annulus) and potentially reduces the amount of aortic insufficiency after dilation. Techniques used to improve balloon stability include adenosine induced asystole popularized by De Giovanni and colleagues,[27] and rapid right ventricular pacing[28,29] first introduced by Ing and colleagues from Texas Children's Hospital. The onset and duration of asystole induced with adenosine is variable and unpredictable, and has been superseded by right ventricular pacing, which is a more controlled option. The goal typically is to reduce the systemic blood pressure by 50%, thus effectively reducing the left ventricular stoke volume and force of ejection. However, in a critically ill neonate, particularly with reduced ventricular function, these maneuvers are not necessary.

Retrograde Approach

Once vascular access has been obtained, there are a variety of tools and techniques that can be used to perform the procedure (**Fig. 2**). In general, the steps to be completed include the following.

1. *Assessment of the transvalvar gradient:* Left ventricular and ascending aorta pressures can be measured simultaneously with a catheter placed in the left ventricle through the patent oval foramen and a catheter in the ascending aorta or nonsimultaneously as the catheter is advanced from the ascending aorta into the left ventricle.
2. *Assessment of aortic insufficiency and valve annulus diameter before the intervention:* Angiography can be performed in the ascending aorta to assess baseline aortic insufficiency and visualize the valve, although this is best assessed by echocardiography. An ascending aortogram can also be helpful in identifying the nonopacified jet of blood from the valve orifice entering the ascending aorta, to help orientate the catheter to cross the vale. Other operators elect to perform a left ventriculogram

for measurement of the valve annulus (**Fig. 3**), because this allows definition of the leaflet attachments to the annulus. In the presence of a bicuspid valve, regardless of angiographic projection, the hinge points are frequently obscured. Sick neonates with poor ventricular function may not tolerate extensive catheter manipulation or angiography, and assessment of aortic insufficiency and annulus diameter can be done by echocardiography.
3. *Guide wire positioning:* The aortic valve can be crossed using any of several different types of catheters (cobra-shaped, right coronary, Amplatzer right, pigtail) and a soft-tipped guide wire. In small neonates, a 0.014-inch coronary guide wire or 0.018-inch hydrophilic wire can be used. If the guide wire used is an appropriate diameter (sufficient backup), the balloon can be advanced over it. If not, it should be exchanged for a J-tipped wire of an appropriate diameter. The wire should be positioned in the apex of the left ventricle (anterior to the mitral valve).
4. *Valve dilation:* Once in position, the balloon is advanced over the wire and positioned across the aortic valve. The balloon is generally inflated by hand, while observing for elimination of a "waist" and full inflation of the balloon. After inflation, the balloon should be quickly deflated. Some balloons do not rewrap around the shaft and deflate in a flattened configuration (like a sting ray), and can obstruct flow to the head and neck vessels if left in the transverse arch. As such, the balloons should always be withdrawn to the descending aorta.
5. *Reassessment*: The gradient across the valve can then be re-assessed. A gradient reduction of 50% or more is typically considered a success. Neonates with poor ventricular function and low cardiac output may not have a significant gradient to begin with and can have a successful dilation procedure without an immediate change in the outflow gradient. Indeed, there are instances where the gradient may increase, as ventricular function improves after relief of the obstruction. An aortogram may or may not be performed to assess the degree of aortic insufficiency and look for any evidence of vascular damage.[30] More often, this is left to echocardiographic review.

Antegrade Approach

A 4- or 5-Fr sheath is placed in the femoral vein and a balloon-tipped angiographic catheter is advanced across the oval foramen through the left atrium and in to the left ventricle. Left ventricular pressure is measured and a ventriculogram

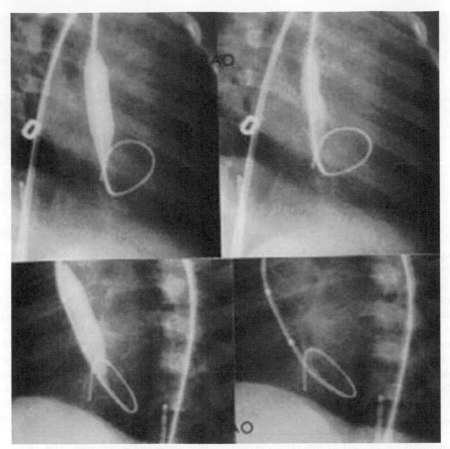

Fig. 2. Retrograde balloon aortic valvuloplasty performed via the femoral artery in a neonate. Note the waist seen at the midpoint of the balloon (at the level of the valve) during inflation.

performed to visualize the valve to determine the annular dimension. The angiographic catheter is removed and an end-hole catheter (usually a right coronary artery shape 2.0 curve) is placed in to the left atrium. From here, a coronary wire can be maneuvered across the mitral valve and turned to cross the aortic valve (**Fig. 4**). Alternatively, the catheter can be placed in the left ventricle for the same maneuver. The wire should be advanced into the descending aorta, but frequently will only go into the right carotid artery. This is not an issue, because the children are heparinized. However, it can be difficult to turn the balloon catheter from the left ventricular apex into the left ventricular

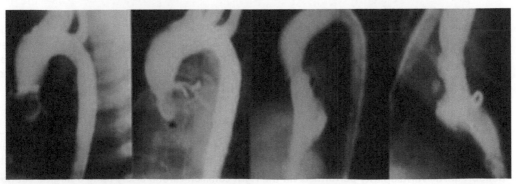

Fig. 3. The aortic valve anatomy and annulus dimensions can be visualized with an ascending aortogram (*two left panels*) or a left ventriculogram (*two right panels*).

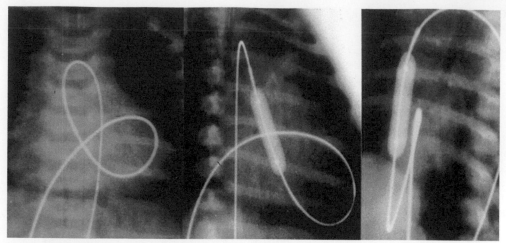

Fig. 4. Antegrade balloon aortic valvuloplasty performed via the femoral vein in a neonate. Note the wire loop formed in the left ventricle to avoid injuring the mitral valve during balloon inflation.

outflow tract, and placing the wire in the descending aorta allows one to pass the wire in to one of the femoral vessels. Here, it can be compressed from the outside improving the wire tractability. Subsequently, the end-hole catheter is removed and the selected balloon can then be advanced for the dilation.

Transcarotid Approach

A 4-Fr sheath can be placed in the right carotid artery through a surgical cut down (**Fig. 5**). Although there is some anecdotal experience with percutaneous entry, no large series has

been published demonstrating the safety of that approach. The valve annulus diameter can be measured by echocardiography or an aortogram to delineate the anatomy. An end-hole catheter is passed through the sheath and directed to the aortic valve, where a soft-tipped wire (0.014 or 0.018 inch) is used to cross the aortic valve. Many operators who use this technique have commented on how easy it is to cross even the most stenotic valve with this approach. That has been our experience as well. The remainder of the procedure is performed as for other vascular approaches. At the end of the procedure, the carotid artery is surgically repaired.

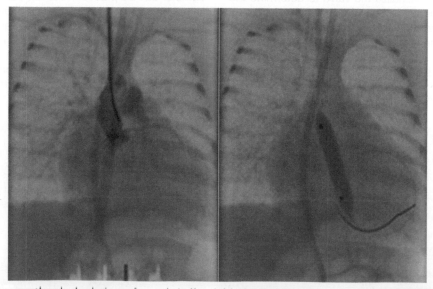

Fig. 5. Balloon aortic valvuloplasty performed via the right common carotid artery using a surgical cut-down in a 1.2-kg, premature infant. Left panel, ascending aortogram; right panel, inflation of a 5-mm-diameter balloon with loss of waist.

POTENTIAL COMPLICATIONS

Balloon aortic dilation in neonates has a higher risk of complications than in older infants and children. Potential complications are listed in **Box 2**.

Acute vascular damage is the most frequently reported complication seen in neonates, with femoral artery occlusion and loss of pulse being reported in up to 43% of procedures[19] in contemporary series. However, a more recent review of more than 1000 patients undergoing balloon dilation reported an overall complication rate of 15% from 334 neonatal procedures.[31] The risk of limb dysfunction later in life is significant[32] and approaches other than the femoral artery should be considered, especially in low birth weight neonates. Studies reporting the use of carotid artery access via a surgical cut down have shown a low risk of vascular complications when compared with femoral arterial access.[19] No neurologic sequelae were seen in these studies and the carotid arteries were patent after repair.[19,33]

Significant aortic insufficiency after balloon dilation has been reported to occur in 1% to 31% of neonates.[31,34–36] Moderate to severe insufficiency is a risk factor for surgical re-intervention[35,37] and progression of the severity of aortic insufficiency over time has been documented.[35] A higher balloon to annulus diameter ratio and the presence of preexisting insufficiency have been shown to be associated with an increased risk of aortic insufficiency after the procedure.[38,39] Acute severe insufficiency can also be because of avulsion or perforation of a valve cusp.[38,40] The antegrade approach has been suggested to result in less aortic insufficiency,[15] because the coronary guide wire can only traverse the outflow through the hemodynamic orifice, whereas retrograde wire manipulation may result in cusp perforation; however, this has not been shown in other studies.[40] The mitral valve may be damaged owing to poor wire position, and this risk may be greater when using an antegrade approach.[15,38,39] Life-threatening arrhythmias[31] as well as cardiac perforation[38,40] have been reported.

Although neonatal balloon aortic valve dilation is an effective procedure resulting in a reduced valve gradient, follow-up studies demonstrate a continuum of risk for major complications, with contemporary series reporting early mortality rates of 9% to 14% (**Table 2**). The increased mortality in neonates compared with older infants and children reflects the severity of the disease, higher incidence of associated anomalies, and technical challenges in small infants. Despite these findings, balloon dilation continues to be a first-line treatment for these infants. There have been no randomized trials comparing surgical and percutaneous therapy in the neonate and few reports retrospectively comparing the 2 procedures. In a recent study comparing such outcomes, from 2 institutions—one that performed balloon aortic valve dilation as the primary intervention, the other primary surgical valvotomy—showed no difference in outcomes 10 years after the procedure (L. Benson, 2012, personal communication). Another study[42] showed that neonates who underwent surgical valvotomy had a higher residual aortic valve gradient, whereas those who underwent percutaneous therapy had a higher incidence of aortic insufficiency. Estimated freedom from re-intervention showed no difference between the 2 approaches. In the majority of neonates re-intervention is required over the ensuing 2 decades for indications, including significant insufficiency and recurrent or inadequate relief of the valve gradient. Those children who have a residual outflow obstruction without significant insufficiency may undergo repeat dilation. Contemporary studies report freedom from re-intervention of 50% to 60% at 5 to 10 years (see **Table 2**).

PERCUTANEOUS INTERVENTIONS FOR NEONATAL COARCTATION OF THE AORTA
Nature of the Problem

Coarctation of the aorta, the 6th most common congenital heart lesion,[43] occurs in 6% to 8% of children with congenital heart disease. Typically, the most common morphologic presentation is a discrete lesion at the level of the arterial duct with or without transverse arch hypoplasia and involvement of the left subclavian artery, but it

---

Box 2
Potential complications of neonatal balloon aortic valve dilation

Aortic insufficiency

Vascular damage

    Acute thrombo-occlusion

    Dissection

    Arteriovenous fistula

    Pseudoaneurysm

Thromboembolism

Arrhythmia

Mitral valve damage

Cardiac perforation

Death

Table 2
Contemporary studies of balloon aortic valve dilation in the neonate

	No. of Neonates	Approach	Gradient Reduction	Periprocedural Mortality	Major Complication	Freedom from Reintervention
Ewert et al[31]	334	Femoral artery n = 251 Femoral vein n = 70 Other n = 13	n/a	n = 29 (8.9%)	15%	70% @ 5 y (surgical)
Crespo et al[41]	33	Predominantly retrograde	60 ± 24% ~60 to ~25 mm Hg (estimated from their **Fig. 3b**)	n = 3 (9.1%)	n = 9 (27%)	n/a
Fratz et al[34]	68	Femoral artery in 'most cases'	~50 to ~25 mm Hg (estimated from their **Fig. 2**)	38% before 1998 3% after 1998	Moderate to severe AI, n = 20 (29%)	47% @ 10 y
McElhinney et al[35]	113 (<60 d) 94 (<30 d)	Retrograde, n = 76 (67%) Antegrade, n = 35 (31%) Both, n = 2 (2%)	57 ± 22 to 24 ± 12 mm Hg	n = 16 (14%) Death within 30 d of procedure	Moderate to severe AI, n = 17 (15%)	58% @ 1 y
McCrindle et al[42]	82	Femoral, n = 52 (65%) Carotid, n = 18 (23%) Umbilical, artery n = 10 (12%)	69–20 mm Hg (mean)	n = 9 (11%) Death before discharge	n = 3 (4%) Moderate to severe AI, n = 18 (21.9%)	48% @ 5 yrs (estimated)

Abbreviation: AI, aortic insufficiency.

may also present as a long segment thoracic obstruction or occur in the abdomen. Associated lesions include bicuspid aortic valve, ventricular septal defect, mitral stenosis, and the spectrum of hypoplastic left heart syndrome. Coarctation of the aorta is also seen in the setting of atrioventricular septal defects, double outlet right ventricle (Taussig-Bing anomaly) and transposition of the great arteries.

Neonates with significant arch coarctation can present with heart failure and shock as the arterial duct closes. Initial management includes initiation of intravenous prostaglandin therapy to re-open or maintain patency of the arterial duct. In neonates with uncomplicated coarctation who stabilize with medical therapy and are of normal weight, first-line treatment is typically surgical repair. Contemporary series show good outcomes for uncomplicated arch repair.[44] However, neonates who are small,[45] premature,[46] unwell, or have other comorbidities are at increased risk for morbidity and mortality from surgical coarctation repair. In a series of 36 infants weighing less than 2.5 kg who underwent surgical coarctation repair,[46] the overall 1-year survival was 67%, although this improved to 90% when considering patients from 1999 onward. Low weight (<2.5 kg) has also been shown to be associated with increased mortality from repair (7.1% vs 2.7% for infants >2.5 kg).[47] Infants with coarctation who are critically ill at presentation are also at risk of a poor outcome. In a review of 326 neonates with coarctation with or without a ventricular septal defect who were severely symptomatic at presentation, 4 infants died before an intervention could be performed, the other 322 neonates underwent primary surgical repair. Follow-up assessment showed only 84% survival at 24 months.[48]

Balloon dilation of native coarctation in neonates was first reported in the 1980s.[49,50] Although primary surgical repair continues to be generally accepted as standard of care, catheter-based interventions may have an important role to play in the palliation of high-risk neonates.

COARCTATION BALLOON DILATION FOR HIGH-RISK NEONATES

There are few reports of palliative balloon dilation of arch coarctation in low birth weight and unwell neonates. Rothman and colleagues[51] reported their experience in 6 premature, low birth weight infants with a median gestational age of 33 weeks and weight 0.79 to 2.5 kg who underwent intervention within the first 3 weeks of life. Three had isolated arch coarctation, one a large ventricular and atrial septal defect, another a large arterial

duct, and the final neonate had a bicuspid aortic valve. Catheterization was performed via the umbilical artery in 2 infants who weighed less than 1.5 kg and through the femoral artery in the others using 3- or 4-Fr sheaths, with balloons 4 or 5 mm in diameter. All procedures were successful with residual gradients of less than 20 mm Hg across the lesion. Two of the neonates catheterized through the femoral artery had transiently diminished pulses, but did not require therapy. Three have not required re-intervention at a mean of 42 months after the initial dilation. The other 3 neonates required repeat balloon dilation at a mean of 71 days after the initial procedure. Two of those have undergone subsequent surgical repair.

Balloon dilation for neonatal coarctation has also been reported as a bridge to surgical repair in infants who present with ventricular dysfunction. Bouzguenda and colleagues[52] performed balloon dilation in 14 neonates presenting with ventricular dysfunction and evidence of end organ hypoperfusion. All procedures were performed via the femoral artery with a 3-Fr sheath. Eight of 14 neonates stabilized and proceeded to surgical coarctation repair. An additional 2 had relief of their obstruction and have not required further intervention. There were no femoral arterial complications seen; however, there were 3 periprocedural deaths. Overall, the outcomes improved when compared with the era before coarctation dilation was available.

COARCTATION STENTING IN HIGH-RISK NEONATES

Although balloon dilation of coarctation in neonates is effective in reducing arch obstruction, the response of each individual to dilation and the durability of the response can be unpredictable. Other operators have reported their experience with stent implantation in low birth weight infants and neonates who are unwell. Gorenflo and colleagues[53] presented a series of 15 premature neonates with or without complex heart lesions, who underwent coarctation stenting over a 10-year period. Eleven of the infants underwent stent placement as the index procedure, whereas 4 had stents placed shortly after failed surgical repair. Mean weight at the time of catheterization was 2.5 kg (range, 1.5–3.8). Fourteen of the procedures were performed via the femoral artery through a 4-Fr sheath. In 1 infant, an antegrade transvenous route was used. Bare metal coronary stents were implanted with diameters of 3.5 to 5 mm, using the shortest lengths possible to cover the narrowed area. All infants had adequate relief of the arch obstruction. Two infants had loss of pulse with documented thrombosis of the femoral artery after the procedure. Nine of the 11 infants who underwent stenting as an initial intervention had successful surgical stent removal and arch repair 2.8 months (range, 0.2–5) after the implantation. One infant was awaiting repair at the time of their report. Three of 4 neonates who had stenting after initial surgical arch repair underwent successful stent removal 61 months (range, 21–78) after catheterization. Two infants (1 from each group) died 3 weeks and 4 months after catheterization from unrelated causes. In this population, palliative stenting of aortic coarctation is a viable treatment strategy.

SUMMARY

Percutaneous balloon aortic valve dilation is an effective procedure for the palliation of aortic valve stenosis in neonates and is a first line treatment consideration in many units. Increasing experience and technical refinements have reduced the risk of procedural complications. However, a significant early mortality and morbidity continues to exist, along with the ongoing hazard for re-intervention.

In the current era, surgical outcomes for "high-risk," small, and unwell neonates with coarctation of the aorta are poor compared with uncomplicated patients. Although few studies are available, percutaneous intervention with balloon dilation or stent implantation can postpone the need for surgical intervention allowing the children to stabilize and grow, so that subsequent surgical repair and outcomes can be improved. Stent implantation provides a stable and predictable method for relief of arch obstruction compared with balloon dilation alone. However, care should be taken to implant stents such that they can be successfully removed at the time of subsequent surgery. In the future, use of bioabsorbable[54] or "breakable" stents[55] may overcome this issue. As our experience increases, the role of percutaneous techniques in the overall management of high risk neonates with coarctation of the aorta will become better defined and improve the outcomes of this patient group.

REFERENCES

1. Freedom RM, Yoo SJ, Mikailian H, et al, editors. The natural and modified history of congenital heart disease. Malden (MA): Blackwell Publishing Inc; 2004.

2. Kitchiner DJ, Jackson M, Walsh K, et al. Incidence and prognosis of congenital aortic valve stenosis in Liverpool (1960-1990). Br Heart J 1993;69:71–9.

3. Lofland GK, McCrindle BW, Williams WG, et al. Critical aortic stenosis in the neonate: a multi-institutional study of management, outcomes, and risk factors. Congenital Heart Surgeons Society. J Thorac Cardiovasc Surg 2001;121:10–27.

4. Colan SD, McElhinney DB, Crawford EC, et al. Validation and re-evaluation of a discriminant model predicting anatomic suitability for biventricular repair in neonates with aortic stenosis. J Am Coll Cardiol 2006;47:1858–65.

5. Lababidi Z, Wu JR, Walls JT. Percutaneous balloon aortic valvuloplasty: results in 23 patients. Am J Cardiol 1984;53:194–7.

6. Rupprath G, Neuhaus KL. Percutaneous balloon valvuloplasty for aortic valve stenosis in infancy. Am J Cardiol 1985;55:1655–6.

7. Lababidi Z, Weinhaus L. Successful balloon valvuloplasty for neonatal critical aortic stenosis. Am Heart J 1986;112:913–6.

8. Feltes TF, Bacha E, Beekman RH 3rd, et al. Indications for cardiac catheterization and intervention in pediatric cardiac disease: a scientific statement from the American Heart Association. Circulation 2011;123:2607–52.

9. Wagner HR, Ellison RC, Keane JF, et al. Clinical course in aortic stenosis. Circulation 1977;56:I47–56.

10. Currie PJ, Hagler DJ, Seward JB, et al. Instantaneous pressure gradient: a simultaneous Doppler and dual catheter correlative study. J Am Coll Cardiol 1986;7:800–6.

11. Lima VC, Zahn E, Houde C, et al. Non-invasive determination of the systolic peak-to-peak gradient in children with aortic stenosis: validation of a mathematical model. Cardiol Young 2000;10:115–9.

12. Beekman RH, Rocchini AP, Gillon JH, et al. Hemodynamic determinants of the peak systolic left ventricular-aortic pressure gradient in children with valvar aortic stenosis. Am J Cardiol 1992;69:813–5.

13. Weber HS. Catheter management of aortic valve stenosis in neonates and children. Catheter Cardiovasc Interv 2006;67:947–55.

14. Kenny D, Hijazi ZM. Percutaneous balloon valvuloplasty for aortic stenosis in newborns and children. Intervent Cardiol Clin 2012;1:121–6.

15. Magee AG, Nykanen D, McCrindle BW, et al. Balloon dilation of severe aortic stenosis in the neonate: comparison of anterograde and retrograde catheter approaches. J Am Coll Cardiol 1997;30:1061–6.

16. Hausdorf G, Schneider M, Schirmer KR, et al. Anterograde balloon valvuloplasty of aortic stenosis in children. Am J Cardiol 1993;71:460–2.

17. Fischer DR, Ettedgui JA, Park SC, et al. Carotid artery approach for balloon dilation of aortic valve

stenosis in the neonate: a preliminary report. J Am Coll Cardiol 1990;15:1633–6.

18. Maeno Y, Akagi T, Hashino K, et al. Carotid artery approach to balloon aortic valvuloplasty in infants with critical aortic valve stenosis. Pediatr Cardiol 1997;18:288–91.

19. Rossi RI, Manica JL, Petraco R, et al. Balloon aortic valvuloplasty for congenital aortic stenosis using the femoral and the carotid artery approach: a 16-year experience from a single center. Catheter Cardiovasc Interv 2011;78:84–90.

20. Beekman RH, Rocchini AP, Andes A. Balloon valvuloplasty for critical aortic stenosis in the newborn: influence of new catheter technology. J Am Coll Cardiol 1991;17:1172–6.

21. Dua JS, Osborne NJ, Tometzki AJ, et al. Axillary artery approach for balloon valvoplasty in young infants with severe aortic valve stenosis: medium-term results. Catheter Cardiovasc Interv 2006;68:929–35.

22. Kim DW, Raviele AA, Vincent RN. Use of a 3 French system for balloon aortic valvuloplasty in infants. Catheter Cardiovasc Interv 2005;66:254–7.

23. Pass RH, Hellenbrand WE. Catheter intervention for critical aortic stenosis in the neonate. Catheter Cardiovasc Interv 2002;55:88–92.

24. Sandhu SK, Silka MJ, Reller MD. Balloon aortic valvuloplasty for aortic stenosis in neonates, children, and young adults. J Interv Cardiol 1995;8:477–86.

25. Helgason H, Keane JF, Fellows KE, et al. Balloon dilation of the aortic valve: studies in normal lambs and in children with aortic stenosis. J Am Coll Cardiol 1987;9:816–22.

26. McCrindle BW. Independent predictors of immediate results of percutaneous balloon aortic valvotomy in children. Valvuloplasty and Angioplasty of Congenital Anomalies (VACA) registry investigators. Am J Cardiol 1996;77:286–93.

27. De Giovanni JV, Edgar RA, Cranston A. Adenosine induced transient cardiac standstill in catheter interventional procedures for congenital heart disease. Heart 1998;80:330–3.

28. Daehnert I, Rotzsch C, Wiener M, et al. Rapid right ventricular pacing is an alternative to adenosine in catheter interventional procedures for congenital heart disease. Heart 2004;90:1047–50.

29. Mehta C, Desai T, Shebani S, et al. Rapid ventricular pacing for catheter interventions in congenital aortic stenosis and coarctation: effectiveness, safety, and rate titration for optimal results. J Interv Cardiol 2010;23:7–13.

30. Brown DW, Chong EC, Gauvreau K, et al. Aortic wall injury as a complication of neonatal aortic valvuloplasty: incidence and risk factors. Circ Cardiovasc Interv 2008;1:53–9.

31. Ewert P, Bertram H, Breuer J, et al. Balloon valvuloplasty in the treatment of congenital aortic valve stenosis–a retrospective multicenter survey of more than 1000 patients. Int J Cardiol 2011;149:182–5.

32. Peuster M, Freihorst J, Hausdorf G. Images in cardiology. Defective limb growth after retrograde balloon valvuloplasty. Heart 2000;84:63.

33. Gasparella M, Milanesi O, Biffanti R, et al. Carotid artery approach as an alternative to femoral access for balloon dilation of aortic valve stenosis in neonates and infants. J Vasc Access 2003;4:146–9.

34. Fratz S, Gildein HP, Balling G, et al. Aortic valvuloplasty in pediatric patients substantially postpones the need for aortic valve surgery: a single-center experience of 188 patients after up to 17.5 years of follow-up. Circulation 2008;117:1201–6.

35. McElhinney DB, Lock JE, Keane JF, et al. Left heart growth, function, and reintervention after balloon aortic valvuloplasty for neonatal aortic stenosis. Circulation 2005;111:451–8.

36. Han RK, Gurofsky RC, Lee KJ, et al. Outcome and growth potential of left heart structures after neonatal intervention for aortic valve stenosis. J Am Coll Cardiol 2007;50:2406–14.

37. Brown DW, Dipilato AE, Chong EC, et al. Aortic valve reinterventions after balloon aortic valvuloplasty for congenital aortic stenosis intermediate and late follow-up. J Am Coll Cardiol 2010;56:1740–9.

38. Rocchini AP, Beekman RH, Ben Shachar G, et al. Balloon aortic valvuloplasty: results of the valvuloplasty and angioplasty of congenital anomalies registry. Am J Cardiol 1990;65:784–9.

39. Sholler GF, Keane JF, Perry SB, et al. Balloon dilation of congenital aortic valve stenosis. Results and influence of technical and morphological features on outcome. Circulation 1988;78:351–60.

40. Egito ES, Moore P, O'Sullivan J, et al. Transvascular balloon dilation for neonatal critical aortic stenosis: early and midterm results. J Am Coll Cardiol 1997;29:442–7.

41. Crespo D, Miro J, Vobecky SJ, et al. Experience in a single centre with percutaneous aortic valvoplasty in children, including those with associated cardiovascular lesions. Cardiol Young 2009;19:372–82.

42. McCrindle BW, Blackstone EH, Williams WG, et al. Are outcomes of surgical versus transcatheter balloon valvotomy equivalent in neonatal critical aortic stenosis? Circulation 2001;104:I152–8.

43. Report of the New England regional infant cardiac program. Pediatrics 1980;65:375–461.

44. Zehr KJ, Gillinov AM, Redmond JM, et al. Repair of coarctation of the aorta in neonates and infants: a thirty-year experience. Ann Thorac Surg 1995;59:33–41.

45. Bacha EA, Almodovar M, Wessel DL, et al. Surgery for coarctation of the aorta in infants weighing less than 2 kg. Ann Thorac Surg 2001;71:1260–4.

46. Karamlou T, Bernasconi A, Jaeggi E, et al. Factors associated with arch reintervention and growth of

the aortic arch after coarctation repair in neonates weighing less than 2.5 kg. J Thorac Cardiovasc Surg 2009;137:1163-7.

47. Curzon CL, Milford-Beland S, Li JS, et al. Cardiac surgery in infants with low birth weight is associated with increased mortality: analysis of the Society of Thoracic Surgeons Congenital Heart Database. J Thorac Cardiovasc Surg 2008;135:546-51.

48. Quaegebeur JM, Jonas RA, Weinberg AD, et al. Outcomes in seriously ill neonates with coarctation of the aorta. A multiinstitutional study. J Thorac Cardiovasc Surg 1994;108:841-51.

49. Finley JP, Beaulieu RG, Nanton MA, et al. Balloon catheter dilatation of coarctation of the aorta in young infants. Br Heart J 1983;50:411-5.

50. Sperling DR, Dorsey TJ, Rowen M, et al. Percutaneous transluminal angioplasty of congenital coarctation of the aorta. Am J Cardiol 1983;51:562-4.

51. Rothman A, Galindo A, Evans WN, et al. Effectiveness and safety of balloon dilation of native aortic coarctation in premature neonates weighing < or = 2,500 grams. Am J Cardiol 2010;105:1176-80.

52. Bouzguenda I, Marini D, Ou P, et al. Percutaneous treatment of neonatal aortic coarctation presenting with severe left ventricular dysfunction as a bridge to surgery. Cardiol Young 2009;19:244-51.

53. Gorenflo M, Boshoff DE, Heying R, et al. Bailout stenting for critical coarctation in premature/critical/complex/early recoarcted neonates. Catheter Cardiovasc Interv 2010;75:553-61.

54. Schranz D, Zartner P, Michel-Behnke I, et al. Bioabsorbable metal stents for percutaneous treatment of critical recoarctation of the aorta in a newborn. Catheter Cardiovasc Interv 2006;67:671-3.

55. Ewert P, Peters B, Nagdyman N, et al. Early and midterm results with the growth stent–a possible concept for transcatheter treatment of aortic coarctation from infancy to adulthood by stent implantation? Catheter Cardiovasc Interv 2008;71:120-6.

Hybrid Procedures in Congenital Heart Disease
Hypoplastic Left Heart Syndrome/Muscular Ventricular Septal Defect/Stenting of Pulmonary Arteries

Ralf J. Holzer, MD, MSc, FSCAI[a],*,
John P. Cheatham, MD, FSCAI[b]

KEYWORDS

- Congenital heart disease • Hybrid procedures • Ventricular septal defect

KEY POINTS

- Hybrid palliation of hypoplastic left heart syndrome (HLHS) is a suitable alternative to conventional Norwood/Sano-type surgical palliation, but patient selection is crucial. Preexisting retrograde aortic arch obstruction is a contraindication to hybrid palliation, especially in patients with limitations to antegrade aortic flow.
- Perventricular closure of ventricular septal defects (VSDs) is a useful therapeutic strategy in infants with muscular VSD and a weight less than 5 kg. Long-term results are excellent and the incidence of significant residual shunts is low.
- Intraoperative pulmonary artery stent is often a quick procedure, avoiding the use of stiff wires and long sheaths, and facilitating stent modifications, which otherwise could not always be achieved in the catheterization laboratory. It does not require a dedicated hybrid suite, but can be performed using a conventional c-arm in the operating room.

INTRODUCTION

Hybrid procedures represent the therapeutic cooperation between interventional cardiologist and cardiothoracic surgeon. They are the result of an increasingly collaborative environment between these 2 specialties, and often combine the advantages of each individual approach to the benefit of the patients. The most common hybrid procedures include intraoperative stent placements,[1] perventricular closure of ventricular septal defects (VSDs),[2,3] as well as hybrid palliation of hypoplastic left heart syndrome (HLHS).[4–6] As awareness of the potential therapeutic advantages of hybrid procedures for selected patients has increased, so has the number of hybrid procedures that are being performed, with the C3PO registry reporting a significant increase in the number of procedures over a 2-year period.[7] This article describes the techniques and therapeutic considerations for each of the 3 most frequently performed hybrid procedures.

a Cardiac Catheterization & Interventional Therapy, Division of Cardiology, The Heart Center, Nationwide Children's Hospital, The Ohio State University, 700 Children's Drive, Columbus, OH 43205, USA; b Cardiac Catheterization & Interventional Therapy, Pediatrics & Internal Medicine, Cardiology Division, The Heart Center, Nationwide Children's Hospital, The Ohio State University, 700 Children's Drive, Columbus, OH 43205, USA
* Corresponding author.
E-mail address: ralf.holzer@nationwidechildrens.org

Intervent Cardiol Clin 2 (2013) 23–38
http://dx.doi.org/10.1016/j.iccl.2012.09.014

HYBRID PALLIATION OF HLHS
Background

Despite progress in the management of patients with hypoplastic left heart syndrome (HLHS), the overall outcome of conventional surgical palliation has remained poor, with multicenter experiences documenting 5-year survival to be as low as 54%.[8] A recent randomized multicenter single-ventricle trial documented a 12-month transplantation-free survival of 74% after Sano-type palliation, and 64% after Norwood-type palliation.[9] In addition to a high overall mortality, studies have documented a significant incidence of neurodevelopmental disabilities associated with conventional surgical palliation of HLHS.[10,11] For these reasons, other strategies for palliation of patients with HLHS have been explored.

Michel-Behnke and colleagues from Giessen in Germany first reported an approach incorporating stenting of the arterial duct with bilateral pulmonary artery banding and balloon atrial septostomy.[4,12] The main concept behind this hybrid approach is to replace an early high-risk surgical procedure, with a lower risk hybrid intervention, thereby allowing the neonate to mature and grow before undergoing a more complex surgical intervention later in the first year of life.

The sequence and combination of the individual procedural components (patent ductus arteriosus [PDA] stent placement, pulmonary artery banding, septostomy) has evolved over time and varies between centers. John Cheatham and Mark Galantowicz from Nationwide Children's Hospital in Columbus have reported extensively on the hybrid approach to palliation of patients with HLHS.[5,13–19] Initial attempts were made at using an all-catheter–based approach, combining percutaneous ductal stent placement and balloon atrial septostomy with placement of a pulmonary artery flow restrictor (St Jude Medical, St Paul, MN). However, because of the stiffness of the delivery cable and the need for long sheaths, this approach was hemodynamically poorly tolerated and therefore abandoned. An alternative approach of performing initially percutaneous PDA stent placement and balloon atrial septostomy, followed by surgical bilateral pulmonary artery banding in a second procedure, created a surgical challenge because of the PDA stent interfering with the ability to place the left pulmonary artery (LPA) band.

A reversal of this approach, placing pulmonary artery bands first, before taking the patient to the catheter laboratory for a second procedure including percutaneous stent placement as well as balloon atrial septostomy is used successfully in many centers.[4,12] Galantowicz and Cheatham

further modified the approach by performing PDA stent placement through a per–main pulmonary artery (per-MPA) procedure directly after bilateral surgical pulmonary artery banding, thereby avoiding the need for long wires and sheaths that would otherwise be needed for antegrade PDA stent placement.[5,16] Balloon atrial septostomy or other atrial septal interventions to create a nonrestrictive atrial septal defect (ASD) are then performed just before hospital discharge. This procedure is then followed at 5 months of age by comprehensive stage II palliation, combining a modified Norwood-type palliation with a bidirectional Glenn.

Stage I Hybrid Palliation

Hybrid stage I palliation includes 3 components: bilateral pulmonary artery banding, placement of a PDA stent, and creation of an unrestrictive ASD.

The procedure is usually performed within the first 2 weeks of life once the patient has been stabilized. One of the weaknesses of the hybrid approach is the potential compromise of flow through the retrograde aortic arch (RAA), which is especially crucial in patients with aortic atresia, in which the coronary and cerebral perfusion depends on the flow through the RAA. Therefore, careful echo Doppler evaluation of the aortic arch should be performed. Any preexisting flow acceleration into the retrograde arch or impingement of the arch at this level (the 3 sign; **Fig. 1**), should be seen as a contraindication to hybrid palliation.[14,19] Placing a stent across the PDA in a patient with a preexisting RAA obstruction can have catastrophic consequences,[5,19] and therefore a more conventional Norwood-type palliation is favored in these patients.

The most common technique of hybrid stage I palliation combines bilateral pulmonary artery banding with per-MPA PDA stent placement in a single procedure through a median sternotomy. Bilateral pulmonary artery bands are placed initially; using 1-mm-wide ends cut from a 3.5-mm Gore-Tex tube graft. Placing the bands usually leads to a small reduction in postductal saturations and an increase of about 10 mm Hg in systemic blood pressure. A purse string suture is subsequently placed at the main pulmonary artery directly above the level of the pulmonary valve. Care has to be taken not to place the purse string too far distal from the valve, especially if a balloon-mounted stent variety is being considered, because the space between MPA puncture site and PDA is limited to accommodate the expansion of the balloon catheter (and its shoulders). A 6-French short sheath is subsequently prepped and a silk suture is placed about 2 mm

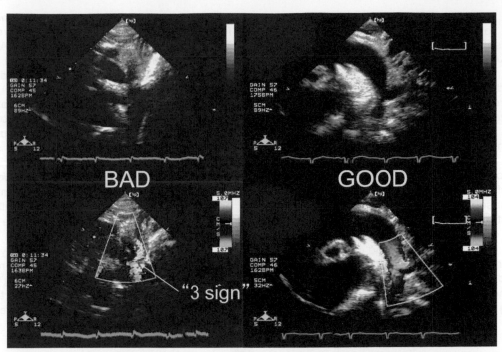

Fig. 1. Echocardiography of the RAA. On the left, the RAA is pinched in at its ductal insertion (3 sign) with flow acceleration across the RAA (unsuitable for hybrid palliation). On the right, the RAA has a wider origin without being pulled in and less flow acceleration (suitable for hybrid palliation).

away from the tip of the sheath, to serve as a marker to avoid inadvertently advancing the sheath too far into the main pulmonary artery. The dilator is then pulled back slightly to protrude by 2 to 3 mm beyond the distal end of the sheath and inserted through the purse string into the main pulmonary artery. Once the sheath is secured in MPA position, the surgeon usually steps to the head end of the patient while maintaining secure control of the sheath. A (ceiling-mounted) c-arm is moved into lateral position. A slightly stiffer 0.46-mm wire (V18, Boston Scientific, Natick, MA) is advanced under fluoroscopic guidance across the sheath and the arterial duct into the descending aorta. At this point, an angiogram is obtained through the side arm of the sheath. To provide appropriate roadmaps, it is important to have the V18 wire in place before performing the angiography, and also to have a temperature probe in the esophagus, which can further aid stent positioning. The diameter of the PDA is measured at the pulmonary arterial end, as well as proximal and distal to the retrograde arch. Additional measurements are obtained of the aortic isthmus, the retrograde arch, as well as the total length of the PDA (**Fig. 2**). Furthermore, adequate tightness and position of the pulmonary artery bands can usually be confirmed on this angiography. Prostaglandins are usually stopped just before stent placement.

Whenever possible, self-expandable stents are preferred because there is a lesser likelihood of stent migration, which can occur when removing a balloon catheter through a nonstenotic PDA. Balloon expandable stents are preferred whenever the PDA is stenotic or if the PDA is particularly

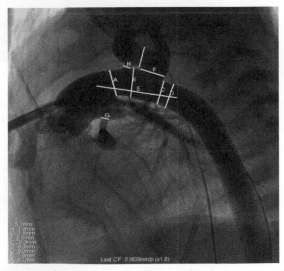

Fig. 2. Pulmonary artery angiography during stage I palliation, documenting dimensions of PDA at the pulmonary and aortic end, the size of the RAA, as well as both pulmonary arterial bands and the small ascending aorta.

short. If balloon expandable stents are used, stents of an open-cell design are preferred, because these more easily facilitate interventions for RAA obstructions, if subsequently needed.

It is helpful to use self-expandable stents that have delivery catheters that are shorter, such as the Protégé stents (EV3, Plymouth, MN), which are available in 80-cm catheter lengths, with the stents 20 mm long. In most normal term infants the most commonly used stent diameter is 8 mm, but other stent diameters should be readily available. Ductal tissue often extends toward the level of the retrograde arch, and therefore, to avoid the subsequent development of a distal stenosis (coarctation), deployment of the stent just distal to the origin of the RAA is usually recommended. If the duct is long, with the potential need for 2 overlapping stents, the first stent should be placed sufficiently distally, and then a second stent added proximally if needed (**Fig. 3**). Compromising on both ends with the need for stent

extensions at either end should be avoided. Furthermore, if a second stent is used, care should be taken to avoid double covering of the RAA with the cells of both stents. Clinicians should err on deploying self-expandable stents too distally, because the stent can be dragged back a little after just 1 row has been deployed. In contrast, once any part of the stent has been uncovered, the stent cannot and should not be pushed forward.

Creating a nonrestrictive atrial communication

Creating an unrestrictive atrial communication is essential for the success of the hybrid palliation. It is important not to overestimate the size of the ASD or the stretched patent foramen ovale (PFO). A low or nonexistent gradient may often develop into a more significant atrial septal restriction during the first 2 to 3 months following hybrid palliation. Holzer and colleagues[18] reported an early experience of atrial septal interventions

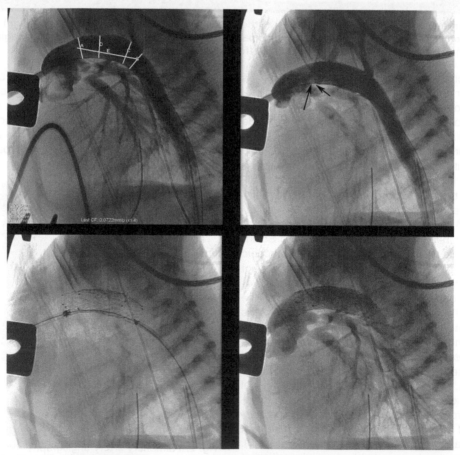

Fig. 3. Neonate with HLHS during hybrid stage 1 palliation. PDA length (*top left*) 20 to 21 mm. The initial (self-expandable) stent was deployed to cover the distal PDA, leaving a small portion of the PDA not covered by the stent (*top right, between arrows*). Subsequent deployment of an additional self-expandable stent (*bottom left*) resulted in complete coverage of the PDA.

following hybrid stage I palliation, with a subsequent need for reinterventions in as many as 26% of patients. This percentage decreased to as little as 13% over the last 2 years, because of the consequent performance of balloon atrial septostomy before hospital discharge in almost all patients.

The success of conventional balloon atrial septostomy is more limited if it is delayed until a gradient develops, because of the increased thickness of the atrial septum. It is therefore recommended to take every patient to the catheterization laboratory before discharge from the hospital. At this point, a baseline hemodynamic evaluation combined with angiographic delineation of the pulmonary arteries (and bands) as well as the PDA stent can be performed, which may be the sole catheter evaluation before comprehensive stage II palliation. At the end of the procedure, balloon atrial septostomy is performed in virtually all patients, irrespective of the baseline mean gradient. Holzer and colleagues[18] described balloon atrial septostomy alone to be successful in as many as 64% of patients, with 36% of patients requiring additional interventions. Noncompliant septostomy balloons, such as the NuMED Z5 septostomy catheters (NuMED, Hopkinton, NY) are usually preferable, and, in most patients, a 2-mL septostomy catheter can be used for balloon atrial septostomy, often completely occupying the small left atrium during inflation. Preshaping the septostomy catheter with a secondary curve may aid in crossing the atrial septum. As an alternative, a stiffer wire can be used to splint open the atrial communication, or an over-the-wire technique can be used.

Additional interventions that may be necessary include static balloon atrial septoplasty, often combining cutting with standard balloon septoplasty; RF perforation of the atrial septum; or atrial septal stent placement. These additional interventions are particularly helpful in patients with very abnormal septal and left atrial anatomy, an intact atrial septum, or an embryonic left atrium. Sometimes static septoplasty may be required before performing balloon atrial septostomy. Static septoplasty through very superior atrial communications should be avoided (**Fig. 4**), because the weakest part of the septum may be the communication with the pulmonary veins, rather than the septum itself, thereby potentially leading to a catastrophic pulmonary vein tear. If RF perforation is required, either because of an intact atrial septum or because of a suboptimal location of the existing defect, any inferior puncture should be avoided, which can be associated with complete heart block (**Fig. 5**). Once the atrial septum has been opened, all patients require careful monitoring

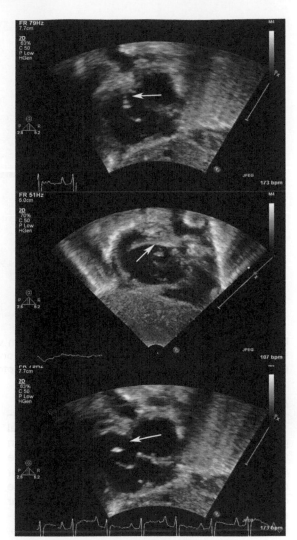

Fig. 4. Infant (2 kg) 2 weeks after hybrid stage I palliation undergoing atrial septal intervention. Echocardiography documented a very aneurysmal atrial septum, with a small communication centrally, and a small communication superiorly at base of the aneurysm (*arrow, top image*). After balloon atrial septostomy of the superior defect a wide-open atrial septum is achieved (*bottom image*).

within an intensive care environment, because of physiologic changes associated with atrial septostomy. Feeding should be delayed by at least 24 hours because the sudden loss of atrial level restriction, combined with pulmonary artery bands that are still loose, may lead to runoff through the pulmonary vascular bed with a concomitant reduction in systemic cardiac output. These patients are at increased risk of necrotizing enterocolitis particularly in the first 1 to 2 days following septostomy. Once feeds are introduced, this should be performed gradually and with caution.

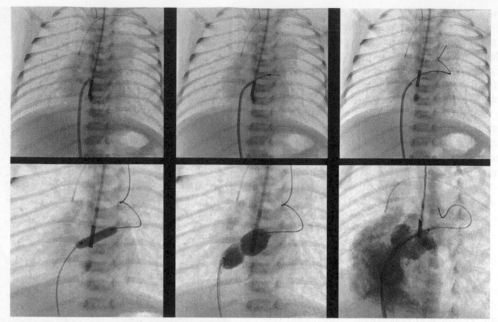

Fig. 5. Neonate with HLHS and intact atrial septum with a decompressing vein. RF perforation of the atrial septum was performed under transesophageal echocardiography (TEE) guidance (using an intracardiac echo probe) followed by cutting and standard balloon septoplasty achieving a wide atrial communication.

Interstage Period

The interstage period carries a variety of potential problems that may require transcatheter evaluation and therapy. These problems include retrograde aortic arch obstruction (RAAO), recurrent or residual stenosis of the PDA stent, as well as the development of an atrial septal restriction. Regular surveillance after hybrid stage 1 palliation is therefore crucial, including weekly clinic visits with echo, electrocardiogram (ECG), oxygen saturations, weight gain, and arm-leg blood pressures, combined with home monitoring, are crucial to identify potential problems early to be able to intervene accordingly. There should be a low threshold to admit these patients for observation, including cardiac catheterization.

RAA obstruction

RAA obstruction (RAAO) is a potentially serious problem, especially in patients with aortic atresia in which the coronary and cerebral perfusion is solely dependent on flow through the retrograde arch. Egan and colleagues[14] reported that 29% of patients developed RAAO at some stage following hybrid stage I palliation. The development of RAAO carries a guarded prognosis, with Stoica and colleagues[19] reporting only a 44% survival to Fontan completion out of 16 patients who required surgical or transcatheter interventions for RAAO. Any concern about the development of a significant

RAAO should lead to hospital admission, as well as transcatheter evaluation and potential therapy, and this should occur before it manifests through deterioration of right ventricular (RV) function as well as increasing tricuspid regurgitation, which are ominous signs in these patients. Increasing Doppler velocities across the RAA as well as ECG changes may occur early and therefore should be evaluated at every clinic visit.

The treatment of RAAO is difficult, and depends on the anatomic diagnosis, associated problems, as well as the age and weight of the patient. If RAAO develops close to comprehensive stage II when the patient is 4 to 5 months of age, then proceeding with stage II palliation a little earlier can be considered with an acceptable risk, provided that RV function is well preserved. However, early stage II palliation is not an option in the presence of poor RV function or new/increasing tricuspid regurgitation. The usual treatment in this situation is retrograde stent placement using a femoral arterial approach, in which a coronary stent is implanted through the cells of the PDA stent into the RAA. In the presence of a closed-cell PDA stent (such as the Palmaz Blue, Cordis, Warren, NJ), balloon angioplasty of the cells may need to be performed before stent implantation. Stenting of the RAA restores blood to the cerebral and coronary circulation and, in patients with reduced RV function, some improvement in RV function combined with a reduction of tricuspid regurgitation can often be observed. However, the clinical benefit is short-lived and often the RAA restenoses because of neointimal proliferation (**Fig. 6**), so this only provides a therapeutic window of about 6 weeks, during which the surgeon should take the patient to the operating room to perform comprehensive stage II palliation. For this reason, clinicians should not only avoid intervening too late for an RAAO but also avoid intervening too early on the RAA. A particular problem is posed by those patients who are less than 3 months of age at the time of development of RAAO, and all clinical and nonclinical data need to be taken into account in the decision-making process for these patients. If RAA stent placement is performed early, this may lead to recurrent obstruction with in-stent stenosis before the patient is old enough for stage II palliation. To avoid this problem, a reverse pulmonary-to-central-aortic shunt has been advocated by Calderone and colleagues.[20] However, results of this technique have been disappointing, likely because of the unpredictable physiology with the potential for steal-away from the coronary and cerebral circulation. An alternative approach in these patients is a conversion to a Norwood-type palliation.

Recurrent or residual PDA stent stenosis

Recurrent or residual stenoses of the PDA are problematic, because this not only reduces the perfusion to the retrograde aortic arch but also adds afterload to the single right ventricle. These problems are readily diagnosed through echo Doppler evaluation, and usually are best treated through implantation of a second stent. It is necessary to be flexible with the angiographic angles, because a standard lateral as well as right anterior oblique projections may not show the stenotic segment. Rotational angiography with three-dimensional (3D) reconstruction can be helpful to further delineate any PDA narrowing (**Fig. 7**). Wherever possible, it is important to avoid double covering the retrograde arch with the newly implanted stent. Stent delivery is usually performed through an antegrade approach from the femoral vein, with an angiographic catheter advanced from the femoral artery to aid stent positioning. It is important to avoid the use of stiff wires or long sheaths because these can splint the tricuspid and pulmonary valves, thereby leading to a significant reduction in blood pressure and cardiac output. ST/T wave changes that occur after placing a wire across the PDA stent indicate this problem, and patients may need to be temporarily supported with inotropes. Balloon expandable stents should be used for these recurrent or residual stenoses, and it is usually sufficient to advance these premounted stents bare across the PDA. The in situ original stent as well as angiographies from an arterial catheter are usually sufficient to facilitate accurate stent positioning. Self-expandable stents are usually inadequate to treat any recurrent or residual narrowing, because a higher radial force is required to expand these lesions.

A combination of PDA in-stent stenosis with extension of the neointimal hyperplasia to the RAA is a particularly difficult management problem (**Fig. 8**). To treat both lesions, it would technically be necessary to stent the PDA first, followed by stenting of the RAA. However, first treating the

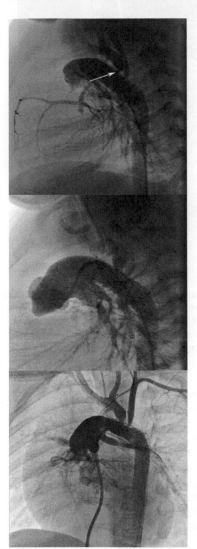

Fig. 6. Six-week-old infant after hybrid stage I palliation with a significant stenosis of the RAA (*arrow, top image*). After stent placement across the RAA an excellent immediate result was achieved (*middle image*). However, the patient developed significant in-stent stenosis involving the RAA stent and the PDA stent (*bottom image*) within 2 month of stenting the RAA.

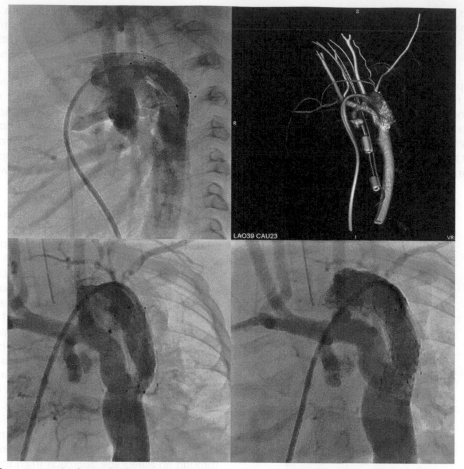

Fig. 7. Infant 1 month after hybrid stage I palliation. An initial angiography in straight lateral projection (*top left*) did not suggest a significant stenosis, despite a notable pressure gradient. Rotational angiography with 3D reconstruction was performed, which documented that part of the distal PDA was not covered by stent (*top right*). Using those (unusual) angles (LAO39, CAU 23) as a roadmap, biplane angiography confirmed the findings (*bottom left*), and an additional stent was placed, eliminating the narrowing (*bottom right*).

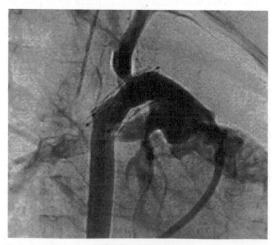

Fig. 8. Three-month-old infant with PDA in-stent stenosis as well as a stenotic RAA.

PDA stenosis through a second stent may temporarily worsen the flow across the retrograde arch, which may be poorly tolerated in a patient who already has RAAO. In contrast, treating the RAAO first prevents any additional stent implantation across the PDA stent. For this reason, if the PDA stent narrowing is mild, it would be more advantageous to treat the RAAO through stent implantation, while not treating the PDA stent stenosis.

Recurrent atrial septal restrictions

The additional problems sometimes seen in the interstage period are recurrent restrictions of the atrial septum. Overall, these problems are rare if a balloon atrial septostomy was performed during the initial hospitalization. Recurrent atrial septal restrictions were more commonly observed during the earlier hybrid experience, when patients with nonrestrictive PFO or small ASD did not undergo any atrial septal intervention. If a patient presents with recurrent atrial septal restriction beyond the neonatal period, balloon atrial septostomy usually does not yield a good result. With increased atrial septal thickness, care is needed not to repeatedly pull a noncompliant balloon against the septum when a significant resistance is encountered, because this may lead to avulsion of pulmonary veins as a potential disastrous complication. Preferred therapeutic options in patients with recurrent atrial septal restrictions include static (cutting) balloon septoplasty or stent placement (**Fig. 9**) across the atrial septum.

Comprehensive Stage II Palliation

Comprehensive stage II palliation is usually performed at 5 months of age at a weight of more than 5 kg. Performing the procedure earlier has been associated with higher morbidity and mortality, caused by immaturity of the pulmonary vascular bed and the small size of the branch pulmonary arteries.[5]

The procedure includes removal of the PDA stent, debanding of the pulmonary arteries, pulmonary artery patch augmentation, a bidirectional Glenn, a Damus-Kaye-Stansel anastomosis, atrial septectomy, as well as arch reconstruction. Although some operators remove the PDA stent en block, others perform a careful dissection. The Toronto group introduced the concept of leaving part of the PDA stent as a reinforcement of the aortic arch reconstruction.

Completion angiography has evolved as an important tool after comprehensive stage II palliation. Holzer and colleagues[21] reported an incidence of 23% of hybrid interventions or surgical revisions resulting from abnormalities identified on exit angiography after comprehensive stage II or Glenn palliation (**Fig. 10**). Not every perceived pulmonary artery narrowing should be treated, because the LPA patch often overemphasizes any LPA stenosis. Furthermore, the nonpulsatile nature of the flow and the open chest changes the images from what is expected when similar angiographies are taken in the catheterization laboratory. Although LPA stent placement may be beneficial if a significant stenosis is identified (**Fig. 11**), isolated balloon angioplasty of the dissected vessels should not be performed, especially of the proximal right pulmonary artery (RPA), because these vessels are often very thin because of surgical dissection and are more susceptible to vascular trauma. Delaying balloon angioplasty of noncritical vascular lesions is often preferred to immediate transcatheter therapy. Further experience with this technique will more clearly define what types of abnormalities require immediate therapy and which should be observed conservatively.

Results of the Hybrid Approach

So far, results of the hybrid approach to palliation of HLHS have been favorable. The difficulty in comparing these results with standard Norwood or Sano-type palliation is related to patient selection, because many centers only consider hybrid palliation for high-risk surgical candidates. Galantowicz and colleagues[16] reported on the outcomes of patients with typical HLHS and uniform risk, describing an overall survival up to and including comprehensive stage II of 87%, which compares well with surgical results from larger centers. Out of the 13% mortality, 2% occurred around hybrid stage I palliation, 5% in the interstage period, and 6% around comprehensive stage II.

Although there is a theoretic neurodevelopmental benefit of delaying major surgical interventions until later in infancy, there is also a concern about the potential impact of reduced cerebral flow

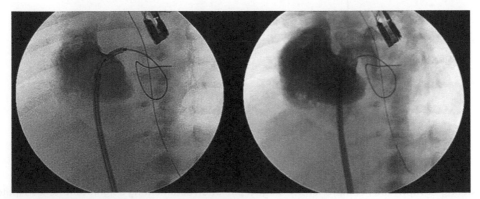

Fig. 9. Atrial septal stent placement after hybrid stage I palliation. (*Left*) Placement of a stent across a restrictive intra-atrial communication. (*Right*) Angiography after stent placement.

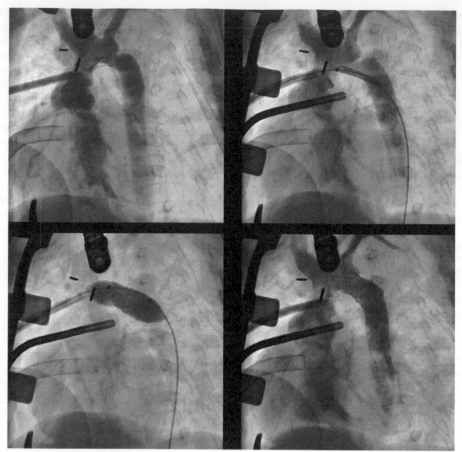

Fig. 10. Exit angiography (aortogram) after comprehensive stage 2 documenting a stenosis of the distal arch (*top left*). Intraoperative stent placement was performed (*top right and bottom left*), with final angiography showing a well-positioned stent (*bottom right*), with complete relief of the stenosis.

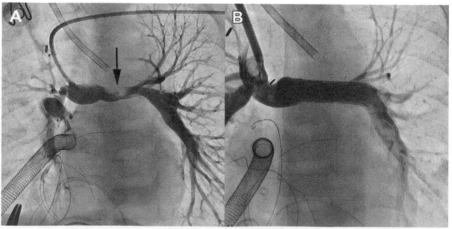

Fig. 11. Exit angiography after comprehensive stage II palliation documenting a significant stenosis (patch infolding) of the midportion of the LPA (*A*). Excellent angiographic result after hybrid intraoperative placement of a Genesis XD stent (*B*).

through the retrograde aortic arch, especially in patients with aortic atresia. Research is presently being undertaken to further study the impact of hybrid palliation on neurodevelopmental outcome.

PERVENTRICULAR CLOSURE OF VSDS

Transcatheter closure of VSDs was introduced as early as 1988 by Lock and colleagues.[22] A variety of devices have since been developed that are suitable for transcatheter closure of VSDs, and the technique has been shown to be safe and effective. However, disadvantages of the transcatheter approach, especially in small children, include the need for an arteriovenous loop, as well as the large and stiff delivery systems in relation to patient size. Holzer and colleagues[23] reported a significantly higher incidence of adverse events, lower procedural success, and a higher incidence of residual shunts when transcatheter closure of muscular VSDs is performed in infants with a weight less than 10 kg. Similar results were reported for device closure of perimembranous ventricular septal defects.[24] Although surgical closure of muscular VSDs is a valuable alternative, the procedure requires cardiopulmonary bypass (CPB) and closure of these defects can be challenging with defects often hidden in the muscular RV trabeculations. These defects are often more difficult to reach surgically, with a higher incidence of residual shunts and higher associated procedural risk.

In contrast, perventricular closure of muscular VSDs has the advantages of an off-pump technique, and avoids the problems seen with percutaneous VSD closure in small infants. The first such procedure using the AMPLATZER Muscular VSD Device was reported by Bacha and colleagues[2] in 2003. A subsequent multicenter experience in 2005 reported successful perventricular VSD closure in 12/13 patients, with only minor residual shunts on follow-up in 2 patients,[3] and Amin and colleagues[25] reported a similar technique for perventricular closure of perimembranous VSDs.

The procedure is performed under general endotracheal anesthesia with access being provided via either a full median sternotomy or a limited subxiphoid incision (depending on the location of the VSD). Transesophageal echocardiography (TEE) is performed to determine the size and location of the VSD. Using gentle manual or instrumental pressure on the RV free wall, a puncture site is determined under TEE guidance that lies in a straight course opposite the VSD. It is important to carefully measure the distance between the RV free wall entry site and the ventricular septum, to obtain a better understanding of how far to advance the

delivery sheath. Using an 18-gauge needle, the RV free wall is punctured through a purse string with the needle directed toward the VSD. A 0.035 angled Glidewire can be used to cross the VSD. To enhance the echogenicity, roughening the tip of the wire on a surgical scratch patch can be helpful. For larger VSDs, the defect may be crossed directly using the 0.9-mm wire that usually comes with a short 7-Fr delivery sheath and that is visible on TEE. Once the wire has crossed the VSD, the needle is removed and a 7-Fr short sheath advanced over the wire, carefully controlling the distance the sheath is advanced to avoid crossing too deeply into the left ventricle (LV). Once the sheath has been visualized on TEE within the LV cavity, the dilator is removed and the sheath flushed with normal saline. The device size chosen is about 1 to 2 mm larger than the size of the VSD by TEE imaging. Most muscular VSDs that are closed using a perventricular approach in infancy require either a 6-mm or 8-mm AMPLATZER Muscular VSD Device. The device is loaded using standard technique, using either an additional short sheath, or the loader supplied with the delivery system with cutting of the distal lock mechanism and attachment of a Tuohy Borst adapter proximally. The device is advanced through the short sheath and this is usually readily visualized by TEE. The LV disk should be deployed just distal to the ventricular septum, taking care not to push the device distally against the LV free wall or to entangle the mitral valve apparatus. The assembly is then pulled back against the septum and the waist and RV disk deployed. Once appropriate device position and the lack of any significant atrioventricular valve regurgitation or residual shunt are confirmed, the device is released and, after a final TEE evaluation (**Fig. 12**), the purse string entry site is closed, followed by surgical closure of the median sternotomy.

Technical variations may need to be used for more difficult VSDs, especially if located below the moderator band. If a VSD cannot be crossed easily from the RV side, it may be beneficial to place a femoral arterial sheath and advance a catheter into the LV with fluoroscopic guidance using a portable c-arm. An LV angiogram can be helpful in outlining the VSD and serving as a roadmap to cross the VSD using a left-sided transcatheter approach. Once a wire has been passed into the pulmonary arteries, a perventricular approach can be used to snare the wire, thereby creating an arterioperventricular loop, which facilitates advancing the short sheath across the VSD into the LV.

Furthermore, configuration of the RV disk can at times be difficult, especially if the defect is located

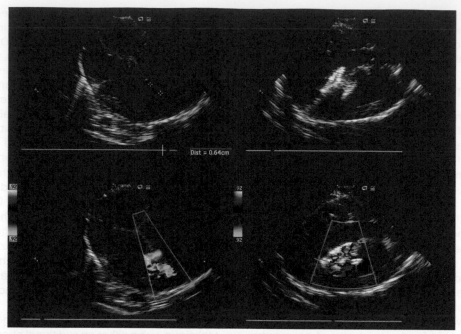

Fig. 12. Perventricular hybrid closure of a moderate-sized muscular VSD in a 3-month-old infant. (*Left*) Four-chamber view documenting a large VSD before closure (*top*, 2D; *bottom*, Doppler). (*Right*) Long-axis view documenting excellent device position after VSD closure (*top*, 2D; *bottom*, Doppler).

with little rim to the apex below the moderator band. In this situation, the surgeon can place a suture through the RV free wall myocardium, capturing and securing some of the nitinol meshwork of the device.

INTRAOPERATIVE STENTING OF BRANCH PULMONARY ARTERIES

Intraoperative pulmonary artery stent placement is one of the most common hybrid procedures performed in the catheterization laboratory, with the C3PO registry reporting it as about 11% of all hybrid procedures performed.[7] The procedure was described as early as 1993 and is used in many centers, with several reports describing experiences of intraoperative stent placement.[26–29]

Little equipment is necessary for intraoperative stent placement, and mainly consists of a portable c-arm (or a hybrid operating room), a surgical endoscope, as well as a power injector (depending on the technique used). The most important ingredient to successful intraoperative stent placement is the cooperation and flexibility of the surgical and catheter teams in combining their individual expertise.

Before performing pulmonary artery stent placement, it is helpful to have some images available that can be used to decide on the length and diameter of the required stent. These images can include an intraoperative angiogram, a cardiac catheterization performed in the recent past, or a computed tomography or MRI study. In addition, Hegar dilators are helpful in determining the tightness of a stenosis, whereas an endoscope can be used to examine the distal vessel.

Intraoperative stent placement can be performed under direct vision with the pulmonary arteries opened (**Fig. 13**), or using angiographic guidance through a sheath that is inserted at the time of surgery (on the beating heart). Sometimes a combination of both approaches is required.

The main advantages of intraoperative stent placement include the avoidance of long sheaths and stiff wires, the ability to deploy adult-sized stents in small infants, and the additional benefit of having the patient on CPB, thereby providing greater control during the procedure. Furthermore, it is easier to trim stents to the desired length to fit any individual lesion. In addition, intraoperative stent placement is usually quicker than transcatheter stenting. However, intraoperative stent placement is usually only performed if a patient requires concomitant surgical correction or palliation of an additional cardiac defect.

If a patient who is expected to require cardiac surgery is found during presurgical cardiac catheterization to have a proximal branch pulmonary artery stenosis, it is important to discuss the

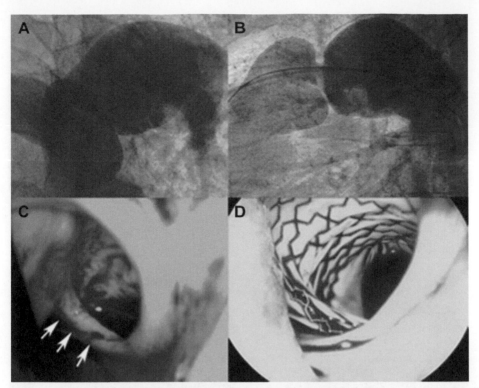

Fig. 13. Intraoperative LPA stent for an LPA kink placement in an adult with a history of tetralogy of Fallot repair, undergoing pulmonary valve replacement. A 42-year-old woman with a previous history of tetralogy of Fallot repair and free pulmonary insufficiency. (*A, B*) LPA angiography documenting an LPA kink with significant post-stenotic dilatation of the LPA. (*C*) Endoscopic image before stent implantation documenting the ridge/fold at the proximal LPA (*arrows*). (*D*) Endoscopic image after stent deployment.

therapeutic strategies with the surgeon at the time of the procedure. In most instances, delaying stent implantation until the time of surgery is the preferred option, not least because it is performed quicker than in the catheterization laboratory. Furthermore, this approach allows the surgeon to inspect the findings at the time of surgery, choosing the best approach for any individual patient or lesion. Pulmonary artery kinking is usually not treated adequately through surgical patch augmentation, and requires stent placement.

For intraoperative stent placement under direct vision, a soft wire is placed under endoscopic guidance in a distal branch pulmonary artery, usually using a larger lower lobe branch. It is important to confirm the wire position with the endoscope, because angiography will not be available during stent positioning. Furthermore, the endoscope can be used to estimate the distance to the offset of the first pulmonary arterial side branch, thereby providing a helpful detail to avoid jailing a side branch. The stent can be trimmed if necessary (unless open-cell design), and is then mounted over a balloon and advanced under direct vision

and endoscopic guidance across the branch pulmonary artery stenosis. It is helpful to inflate the balloon not just under direct vision and endoscopic guidance but also using fluoroscopy whenever feasible, because this better shows whether a balloon is accidentally engaging a side branch or whether the stent milks off the balloon. Once the stent is deployed and the balloon removed, the endoscope is used to evaluate the result, followed by molding the overlapping and protruding stent struts to create a smooth entry to the branch pulmonary artery (**Fig. 14**), which aids any future transcatheter rehabilitation that may be required.

If an approach with angiographic guidance is used, a sheath is inserted in close proximity to the lesion that requires treatment, leaving sufficient distance to expand the shoulders of the balloon catheter. Angiographies are usually performed before wire positioning, as well as after positioning a (softer) wire. The mounted adult stent is usually advanced directly through the sheath and it is usually not necessary to push the sheath across the lesion. In smaller patients with freshly dissected vasculature, using larger sheaths to advance across

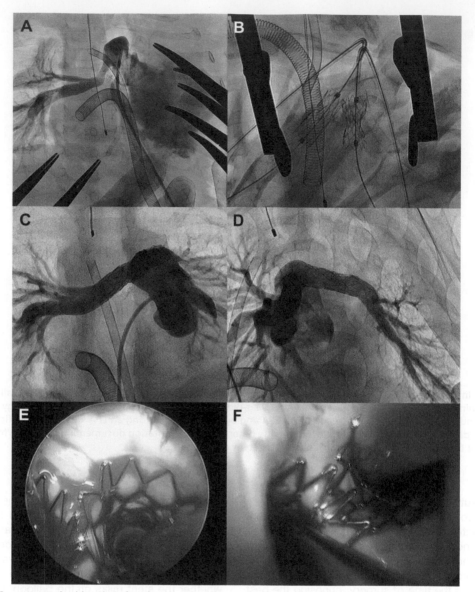

Fig. 14. Seven-month-old male infant born with pulmonary artery VSD after complete repair. The patient developed a large RV outflow tract pseudoaneurysm and had bilateral stenotic and hypoplastic branch pulmonary arteries. Hybrid stent therapy was delivered to both branch pulmonary arteries, using a per-MPA approach, followed by resection of the aneurysm, and molding of the stents under endoscopic guidance. (*A*) Intraoperative angiography documenting hypoplastic and stenotic branch PAs. (*B*) Simultaneous expansion of both LPA and RPA stents; the LPA stent required the use of higher pressure balloons to fully expand. (*C, D*) Angiography of LPA and RPA after stent deployment, documenting a good angiographic result. (*E, F*) Endoscopic image of both PA stents before (*E*) and after (*F*) molding the edges to create a smother surface.

the area of stenosis should be avoided because it can easily damage the vessel wall. The combination of hand injections of contrast as well as surgical roadmaps is usually sufficient to appropriately position and expand the stent. In most patients, a completion angiogram is helpful at the end of the procedure once the patient is weaned off CPB. Techniques used for intraoperative stent placement in branch pulmonary arteries can equally be used to

place intraoperative stents in any other vascular location.

SUMMARY

Hybrid therapies have increased and offer a valuable alternative to standard catheter or surgical therapies in selected patient. These hybrid therapies often combine the best of both techniques, in particular for VSD closure and intraoperative pulmonary artery stent placement.

For patients with HLHS, the hybrid approach is an important alternative therapeutic strategy, providing similar results to conventional Norwood-type palliation. Further studies are needed and are underway to evaluate the neurodevelopmental outcome in these patients.

REFERENCES

1. Hjortdal VE, Redington AN, de Leval MR, et al. Hybrid approaches to complex congenital cardiac surgery. Eur J Cardiothorac Surg 2002;22(6):885–90.

2. Bacha EA, Cao QL, Starr JP, et al. Perventricular device closure of muscular ventricular septal defects on the beating heart: technique and results. J Thorac Cardiovasc Surg 2003;126(6):1718–23.

3. Bacha EA, Cao QL, Galantowicz ME, et al. Multicenter experience with perventricular device closure of muscular ventricular septal defects. Pediatr Cardiol 2005;26(2):169–75.

4. Michel-Behnke I, Akintuerk H, Marquardt I, et al. Stenting of the ductus arteriosus and banding of the pulmonary arteries: basis for various surgical strategies in newborns with multiple left heart obstructive lesions. Heart 2003;89(6):645–50.

5. Galantowicz M, Cheatham JP. Lessons learned from the development of a new hybrid strategy for the management of hypoplastic left heart syndrome. Pediatr Cardiol 2005;26(2):190–9.

6. Galantowicz M, Cheatham JP. Fontan completion without surgery. Semin Thorac Cardiovasc Surg Pediatr Card Surg Annu 2004;7:48–55.

7. Holzer R, Marshall A, Kreutzer J, et al. Hybrid procedures: adverse events and procedural characteristics–results of a multi-institutional registry. Congenit Heart Dis 2010;5(3):233–42.

8. Ashburn DA, McCrindle BW, Tchervenkov CI, et al. Outcomes after the Norwood operation in neonates with critical aortic stenosis or aortic valve atresia. J Thorac Cardiovasc Surg 2003;125(5):1070–82.

9. Ohye RG, Sleeper LA, Mahony L, et al. Comparison of shunt types in the Norwood procedure for single-ventricle lesions. N Engl J Med 2010;362(21):1980–92.

10. Mahle WT, Clancy RR, Moss EM, et al. Neurodevelopmental outcome and lifestyle assessment in school-aged and adolescent children with hypoplastic left heart syndrome. Pediatrics 2000;105(5):1082–9.

11. Tabbutt S, Nord AS, Jarvik GP, et al. Neurodevelopmental outcomes after staged palliation for hypoplastic left heart syndrome. Pediatrics 2008;121(3):476–83.

12. Akintuerk H, Michel-Behnke I, Valeske K, et al. Stenting of the arterial duct and banding of the pulmonary arteries: basis for combined Norwood stage I and II repair in hypoplastic left heart. Circulation 2002;105(9):1099–103.

13. Cua CL, Galantowicz ME, Turner DR, et al. Palliation via hybrid procedure of a 1.4-kg patient with a hypoplastic left heart. Congenit Heart Dis 2007;2(3):191–3.

14. Egan MJ, Hill SL, Boettner BL, et al. Predictors of retrograde aortic arch obstruction after hybrid palliation of hypoplastic left heart syndrome. Pediatr Cardiol 2011;32(1):67–75.

15. Fenstermaker B, Berger GE, Rowland DG, et al. Interstage echocardiographic changes in patients undergoing hybrid stage I palliation for hypoplastic left heart syndrome. J Am Soc Echocardiogr 2008;21(11):1222–8.

16. Galantowicz M, Cheatham JP, Phillips A, et al. Hybrid approach for hypoplastic left heart syndrome: intermediate results after the learning curve. Ann Thorac Surg 2008;85(6):2063–70 [discussion: 2070–61].

17. Holzer RJ, Green J, Bergdall V, et al. An animal model for hybrid stage I palliation of hypoplastic left heart syndrome. Pediatr Cardiol 2009;30(7):922–7.

18. Holzer RJ, Wood A, Chisolm JL, et al. Atrial septal interventions in patients with hypoplastic left heart syndrome. Catheter Cardiovasc Interv 2008;72(5):696–704.

19. Stoica SC, Philips AB, Egan M, et al. The retrograde aortic arch in the hybrid approach to hypoplastic left heart syndrome. Ann Thorac Surg 2009;88(6):1939–46 [discussion: 1946–37].

20. Caldarone CA, Benson LN, Holtby H, et al. Main pulmonary artery to innominate artery shunt during hybrid palliation of hypoplastic left heart syndrome. J Thorac Cardiovasc Surg 2005;130(4):e1–2.

21. Holzer RJ, Sisk M, Chisolm JL, et al. Completion angiography after cardiac surgery for congenital heart disease: complementing the intraoperative imaging modalities. Pediatr Cardiol 2009;30(8):1075–82.

22. Lock JE, Block PC, McKay RG, et al. Transcatheter closure of ventricular septal defects. Circulation 1988;78(2):361–8.

23. Holzer R, Balzer D, Cao QL, et al. Amplatzer muscular ventricular septal defect I. Device closure of muscular ventricular septal defects using the Amplatzer muscular ventricular septal defect occluder: immediate and mid-term results of a U.S. registry. J Am Coll Cardiol 2004;43(7):1257–63.

24. Holzer R, de Giovanni J, Walsh KP, et al. Transcatheter closure of perimembranous ventricular septal defects using the Amplatzer membranous VSD occluder: immediate and midterm results of an international registry. Catheter Cardiovasc Interv 2006;68(4):620–8.

25. Amin Z, Danford DA, Lof J, et al. Intraoperative device closure of perimembranous ventricular

septal defects without cardiopulmonary bypass: preliminary results with the perventricular technique. J Thorac Cardiovasc Surg 2004;127(1): 234–41.

26. Mendelsohn AM, Bove EL, Lupinetti FM, et al. Intraoperative and percutaneous stenting of congenital pulmonary artery and vein stenosis. Circulation 1993;88(5 Pt 2):II210–7.

27. Mitropoulos FA, Laks H, Kapadia N, et al. Intraoperative pulmonary artery stenting: an alternative technique for the management of pulmonary artery stenosis. Ann Thorac Surg 2007;84(4):1338–41 [discussion: 1342].

28. Ing FF. Delivery of stents to target lesions: techniques of intraoperative stent implantation and intraoperative angiograms. Pediatr Cardiol 2005;26(3): 260–6.

29. Holzer RJ, Chisolm JL, Hill SL, et al. "Hybrid" stent delivery in the pulmonary circulation. J Invasive Cardiol 2008;20(11):592–8.

Outcomes After Transcatheter ASD Closure

Alejandro Román Peirone, MD, FSCAI[a],*,
Simone Fontes Pedra, MD, PhD[b],
Carlos Augusto Cardoso Pedra, MD, PhD[c,d]

KEYWORDS

• Atrial septal defect • Percutaneous device closure • Outcomes • Complications

KEY POINTS

• Surgical and interventional closure of an ostium secundum–type atrial septal defect (ASD-II) are equally effective.

• Percutaneous closure shows lower major and minor complication rates compared with surgical closure.

• Although rare, the most frequent complications described for device closure are embolization, erosion/perforations, and arrhythmias.

• Transcatheter closure has proved safe and effective, becoming the standard treatment of ASD-II.

INTRODUCTION

The ASD-II represents approximately 10% of all congenital heart disease and, with the exception of bicuspid aortic valve, is the most common congenital heart defect in adulthood.[1] Although recognized as a benign form of heart lesion, if left untreated, it can eventually contribute to significant morbidity and mortality, as reported by the natural history studies.[2,3] Over the past 4 decades, pediatric interventional cardiology has evolved enormously. The use of novel materials, technologies, and imaging modalities has opened new possibilities in the field and has had a significant impact on the outcomes of old and new procedures. As such, percutaneous closure of the ASD-II had evolved to become the standard treatment modality in lieu of cardiac surgery with cardiopulmonary bypass. Since the initial report by King and colleagues[4] of nonoperative closure of secundum ASD during cardiac catheterization,[4] several devices constructed in different shapes and materials have been introduced in the interventional arena. Some of these devices have undergone modifications and redesign and some have even disappeared from the market due to problems detected in the original models. This article presents the current clinical outcomes after ASD-II transcatheter closure as well as the complications encountered and future directions.

THERAPEUTIC OPTIONS AND/OR SURGICAL TECHNIQUES

Percutaneous device implantation has emerged as an attractive and effective alternative to surgical approach for ASD-II closure. Current devices have significantly improved the safety and success rate of the procedure, resulting in an expansion of the indications of the technique for more complex cases.[5,6] Currently, it has been estimated that more than 85% to 90% of all ASD-II are amenable to transcatheter closure and include fenestrated defects (associated or not with an aneurysm of the interatrial septum), multiple distant defects, and

[a] Pediatric Cardiology Section, Hospital Privado de Córdoba, Naciones Unidas 346, Córdoba 5016, Argentina; [b] Echocardiography Laboratory for Congenital Heart Disease, Instituto Dante Pazzanese de Cardiología, Av Dr Dante Pazzanese 500 CEP 04012-180, Sao Paulo, Brazil; [c] Catheterization Laboratory for Congenital Heart Disease, Instituto Dante Pazzanese de Cardiología, Avenida Doutor Dante Pazzanese 500 CEP 04012-180, Sao Paulo, Brazil; [d] Catheterization Laboratory for Congenital Heart Disease, Hospital do Coração, Sao Paulo, Brazil
* Corresponding author.
E-mail address: alepeirone@yahoo.com

Intervent Cardiol Clin 2 (2013) 39–49
http://dx.doi.org/10.1016/j.iccl.2012.09.004
2211-7458/13/$ – see front matter © 2013 Elsevier Inc. All rights reserved.

large ASDs (**Figs. 1–5**).[7–9] Device and surgical closures have low risks, equal effectiveness, and comparable cost. A recently published meta-analysis[10] compared the 2 methods of closure for occurrence of death and major complications. Thirteen original nonrandomized studies, including 3082 patients, searched in electronic databases, journals, and major international conference proceedings were reviewed until December 2008. Only 1 death was reported in the surgical group. Analysis of postprocedural complications showed a 31% rate in surgical patients and a 6.6% rate in patients who received a device (odds ratio [OR] 5.4; 95% CI, 2.96–9.84; $P<.0001$). The postprocedural major

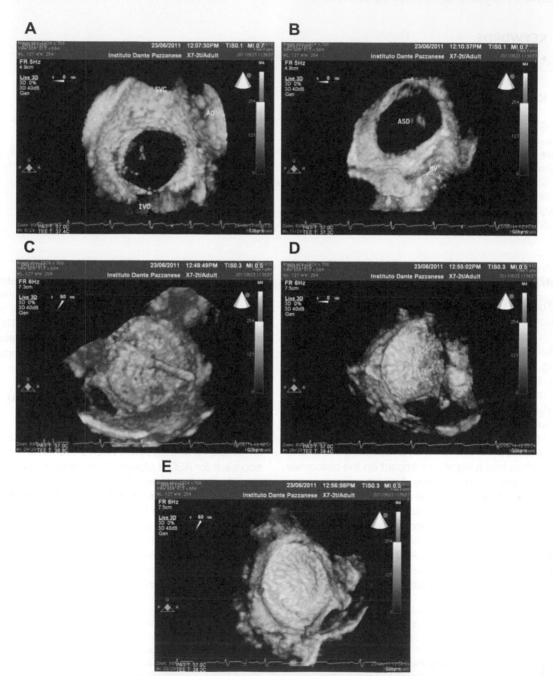

Fig. 1. Very large ASD-II (33 mm) seen on 3-D transesophageal echocardiogram. (*A*) Right atrial view. (*B*) Left atrial view. (*C*) An Occlutech device still attached to the delivery cable (right atrial view). Final aspect after device release with adequate device position and no residual defect seen from right atrial (*D*) and left atrial aspects (*E*). AO, aorta; ASD, atrial septal defect; IVC, inferior vena cava; MV, mitral valve; SVC, superior vena cava.

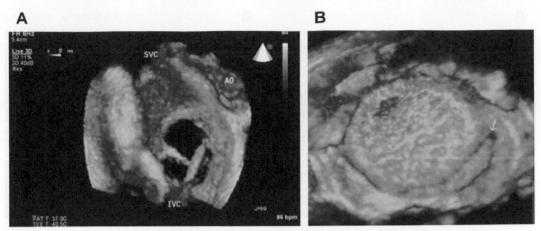

Fig. 2. Two close ASDs divided by a flimsy tongue of tissue seen on 3-D transesophageal echocardiogram (right atrial view). The catheter crosses through the superior hole (*A*). Both ASDs were closed with a single Occlutech device: final aspect after device release with a tiny residual leak (*arrow*) in the posteroinferior portion of the interatrial septum (left atrial view) (*B*). AO, aorta; IVC, inferior vena cava; SVC, superior vena cava.

complication rate was 6.8% in the surgical group and 1.9% for catheter-based closure (OR 3.81; 95% CI, 2.7–5.36; *P* = .006), again favoring percutaneous closure.

Another cohort of patients comparing both methods, including 1268 consecutive patients with isolated ASD-II, was published by the same group, with emphasis on mortality, morbidity, hospital stay, and efficacy.[11] There were no postoperative deaths. The overall rate of complications was higher in the surgical group than in the interventional group: 44% (95% CI, 39.8%–48.2%) versus 6.9% (95% CI, 5%–8.7%) (*P*<.0001). Major complications were also more frequent among surgical patients: 16% (95% CI, 13%–19%) versus 3.6% (95% CI, 2.2%–5.0%) (*P* = .002). Multiple

logistic regression analysis showed that surgery was independently strongly related to the occurrence of total complications (OR 8.13; 95% CI, 5.75–12.20) and of major complications (OR 4.03; 95% CI, 2.38–7.35). The occurrence of minor complications was also independently related to surgery. Hospital stay was shorter in the interventional group (3.2 ± 0.9 vs 8.0 ± 2.8 days, *P*<.0001).

A multicenter, nonrandomized concurrent study comparing both techniques with the purpose of looking for differences in safety, efficacy, and clinical utility was presented by Du and colleagues[12] in 2002. Among 596 patients, the total complication rate was 7.2% for the device group and 24.0% for the surgical group (*P*<.001). There were no deaths. The success rates for both groups were

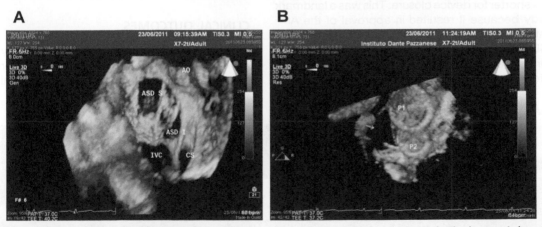

Fig. 3. Two distant ASDs as seen by 3-D transesophageal echocardiogram (right atrial view). The largest is located in the anterosuperior portion of the interatrial septum and the smaller is located in the posteroinferior interatrial septum. The distance between the defects is 10–12 mm (*A*). Two Occlutech devices (P1 – P2) were used to close the holes and there is some interposition between the two. Despite that, there is a tiny residual leak (*arrow*) between the 2 disks (left atrial view) (*B*). AO, aorta; ASD I, atrial septal defect–inferior; ASD S, atrial septal defect–superior; CS, coronary sinus; IVC, inferior vena cava.

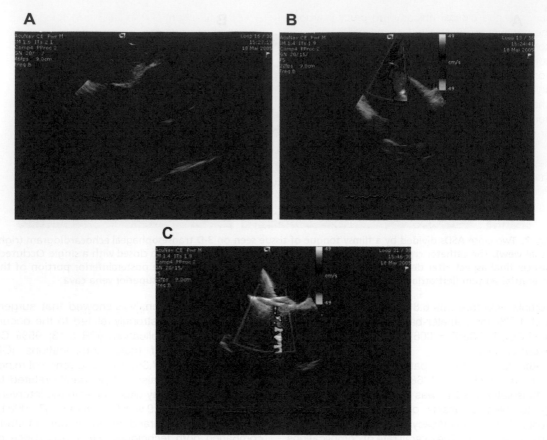

Fig. 4. Multifenestrated aneurismal septum seen on intracardiac echocardiography. On home view, the redundant and aneurismatic interatrial septum is seen (*A*). On short-axis view, color flow Doppler shows a multifenestrated interatrial septum with left-to-right shunt (right atrial, superior portion of the screen) (*B*). One single Amplatzer cribiform device was used to close the multifenestrations. It is seen still attached to the delivery cable (*C*).

not statistically different; however, the complication rate was lower and the length of hospital stay was shorter for device closure. This was a landmark study because it resulted in approval of the Amplatzer device for transcathter closure of the ASD-II by the Food and Drug Administration (FDA).

In several other smaller studies, the overall safety and effectiveness of the percutaenous technique have compared favorably with surgical repair.[11–14]

CLINICAL OUTCOMES

In the proper assessment of outcomes after any interventional procedure, especially with insertion of a device in the heart, the definitions of clinical

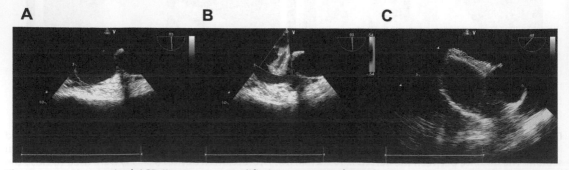

Fig. 5. A moderate-sized ASD-II seen on a modified 91° transesophageal echocardiogram view in 2-D (*A*) and color Doppler (*B*). The defect was closed using a Nit-Occlud ASD-R device, which is seen after release in a correct position without residual shunting (*C*). V, a mark for orientation of the side of the echo image.

success and clinical efficacy are crucial. Among the multiple goals pursued during ASD-II closure, complete defect occlusion, right ventricular (RV) volume normalization, absence of late complications (erosion, perforation, and fractures), and no significant arrhythmias or deleterious ECG changes are the most important. Absence of additional interventions after closure and no infectious or thrombotic events are also key issues.

The success rate of implantation of devices depends on the experience of the operator and the anatomy of the defect (presence of large defects, multiple defects, inadequate rims of septal tissue, atrial septal aneurysm, or combination of those factors).[6] Due to its design and easier-to-use system, the Amplatzer septal occluder results in higher rates of successful implantation, approaching 99% in experienced hands.[12,15] Although this device can close a broad range of ASD dimensions, including the large ones, the Helex device is only recommended for small-to-moderate size defects (up to 18 mm of stretched diameter).[13]

RV volume overload is a well-known cardiac consequence of ASD-II left-to-right shunt, accounting for most of its long-term complications. Thus, cardiac volumetric unloading is a major aim of percutaneous intervention. Transcatheter closure of ASD-II results in a rapid normalization of RV volume overload and improvement of RV function, as demonstrated by the decrease of RV end-diastolic and end-systolic volumes, the decrease of the RV myocardial performance index, and the increase of the RV ejection fraction after device insertion.[16–18] Percutaneous closure leads to a progressive decrease in size of the RV, usually taking 6 to 12 months (or even more) to attain normal dimensions. In some patients, however, especially those with higher pulmonary blood flow and operated at older ages, the RV remains enlarged. Although this residual dilatation has been termed, cardiomyopathy of volume loading, its clinical impact on exercise performance is limited. By the same token, the left ventricular volume increases due to the shift of the septum toward the decompressed RV and this plays a major role in the improved exercise response. Echocardiography, CT, and functional studies have shown better RV improvement in younger than older patients and those undergoing closure by interventional catheterization rather than by surgery.[19–28]

Complete closure of the defect depends on the type of device, size of the defect, and timing of evaluation. An immediate residual shunt may be seen in up to 10% to 30% of patients immediately after device release.[12,13] With progressive endothelialization of the devices, closure rates reach 92% to 99% after a year of follow-up, higher for the Amplatzer device and smaller defects.[7] Due to its non–self-centering mechanism, residual leaks are more frequently observed with the Helex device.[13,29] The vast majority, if not all, of these residual leaks seen with either device, however, are trivial or small in size (<3–4 mm) and do not result in any hemodynamic burden to the RV. Therefore, clinical cure is achieved in virtually 100% of patients.

Several publications showing long-term outcomes after ASD-II closure in children and adults have confirmed the safety and effectiveness of the procedure.[7,15,30–32] Successful interventions associated with high closure rate and improvement in both RV dilatation and supraventricular arrhythmias are commonly reported.[5,30,33] Moreover, a recent analysis of the FDA Manufacturer and User Facility Device Experience (MAUDE database) revealed that there was no difference between clinical outcomes and overall mortality comparing surgical and device closure.[34,35] Device embolization was the most prevalent adverse event for the percutaneous procedure, with an estimated rate between 0.55% and 0.62%.[36,37]

A report showing long-term outcomes (5–20 years) after surgical or device ASD-II closure was recently published.[31] Outcomes for either method were excellent and no significant differences were found with regards to survival, functional capacity, atrial arrhythmias, or embolic neurologic events. Age and pre-existing arrhythmia, but not surgery or percutaneous closure, were identified as independent risk factors for late arrhythmia.

Patients with ASD-II associated with pulmonary arterial hypertension constitute a challenging group to manage.[14,38,39] The clinical outcomes in 54 patients with moderate or severe pulmonary arterial hypertension who underwent successful device implantation for ASD-II closure have been recently examined by the group in Toronto.[40] During early follow-up, all patients were alive and the RV systolic pressure decreased significantly. At the late follow-up, 2 patients had died and the baseline RV systolic pressure continued to decrease significantly. Nevertheless, only 43.6% of patients had normalization (<40 mm Hg) of RV pressure during the last clinical visit. In patients showing severe pulmonary arterial hypertension with a partial fall of pressure after compliant balloon occlusion test, implantation of a home-made fenestrated Amplatzer septal occluder device has been reported to decrease the left-to-right shunt and promote further decrease of pulmonary arterial pressure in the long-term.[41]

The diameter of the modified fenestration decreases significantly in size during follow-up, although applying this technique the selected patients avoid acute decompensation and benefit from gradual diminution of RV volume overload.[42] Additionally, the group in Mexico[14] showed that the efficacy for ASD-II closure was similar in both a percutaneous and a surgical group, although a higher rate of events was significantly associated with age greater than 40 years, pulmonary arterial hypertension, and low oxygen saturations.[43]

Perhaps the elderly patients with ASD-II are the ones who are at a higher risk of surgical complications and may benefit from the interventional procedure the most. In this regard, a group in Edmonton, Canada, has recently reported the clinical outcomes after device (81%) or surgical (19%) ASD-II closure in such groups of patients (older than 60 years). During follow-up (3.3 years), the quality of life was comparable to age-matched healthy controls, and RV and left ventricular end-diastolic dimensions, RV function, and New York Heart Association class showed significant improvement ($P<.001$) in both groups. The prevalence of atrial arrhythmias, however, was unchanged. Morbidity was higher for the surgical group (23% vs 7%).[44]

Although chronic right heart volume overload and right heart failure are abolished over time after transcatheter closure of ASD-II, acute pulmonary venous congestion may be occasionally observed in older patients with large defects immediately after device closure. The main mechanism of this complication is probably an age-related left ventricular diastolic dysfunction, although other factors, such as left systolic dysfunction, ventricular wall and vascular stiffening, and increased incidence of comorbidities (diabetes, systemic hypertension, and coronary artery disease), may also play a role. The resultant effect of ASD closure is an acute volume loading of the noncompliant left chambers and subsequent pulmonary edema, which may require positive pressure ventilation for 24 to 48 hours until it subsides. Accurate assessment of preclosure diastolic function, especially after test ASD-II occlusion to unmask possible abnormalities, may help identify high-risk patients for postclosure pulmonary edema. Anticongestive therapy (dopamine, milrinone, and furosemide) for 48 to 72 hours before definitive device closure or the use of fenestrated device seems effective in preventing this complication in high-risk patients. Long-term outcome of such patients needs further studies.[45–47]

In conclusion, excellent quality of life, functional class improvement, and ventricular remodeling are the rule after percutaneous ASD-II closure.

COMPLICATIONS AND CONCERNS

Both pivotal studies for the FDA-approved devices (Amplatzer Septal Occluder and Helex Septal Occluder) showed that the rate of major adverse events was lower in the device group compared with the surgical group.[12,13] The Mid-Atlantic Group of Interventional Cardiology (MAGIC) reported the results of unrestricted multiinstitution routine use of an ASD device in 478 patients from 2004 to 2007. This ASD study showed a major adverse event rate of only 1.1%.[48] Although these complications are rare, they can be life threatening (discussed later).

MALPOSITION AND EMBOLIZATION

The major adverse events attributed to the transcatheter group in the pivotal Amplatzer Septal Occluder study included device embolization requiring surgical (0.7%) or percutaneous retrieval (0.2%).[12] In the pivotal Helex Septal Occluder study, device embolization also represents the most frequent major adverse events (1.7%).[13] If an embolization does happen, devices can usually be retrieved from the heart using transcatheter techniques, with the exception of devices that are entangled with the tricuspid or mitral valve chordae. Surgical removal is recommended in such cases. The overall published embolization rate is approximately 0.55% and the mortality rate for surgical management of a device adverse event increases to 1.8% to 2.6%.[34,36] Most embolizations occurred because of inadequate rim or undersized devices. Among the various causes of device embolization, the most common is the absence or inadequacy of an inferior vena cava rim. Large and eccentric defects, other rim deficiencies, and technical problems during the procedure (improper sizing of the defect and suboptimal placement of the device) are also risk factors related to embolization. More than 90% of these events occur within the first 24 hours of implantation, typically while the patients are being observed in the hospital setting, although late embolizations have been reported.[49] Because of its design and configuration, the Helex device is, perhaps, the easiest device to be retrieved using snares and bioptomes.

DEVICE MALFUNCTION (EROSION/ PERFORATION AND FRACTURE)

Injury to either the atrial wall or the aorta has been described as a consequence of device implantation in the interatrial septum. The mechanisms of device erosion/perforation after ASD-II device implantation have not been established with certainty, but several clinical observations merit discussion. In 2002, AGA Medical Corporation focused on the issue of cardiac perforation and selected an expert panel to review all cases of hemodynamic compromise after device implantation with the objective of dictate recommendations to minimize its occurrence. The incidence of device erosion was 0.1%. Twenty-eight cases were reported to AGA Medical Corporation and all erosions occurred at the dome of the atria, near the aortic root (5 involved perforation of the roof of the left atrium and the aorta, 6 involved perforation of the roof of the right atrium and the aorta, both atria were involved in 1 case, no atrial perforation in were involved in 3 cases, and, in 3 cases with aortic perforations, a fistulous communication was noted). Deficient aortic rim was seen in 89% and the defect was described as a high ASD-II, suggesting deficient superior rim. Device to unstretched ASD ratio was significantly larger in the adverse event patients. The panel concluded that a deficient aortic rim and/or superior rim, an overstretching during balloon sizing, and use of oversized devices were all possible risks factors for erosion.[50] Nevertheless, other poorly understood mechanisms of erosion may also play a role and may include older age, extensive device manipulation during prolonged procedures, and alternative techniques to anchor the device (coming from pulmonary veins).

A retrospective review of all adverse events reported to the FDA (MAUDE database) and Health Canada published in the literature, including a review presented by Divekar and colleagues,[51] found 24 cardiac perforations occurring early in 20.8% and late in 66.6%. Five events occurred within 1 day, 10 within 3 days, and 6 after 3 days (3 weeks to 3 years). Cardiac perforation occurred predominantly in the anterosuperior atrial walls and/or adjacent aorta. The relationship of device size, patient size, or atrial dimensions have not been clearly associated with the occurrence of device erosion. What is unknown is the extent of rim deficiency that would result in an unsecure placement and whether this contributes to erosion risks. The most important action to minimize future risks of this adverse event is to identify high-risk cases, alert for early recognition of complications, and prompt adequate intervention.

Alternatively, wire frame or wire wings/arms fractures are potential structural problems in other types of devices. This complication has been reported for the Clamshell family of devices,[32,52,53] the Helex device,[29] and the Solysafe device[54] and has occurred even after some modifications were implemented to overcome this problem. The incidence of wire frame fracture for the more compliant and less rigid Helex device was approximately 6.4% and it was most commonly observed in larger devices. Although this is usually benign, mitral valve perforation by a fractured wire has been reported.[29] Because wire fracture on the Solysafe device could lead to cardiac perforation and tamponade,[54] this device was withdrawn from the market recently.

ARRHYTHMIAS

Conduction abnormalities and new-onset arrhythmias are some of the most important complications after device insertion, most frequent in the adult population, with an estimated incidence of approximately 1.5% of the patients.[44,55] Whether conduction abnormalities and new-onset arrhythmias is caused or just triggered by the device in a subpopulation who already has an underlying anatomic substrate for this occurrence is debatable.

An acute increase in supraventricular ectopy and a small risk of atrioventricular conduction abnormalities, including complete heart block, has been rarely reported among patients undergoing ASD-II percutaneous closure.[56] Occasionally, the use of larger devices in young patients may result in a higher than expected incidence of postprocedural heart block.[57] The group at the Mayo Clinic, Rochester, Minnesota, has presented a study comparing ECGs registered before and after ASD-II or PFO device closure. Although uncommon, significant heart block episodes, changes in several markers of atrial conduction, and new-onset atrial tachyarrhytmias were found. Moreover, a low risk of clinically significant postprocedure arrhythmias suggesting an effect of device closure on intra-atrial conduction was encountered.[58] It has been postulated that patients with prolonged PR interval before device closure are at a higher risk of developing complete heart block after the procedure.

In the majority of cases, the rhythm abnormality improves after the device is removed. It is recommended that a device should be electively removed even if the heart block episode is intermittent. A large device related to the defect diameter seems associated to arrhythmias, suggesting mechanical compression of the disk as etiology of the complication.[59]

THROMBOEMBOLISM

According to the published literature, the incidence of thrombus formation on closure devices is low, and if it does occur, usually resolves under anticoagulation therapy. In a major study presented by Krumsdorf and colleagues,[60] a total of 1000 consecutive patients were investigated using transesophageal echocardiography after patent foramen ovale (PFO) or ASD-II closure at 1 and 6 months postprocedure. Thrombus formation was detected in 1.2% of the ASD-II patients and in 2.5% of the PFO patients (P = NS). The majority of the diagnoses were made after the first 4 weeks. The incidence distributed by device type was 7.1% in the CardioSEAL device (NMT Medical, Boston, Massachusetts); 5.7% in the StarFLEX device (NMT Medical); 6.6% in the PFO-Star device (Applied Biometrics, Burnsville, Minnesota); 3.6% in the ASDOS device (Dr Ing, Osypka Corp., Grenzach-Wyhlen, Germany); 0.8% in the Helex device (W.L. Gore and Associates, Flagstaff, Arizona); and 0% in the Amplatzer device (St Jude Medical, St Paul, Minnesota). A prethrombotic disorder as a possible cause of the thrombus was found in 2 PFO patients. Postprocedure atrial fibrillation and persistent atrial septal aneurysm were shown as significant predictors for thrombus formation (P<.05). In the vast majority of patients, the thrombus resolved under anticoagulation therapy using heparin or warfarin.

Also, periprocedural events with detection of acute thrombi formation in both the device and the sheath have been described, despite proper preprocedural anticoagulation.[61,62] Meticulous flushing of catheters and sheaths is imperative to avoid this complication.

Finally, a routine and standard cardiac catheterization should be performed before devices are implanted. As such, it has the potential of causing some complications, including hematoma formation, vascular damage, air embolism, catheter-related arrhythmia, pericardial effusion, and/or tamponade and infection. The occurrence of these events is low and may need a specific treatment.[63,64]

FUTURE CONSIDERATIONS

During past decades, there has been a great deal of effort to design and develop the "perfect" device for ASD-II closure. Ideally, this device should be easy to implant and retrieve, show 100% closure rate and no potential for erosion or embolization, require small-size sheath for implantation, and maintain a low profile in the atrial septum as well as be manufactured in biocompatible and bioabsorbable[65–67] materials to optimize biologic response and mechanical integrity. Alternative methods of device fixation that do not rely on device dimensions exceeding the defect itself for closure would also be beneficial. The years to come will surely witness the application of new technologies for the imaging diagnosis and treatment of ASD-II. Evolving imaging technology will be applied not only for the accurate diagnosis of all types of ASDs but also mainly for the guidance of transcather closure. Real-time 3-D intracardiac echocardiography will probably be helpful in this regard. MRI-guided interventions is an exciting field that may have an impact on abolishing the need for radiation exposure in the catheterization laboratory for ASD-II closure. With the rapid development of new devices to close the left atrial appendage in high-risk elderly patients with atrial fibrillation and to repair functional mitral valve insufficiency percutaneously, the development of devices manufactured using bioabsorbable materials is of paramount importance to allow free transseptal access to the left atrium in the future.

SUMMARY

ASD-II closure has evolved from a surgical procedure requiring cardiopulmonary bypass to a percutaneous, catheter-based procedure usually requiring only an overnight hospital stay. The overall safety and effectiveness have compared favorably with surgical repair. Although rare, complications have been described, including device embolization, malfunction, and arrhythmias. The overall long-term clinical outcomes have been excellent: good quality of life, functional class improvement, and ventricular remodeling have been the rule after the procedure. It is mandatory to recommend indefinite follow-up of patients undergoing this procedure for potential long-term complications.

REFERENCES

1. Carlgren LE. The incidence of congenital heart disease in children born in Gothenburg 1941-1950. Br Heart J 1959;21:40–50.
2. Campbell M. Natural history of atrial septal defect. Br Heart J 1970;32:820.
3. Craig RJ, Selzer A. Natural history and prognosis of atrial septal defect. Circulation 1968;37:805.
4. King T, Thompson S, Steiner C, et al. Secundum atrial septal defect: nonoperative closure during cardiac catheterization. JAMA 1976;235:2506–9.
5. Pedra CA, Pedra SR, Esteves CA, et al. Transcatheter closure of secundum atrial septal defects with complex anatomy. J Invasive Cardiol 2004;16:117–22.
6. Butera G, Romagnoli E, Carminati M, et al. Treatment of isolated secundum atrial septal defects: impact of age and defect morphology in 1,013 consecutive patients. Am Heart J 2008;156:706–12.
7. Diab KA, Cao QL, Bacha EA, et al. Device closure of atrial septal defects with the Amplatzer septal

occluder: safety and outcomes in infants. J Thorac Cardiovasc Surg 2007;134:960–6.

8. Awad SM, Garay FF, Cao QL, et al. Multiple Amplatzer septal occluder devices for multiple atrial communications: immediate and long-term follow-up results. Catheter Cardiovasc Interv 2007;70:265–73.

9. Pedra SR, Pontes SC Jr, Cassar Rde S, et al. The role of echocardiography in the percutaneous treatment of septal defects. Arq Bras Cardiol 2006;86:87–96 [in Portuguese].

10. Butera G, Biondi-Zoccai G, Sangiorgi G, et al. Percutaneous versus surgical closure of secundum atrial septal defects: a systematic review and meta-analysis of currently available clinical evidence. EuroIntervention 2011;7:377–85.

11. Butera G, Carminati M, Chessa M, et al. Percutaneous versus surgical closure of secundum atrial septal defect: comparison of early results and complications. Am Heart J 2006;151:228–34.

12. Du ZD, Hijazi ZM, Kleinman CS, et al. Comparison between transcatheter and surgical closure of secundum atrial septal defect in children and adults: results of a multicenter nonrandomized trial. J Am Coll Cardiol 2002;39:1836–44.

13. Jones TK, Latson LA, Zahn E, et al, Multicenter Pivotal Study of the HELEX Septal Occluder Investigators. Results of the U.S. multicenter pivotal study of the HELEX septal occluder for percutaneous closure of secundum atrial septal defects. J Am Coll Cardiol 2007;49:2215–21.

14. Rosas M, Zabal C, Garcia-Montes J, et al. Transcatheter versus surgical closure of secundum atrial septal defect in adults: impact of age at intervention. A concurrent matched comparative study. Congenit Heart Dis 2007;2:148–55.

15. Masura J, Gavora P, Podnar T. Long-term outcome of transcatheter secundum-type atrial septal defect closure using Amplatzer septal occluders. J Am Coll Cardiol 2005;45:505–7.

16. Ding J, Ma G, Huang Y, et al. Right ventricular remodeling after transcatheter closure of atrial septal defect. Echocardiography 2009;26:1146–52.

17. Wu ET, Akagi T, Taniguchi M, et al. Differences in right and left ventricular remodeling after transcatheter closure of atrial septal defect among adults. Catheter Cardiovasc Interv 2007;69:866–71.

18. Pawelec-Wojtalik M, Wojtalik M, Mrowczynski W, et al. Comparison of cardiac function in children after surgical and Amplatzer occluder closure of secundum atrial septal defects. Eur J Cardiothorac Surg 2006;29:89–92.

19. Berbarie RF, Anwar A, Dockery WD, et al. Measurement of right ventricular volumes before and after atrial septal defect closure using multislice computed tomography. Am J Cardiol 2007;99:1458–61.

20. Di Salvo G, Drago M, Pacileo G, et al. Atrial function after surgical and percutaneous closure of atrial septal defect: a strain rate imaging study. J Am Soc Echocardiogr 2005;18:930–3.

21. Eerola A, Pihkala JI, Boldt T, et al. Hemodynamic improvement is faster after percutaneous ASD closure than after surgery. Catheter Cardiovasc Interv 2007;69:432–41.

22. Giardini A, Donti A, Formigari R, et al. Determinants of cardiopulmonary functional improvement after transcatheter atrial septal defect closure in asymptomatic adults. J Am Coll Cardiol 2004;43:1886–91.

23. Pascotto M, Santoro G, Cerrato F, et al. Time-course of cardiac remodeling following transcatheter closure of atrial septal defect. Int J Cardiol 2006;112:348–52.

24. Santoro G, Pascotto M, Caputo S, et al. Similar cardiac remodelling after transcatheter atrial septal defect closure in children and young adults. Heart 2006;92:958–62.

25. Schussler JM, Anwar A, Phillips SD, et al. Effect on right ventricular volume of percutaneous Amplatzer closure of atrial septal defect in adults. Am J Cardiol 2005;95:993–5.

26. Thilén U, Persson S. Closure of atrial septal defect in the adult. Cardiac remodeling is an early event. Int J Cardiol 2006;108:370–5.

27. Kort HW, Balzer DT, Johnson MC. Resolution of right heart enlargement after closure of secundum atrial septal defect with transcatheter technique. J Am Coll Cardiol 2001;38:1528–32.

28. Brochu MC, Baril JF, Dore A, et al. Improvement in exercise capacity in asymptomatic and mildly symptomatic adults after atrial septal defect percutaneous closure. Circulation 2002;106:1821–6.

29. Fagan T, Dreher D, Cutright W, et al, GORE HELEX Septal Occluder Working Group Catheter. Fracture of the Gore Helex septal occluder: associated factors and clinical outcomes. Catheter Cardiovasc Interv 2009;73:941–8.

30. Wilson NJ, Smith J, Prommete B, et al. Transcatheter closure of secundum atrial septal defects with the Amplatzer septal occluder in adults and children-follow-up closure rates, degree of mitral regurgitation and evolution of arrhythmias. Heart Lung Circ 2008;17:318–24.

31. Kutty S, Hazeem AA, Brown K, et al. Long-term (5- to 20-year) outcomes after transcatheter or surgical treatment of hemodynamically significant isolated secundum atrial septal defect. Am J Cardiol 2012;109:1348–52.

32. Law MA, Josey J, Justino H, et al. Long-term follow-up of the STARFlex device for closure of secundum atrial septal defect. Catheter Cardiovasc Interv 2009;73:190–5.

33. Vecht JA, Saso S, Rao C, et al. Atrial septal defect closure is associated with a reduced prevalence of

atrial tachyarrhythmia in the short to medium term: a systematic review and meta-analysis. Heart 2010;96:1789–97.

34. DiBardino DJ, McElhinney DB, Kaza AK, et al. Analysis of the US Food and Drug Administration Manufacturer and User Facility Device Experience database for adverse events involving Amplatzer septal occluder devices and comparison with the Society of Thoracic Surgery congenital cardiac surgery database. J Thorac Cardiovasc Surg 2009; 137:1334–41.

35. U.S. Food and Drug Administration Web site. Available at: http://www.fda.gov/default.htm.

36. Levi DS, Moore JW. Embolization and retrieval of the Amplatzer Septal Occluder. Catheter Cardiovasc Interv 2004;61:543–7.

37. Delaney JW, Li JS, Rhodes JF. Major complications associated with transcatheter atrial septal occluder implantation: a review of the medical literature and the manufacturer and user facility device experience (MAUDE) database. Congenit Heart Dis 2007;2: 256–64.

38. de Lezo JS, Medina A, Romero M, et al. Effectiveness of percutaneous device occlusion for atrial septal defect in adult patients with pulmonary hypertension. Am Heart J 2002;144:877–80.

39. Yong G, Khairy P, De Guise P, et al. Pulmonary arterial hypertension in patients with transcatheter closure of secundum atrial septal defects: a longitudinal study. Circ Cardiovasc Interv 2009;2:455–62.

40. Balint OH, Samman A, Haberer K, et al. Outcomes in patients with pulmonary hypertension undergoing percutaneous atrial septal defect closure. Heart 2008;94:1189–93.

41. Dell'avvocata F, Rigatelli G, Cardaioli P, et al. Homemade fenestrated amplatzer occluder for atrial septal defect and pulmonary arterial hypertension. J Geriatr Cardiol 2011;8:127–9.

42. Schneider HE, Jux C, Kriebel T, et al. Fate of a modified fenestration of atrial septal occluder device after transcatheter closure of atrial septal defects in elderly patients. J Interv Cardiol 2011;24:485–90.

43. Rosas M, Attie F, Sandoval J, et al. Atrial septal defect in adults > or =40 years old: negative impact of low arterial oxygen saturation. Int J Cardiol 2004; 93:145–55.

44. Hanninen M, Kmet A, Taylor DA, et al. Atrial septal defect closure in the elderly is associated with excellent quality of life, functional improvement, and ventricular remodelling. Can J Cardiol 2011;27: 698–704.

45. Masutani S, Senzaki H. Left ventricular function in adult patients with atrial septal defect: implication for development of heart failure after transcatheter closure. J Card Fail 2011;17:957–63.

46. Schubert S, Peters B, Abdul-Khaliq H, et al. Left ventricular conditioning in the elderly patient to prevent congestive heart failure after transcatheter closure of atrial septal defect. Catheter Cardiovasc Interv 2005;64:333–7.

47. MacDonald ST, Arcidiacono C, Butera G. Fenestrated Amplatzer atrial septal defect occluder in an elderly patient with restrictive left ventricular physiology. Heart 2011;97:438.

48. Everett AD, Jennings J, Sibinga E, et al. Community use of the amplatzer atrial septal defect occluder: results of the multicenter MAGIC atrial septal defect study. Pediatr Cardiol 2009;30:240–7.

49. Teoh K, Wilton E, Brecker S, et al. Simultaneous removal of an Amplatzer device from an atrial septal defect and the descending aorta. J Thorac Cardiovasc Surg 2006;131:909–10.

50. Amin Z, Hijazi ZM, Bass JL, et al. Erosion of Amplatzer septal occluder device after closure of secundum atrial septal defects: review of registry of complications and recommendations to minimize future risk. Catheter Cardiovasc Interv 2004;63: 496–502.

51. Divekar A, Gaamangwe T, Shaikh N, et al. Cardiac perforation after device closure of atrial septal defects with Amplatzer septal occluder. J Am Coll Cardiol 2005;45:1213–8.

52. Carminati M, Chessa M, Butera G, et al. Transcatheter closure of atrial septal defects with the STAR-Flex device: early results and follow-up. J Interv Cardiol 2001;14:319–24.

53. Pedra C, Pihkala J, Lee KJ, et al. Transcathter closure of atrial septal defects using the Cardioseal implant. Heart 2000;84:320–6.

54. Cabrera M, Contreras A, Peirone A. Late cardiac perforation following percutaneous atrial septal defect closure using the Solysafe device. J Invasive Cardiol 2011;23:E139–41.

55. Sadiq M, Kazmi T, Rehman AU, et al. Device closure of atrial septal defect: medium-term outcome with special reference to complications. Cardiol Young 2012;22:71–8.

56. Hill SL, Berul CI, Patel HT, et al. Early ECG abnormalities associated with transcatheter closure of atrial septal defects using the Amplatzer septal occluder. J Interv Card Electrophysiol 2000;4: 469–74.

57. Suda K, Raboisson MJ, Piette E, et al. Reversible atrioventricular block associated with closure of atrial septal defects using the Amplatzer device. J Am Coll Cardiol 2004;43:1677–82.

58. Johnson JN, Marquardt ML, Ackerman MJ, et al. Electrocardiographic changes and arrhythmias following percutaneous atrial septal defect and patent foramen ovale device closure. Catheter Cardiovasc Interv 2011;78:254–61.

59. Amin Z. Complications of device closure of ASD's and PFO's. In: Hijazi ZM, Feldman T, Al-Qbandi MH, et al, editors. Transcatheter closure of ASDs and

PFOs. Minneapolis (MN): Cardiotext Publishing, LLC; 2010. p. 271–81.

60. Krumsdorf U, Ostermayer S, Billinger K, et al. Incidence and clinical course of thrombus formation on atrial septal defect and patient foramen ovale closure devices in 1,000 consecutive patients. J Am Coll Cardiol 2004;43:302–9.

61. Yorgun H, Canpolat U, Kaya EB, et al. Thrombus formation during percutaneous closure of an atrial septal defect with an Amplatzer septal occluder. Tex Heart Inst J 2011;38:427–30.

62. Eren NK, Akyildiz ZI, Acet H, et al. Thrombus formation on the delivery sheath during transcatheter atrial septal defect closure. Tex Heart Inst J 2009;36:624–5.

63. Balasundaram RP, Anandaraja S, Juneja R, et al. Infective endocarditis following implantation of Amplatzer atrial septal occluder. Indian Heart J 2005; 57:167–9.

64. Bullock AM, Menahem S, Wilkinson JL. Infective endocarditis on an occluder closing an atrial septal defect. Cardiol Young 1999;9:65–7.

65. Jux C, Bertram H, Wohlsein P, et al. Interventional atrial septal defect closure using a totally bioresorbable occluder matrix: development and preclinical evaluation of the BioSTAR device. J Am Coll Cardiol 2006;48:161–9.

66. Mullen MJ, Hildick-Smith D, De Giovanni JV, et al. BioSTAR Evaluation Study (BEST): a prospective, multicenter, phase I clinical trial to evaluate the feasibility, efficacy, and safety of the BioSTAR bioabsorbable septal repair implant for the closure of atrial-level shunts. Circulation 2006;114:1962–7.

67. Hoehn R, Hesse C, Ince H, et al. First experience with the BioSTAR device for various applications in pediatric patients with congenital heart disease. Catheter Cardiovasc Interv 2010;75:72–7.

Influence of PFO Anatomy on Successful Transcatheter Closure

Eustaquio Onorato, MD, FSCAI[a,b,*], Francesco Casilli, MD[c]

KEYWORDS

- Patent foramen ovale anatomy • Atrial septal morphology • Atrial septal aneurysm
- Transcatheter closure of patent foramen ovale • Outcomes • Complications • Paradoxic embolism
- Cryptogenic stroke

KEY POINTS

- Patent foramen ovale (PFO) is considered a risk factor for serious clinical syndromes, the most important of which is cryptogenic stroke in the setting of paradoxic embolism.
- The safety and feasibility of transcatheter PFO closure have been addressed in several studies; nowdays, this procedure is performed worldwide in many centers with excellent results.
- The various PFO devices are inserted percutaneously with a high degree of success and a low complication rate.
- Nevertheless, variations in the atrial septal configuration and PFO are frequent and their impact on the technical aspects and success in transcatheter PFO closure is noteworthy.
- To minimize the rate of complications of percutaneous closure of PFO, patients must be carefully selected on the basis of morphology and location of the interatrial defect.

PFO ANATOMY FOR THE INTERVENTIONALIST

Failure of the primum and secundum septa to fuse postnatally results in a PFO, a vestige of fetal circulation, usually with a tunnel-like shape that is observed in more than 25% of the adult population.[1] The risk of recurrent cerebrovascular events is further elevated if the PFO is associated with atrial septal aneurysm (ASA).[2,3] A PFO is defined as a valve-like opening between the fibrous, thin, and mobile septum primum and the muscular septum secundum without evidence of an anatomic defect in the septa by transthoracic echocardiography (TTE) and/or transesophageal echocardiography (TEE). Anatomic features of the interatrial septum, the morphology of the PFO valve-like opening, the degree of mobility of the septum primum, and the size of the PFO defects are all variable and require careful evaluation by the operator before implantation of the closure device (**Fig. 1**).[4] The relationship of PFO to the surrounding structures has to be considered when choosing the correct closure device. The upper margin of the septum primum is a crescent that forms the lower boundary of the foramen ovale. The average distance from PFO to the superior vena cava is 12.2 mm and 8.1 mm to the aortic annulus.[5] From autopsy series, PFO has a circular to elliptical shape and is located in the anterosuperior portion of interatrial septum (see **Fig. 1**).[6] The extent to which the dynamic components of the atrial septum overlap determines the length of

---

Disclosures: The authors have nothing to disclose regarding the content of this article.
[a] Clinica Montevergine, Via M. Malzoni, 83013 Mercogliano (Av), Italy; [b] Humanitas Gavazzeni, Bergamo, Italy; [c] Emodinamica e Radiologia Cardiovascolare, Policlinico San Donato, Piazza Edmondo Malan–20097 San Donato Milanese, Milano, Italy
* Corresponding author. Via Mirabella, 7 – 25064 Gussago (Brescia), Italy.
E-mail address: eonorato@libero.it

interventional.theclinics.com

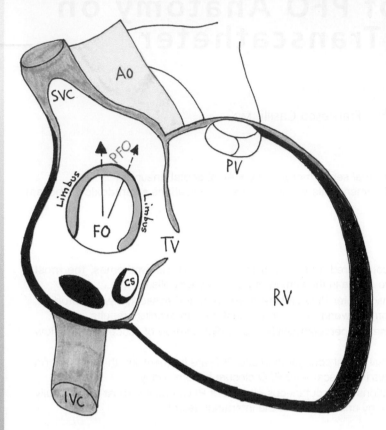

Fig. 1. Atrial septal anatomy. The fossa ovalis (FO) does not lie exactly in the middle of the atrial septum but instead is displaced a little infero-posteriorly. Inferior to the FO is the IVC and inferoanteriorly, the CS. The SVC enters from above along the posterior aspect of the atrial septum. The tricuspid valve lies anteriorly. The aortic valve and root lie centrally in the heart, wedged between the 2 atria and resting on the atrial septum. Thus the anterosuperior border of the FO is related to the aortic root. There is a complex anatomic relationship between the FO and the structures adjacent. The atrial septal tissue between each structure and the FO is called a rim, of which there are 5 on the right atrial side (SVC rim, aortic rim, IVC rim, CS rim, and tricuspid valve rim) and 2 on the left atrial side (mitral valve rim and right upper pulmonary vein rim). AO, aorta; FO, fossa ovalis; PV, pulmonary valve; RV, right ventricle; TV, tricuspid valve.

this tunnel. The distance of nonfusion between the septa determines its width or size. All these anatomic features may be characterized by different imaging modalities in the preoperative morphologic and functional assessment: TTE/TEE, 3-D TEE, cardiac CT, and cardiac MRI. In clinical practice TEE is the preferred tool to define this complex anatomic structure because it provides the ability to measure both the size (the largest separation between the primum and secundum septa) and the length of the tunnel.

PFO Size

The PFO size increases with each decade of life. In an autopsy study[5] performed on 100 samples representative of the 10 decades of life, it was confirmed that PFO has a mean diameter of 5.1 mm, ranging from 3.4 mm in the first decade to 5.8 mm in the tenth decade (**Table 1**). Furthermore, PFO diameter was larger in women than men (5.56 mm vs 4.7 mm; $P = .028$). It has been proposed that PFOs larger than 4 mm in diameter convey a greater risk for recurrent stroke compared with smaller defects.[7] Heterogeneity of size and morphology are also pertinent to interventional device closure selection.[8] Studies that have been published to date have emphasized a single

measurement of the PFO, typically made by TTE/TEE and using either the maximum separation between the rims of the defect or the largest diameter of a balloon that can be pulled or pushed through the defect (stretched diameter by sizing balloon [SB]). Stretchability index has been calculated as the ratio of stretched to unstretched diameter. The variable thickness and aneurismal nature of the atrial septum may lead to wide variation in the stretchability of defects of the same unstretched diameter. The nonstreched PFO diameters were significantly smaller than stretched ones. The device size–to–stretched diameter ratio was significantly increased in patients with septal

Table 1 Anatomic characteristics and relationship of PFO to the surrounding structures	
PFO diameter	Range: 1–19 mm; mean 4.9 mm
PFO tunnel length	Range: 3–18 mm; mean 8 mm
PFO distance from SVC	Average: 12.2 mm
PFO distance from aortic annulus	Average: 8.1 mm

aneurysm and complex PFO compared with those patients with simple PFO morphology (mean 3.9:1 vs 2.6:1; $P<.05$).[9]

Tunnel Length

The usually tunnel-like shape of the PFO is determined by the extent to which the thin fibrous septum primum and the thick muscular secundum overlap.

As described by McKenzie and colleagues,[5] the length of PFO overlap ranged between 3 mm and 18 mm with an average length equal to 8 mm (see **Table 1**). The same result was highlighted by Marshall and Lock,[10] who described a tunnel length varying widely between 2.4 and 19.5 mm.

As previously reported,[9–11] a schematic classification of PFO anatomy based on a separate analysis of the PFO and atrial septal morphology is proposed (**Table 2**).

Simple PFO

A simple PFO is defined as a short tunnel (up to 8 mm), not associated with ASA or prominent eustachian valve (EV), and with a thickness of the muscular septum up to 6 mm; it is present in approximately 45% of the cases submitted to catheter closure (**Fig. 2**).

Complex PFO

Atrial septal aneurysm

ASA refers to a redundancy of septum primum tissue bulging into the right and/or the left atrium. The prevalence of ASA in the general population ranges from 1% in autopsy studies[12] to 2.2% to 4.9% in TEE series.[13] A significantly higher percentage has been reported in preselected

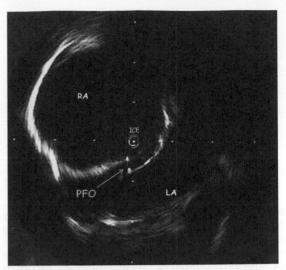

Fig. 2. Rotational intracardiac echocardiography (Ultra ICE) showing the usual tunnel-like shape of the PFO (*arrow* is pointing at the tunnel). Long-axis 4-chamber parasagittal view (author's experience). LA, left atrium; RA, right atrium.

patient populations with otherwise unexplained transient ischemic attack and stroke (7.9%).[14] ASA is frequently (50%–89%) associated with a PFO: this association has emerged as potentially increasing the risk of stroke occurrence or relapse.[2] Furthermore, PFOs seen in the presence of ASA tend to be larger compared with the those seen without ASA; thus, the association of ASA with embolic events is likely based on the high prevalence of a large PFO.[15] ASA is defined according to criteria previously published by Hanley and colleagues[16] (**Fig. 3**). The presence of ASA is not associated with an increased rate of complications or decreased success rate of PFO closure[17]; however, a large ASA may be problematic and needs to be individually considered when selecting the type or size of the device for adequate closure. This anatomic variant is present up to 20% to 25% of cases submitted to catheter closure.

Long tunnel

A long-tunnel PFO is defined by an overlap between septum primum and secundum of more than 8 mm.[5,18] Recently, it has been suggested to further characterize the overlap by taking into consideration the so-called functional tunnel length[19,20]: type I, when septum primum and secundum overlapping is greater than or equal to 4 mm, without redundant or aneurismatic septum primum (**Fig. 4**); and type II, in the presence of PFO with floppy redundant septum primum and tunnel length at maximal excursion of at least 4 mm (**Fig. 5**). A long tunnel is present in

Table 2 PFO categories and anatomic characteristics	
SIMPLE PFO	Standard anatomy, apparent short tunnel, no ASA
COMPLEX PFO	1. Association with ASA 2. Long tunnel (length ≥8 mm) 3. Association with lipomatous hypertrophy of septum secundum 4. Association with CN/EV 5. Multifenestrated ASA or association with additional defects on the fossa ovalis (small ASDs) 6. Presence of distorted anatomy (aortic root enlargement, septal rim deficiency)

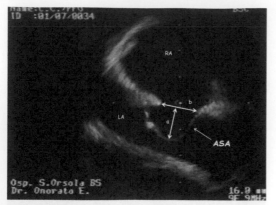

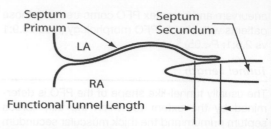

Fig. 5. Schematic representation of a long-tunnel PFO (functional tunnel length classification type II). Vertical arrows refers to functional tunnel length. RA, right atrium; LA, left atrium.

Fig. 3. Rotational intracardiac echocardiography (Ultra ICE) showing PFO with ASA according to criteria published by Hanley and colleagues: protrusion of interatrial septum, or part of it, ≥15 mm beyond plane of interatrial septum (a, ≥15 mm) or phasic excursion of interatrial septum during cardiorespiratory cycle. Long-axis 4-chamber parasagittal view (author's experience). *arrow* a is the excursion of interatrial septum, *arrow* b is the Plane of interatrial septum, *arrow* ASA is pointing at the atrial septal aneurysm. LA, left atrium; RA, right atrium. (*Data from* Hanley PC, Tajik AJ, Hynes JK, et al. Diagnosis and classification of atrial septal aneurysm by two-dimensional echocardiography: report of 80 consecutive cases. J Am Coll Cardiol 1985;6:1370–82.)

approximately 10% of the cases submitted to catheter closure. In the presence of these anatomic variants, SB could represent an important technique helping in the assessment of the shape of the defect, especially in the presence of a tunnel when a longer indentation is well visualized on the inferior edge of the balloon. By using a compliant balloon with static inflation, a waist is well delineated and it is thus easier to accurately measure the tunnel length (**Fig. 6**).

Lipomatous hypertrophy of the atrial septum

Lipomatous hypertrophy of the atrial septum (LHAS) is a histologically benign proliferation of adipose tissue with deposition of nonencapsulated fat cells in the atrial septum.[21] Lipomatous

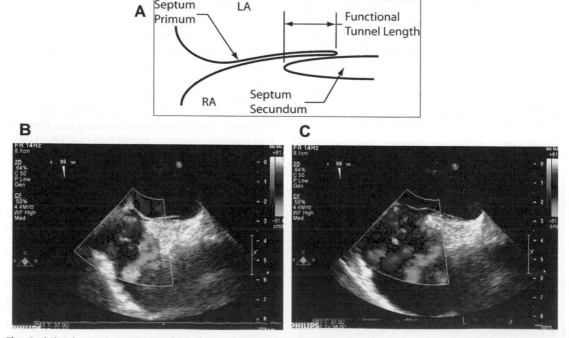

Fig. 4. (*A*) Schematic representation of a long-tunnel PFO (functional tunnel length classification type I); (*B*) and (*C*) TEE showing PFO with long-tunnel (type I) (author's experience). LA, left atrium; RA, right atrium.

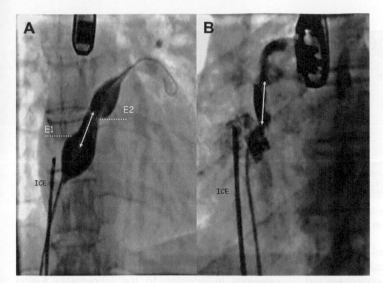

Fig. 6. SB (*A*) and angiography (*B*) of a long-tunnel PFO (author's experience). The balloon takes the characteristic dog bone appearance due to longer indentation on the inferior edge of the SB in the presence of an unmodifiable tunnel. The angiography by 6F multipurpose cathetere delineates the tunnel features. E1, tunnel entrance; E2, tunnel exit; yellow arrow refers to the longitude of the PFO tunnel.

hypertrophy of the cardiac interatrial septum was first described at a postmortem examination in 1964.[22] The reported incidence of LHAS at autopsy is approximately 1% and up to 8% in the general population.[23] The precise cause is unknown but it has been suggested that LHAS is typically associated with obesity and aging. The LHAS appears on TEE as a hyperechogenic enlargement of the upper and lower part of the interatrial septum but sparing the fossa ovalis, resulting in a characteristic bilobar, dumbbell-shaped morphology.[24–26] Although rarely associated with obstruction or arrhythmias, LHAS is of primary interest to echocardiographers in that it must be distinguished from other potential causes of intracardiac mass. Lipomatous hypertrophy may occasionally extend beyond the atrial septum and may simulate an atrial mass. The ability of other noninvasive imaging techniques (cardiac CT and cardiac MRI) to recognize the entity of

LHAS, including tissular characterization as fatty nature, makes them the preferred imaging tools to confidently recognize this benign disorder, avoiding the need for tissue biopsy.[27]

Hypertrophy of the atrial septum has been defined as a thickness between 6 mm and 14 mm, whereas in the case of the LHAS, characterized by massive fatty deposits in the secundum atrial septum, the thickness is greater than or equal to 15 mm (**Fig. 7**).[23,28]

Chiari network and eustachian valve

The right valve of the sinus venosus usually regresses between the ninth and the fifteenth week of gestation. Its persistence has been reported to have an incidence of 1.4% and may develop in 2 different patterns: (1) Chiari network (CN),[29] defined as a reticolous membrane with attachment to the upper wall of the right atrium or atrial septum; it often appears as a web-like

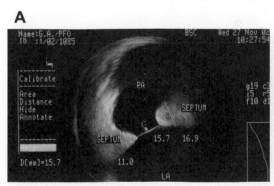

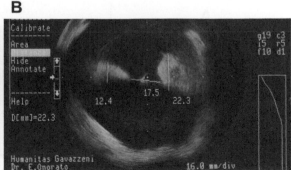

Fig. 7. Lipomatous LHAS. Massive fatty deposits in the secundum atrial septum (septum secundum ≥15 mm thick) in a case of LHAS, identified by rotational ICE (Ultra ICE) (*A*) and (*B*) long-axis 4-chamber parasagittal view (personal experience). LA, left atrium; RA, right atrium; SEPTUM, thick septum secundum.

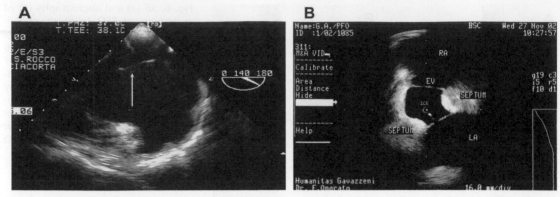

Fig. 8. TEE showing a redundant EV (*yellow arrow*) (*A*); rotational ICE (Ultra ICE) showing a PFO with LHAS associated with prominent EV (*B*). LA, left atrium; RA, right atrium.

structure with a variable number of thread-like components[30]; or (2) EV (so called valvula venae cavae inferioris), which is characterized by a mobile and fenestrated membrane without any anatomic connection.[31] Limacher and colleagues[32] found an incidence of EV in approximately 70% in children of various ages. Although no data exist on the real incidence of prominent EV, the features and the physiology of the valve have been well described by 2-D echocardiography (**Fig. 8**)[33,34] and more recently by 3-D echocardiography.[35] CN/EV are frequently found in adult patients with septal abnormalities and mainly PFO, and they may participate in the mechanism of a paradoxic embolism by maintaining an embryonic right atrial flow pattern into adult life and directing the blood from the IVC toward the interatrial septum. Therefore, the presence of such anatomic variants may increase the chance of paradoxic embolization beyond that associated with PFO size.

Multifenestrated ASA and/or PFO associated with a small atrial setpal defect
Additional defects on the fossa ovalis in the form of small or discrete or single or multiple defects are associated with PFO and ASA (**Fig. 9**). The septum primum aneurysm may have single or multiple openings in addition to the incomplete fusion with the septum secundum, which is the actual PFO. Ewert and colleagues[36] classified the perforated aneurysms as follows: type A, ASA with patent foramen; type B, ASA with single atrial septal defect (ASD); type C, ASA with 2 perforations or few perforations located in not more than 2 clusters; and type D, ASA with multiple perforations located in more than 3 areas of the atrial septum (**Fig. 10**).

PFO with distorted anatomy
Aortic root enlargement Bertaux and colleagues[37] demonstrated that enlargement of the aortic root may decrease the size of the atrial septum and proportionally increase its mobility. In PFO patients, this atrial septal distortion can favor platypnea-orthodeoxia syndrome by enhancing the amount of right-to-left shunt (RLS) (**Fig. 11**). It has been hypothesized that in PFO patients an interaction exists between PFO size, RLS amount, and body position (standing or recumbent position). This interaction may be considered not only the result of dynamic changes in venous

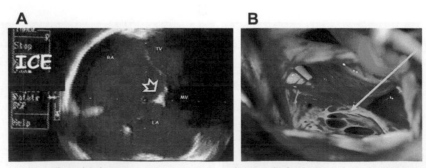

Fig 9 A case of ASA with multiple septal defects and rim deficiency (inferoanterior rim [*yellow arrow*]) identified by rotational ICE (Ultra ICE) (*A*) with corresponding intraoperative image (*B*) after unsuccessful percutaneous closure (author's experience). LA, left atrium; MV, mitral valve; RA, right atrium; TV, tricuspid Valve; Panel A, arrow point at inferoanterior rim; Panel B, arrow point at additional defects of the fossa ovalis.

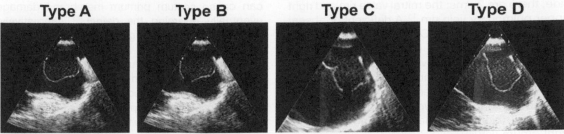

Fig. 10. Ewert and colleagues multifenestrated ASA classification is shown with echocardiograms taken from the authors' patients: *type A*, ASA with patent foramen; *type B*, ASA with single ASD; *type C*, ASA with 2 perforations or few perforations located in not more than 2 clusters; and *type D*, ASA with multiple perforations located in more than 2 areas of the atrial septum. (*Data from* Ewert P, Berger F, Vogel M, et al. Morphology of perforated atrial septal aneurysm suitable for closure by transcatheter device placement. Heart 2000;84:327–31.)

blood return to right atrium but also possibly a consequence of the anatomic relationship between the interatrial septum and the great vessels, mainly the aorta.[38]

Deficient septal rims There are 5 rims on the right atrial side: superior vena cava rim (SVC rim), aortic rim, inferior vena cava (IVC) rim, coronary sinus (CS) rim, and tricuspid valve rim. On the left atrial

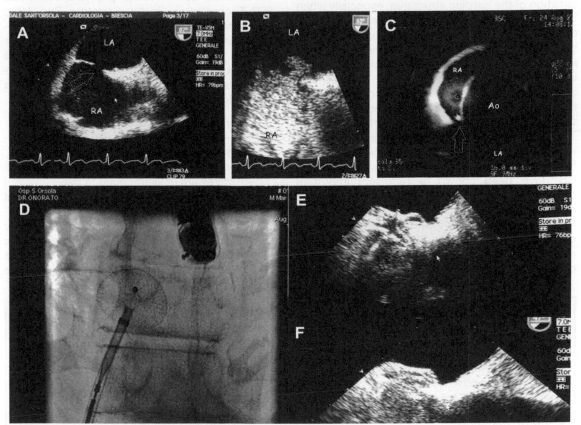

Fig. 11. Case report of PFO with distorted anatomy. A 53-year-old man with a large PFO and a significant bidirectional shunt, prominent EV, aortic root (58 mm) and the ascending aorta (42 mm) enlargement associated with moderate aortic insufficiency and normal left ventricular systolic function was admitted to our center for platypnea-orthodeoxia syndrome showing an O_2 saturation 66% versus 94% from upright to supine position. (*A*) TEE showing large PFO (vs small ASD) (*orange arrow*); (*B*) significant RLS on bubble test during normal breathing; (*C*) rotational ICE (Ultra ICE) showing the distortion of the septal anatomy (*orange arrow*) due to a significant enlarged aortic root. Effective atrial septal repair using an Amplatzer Septal Occluder (18 mm) under fluoroscopic (*D*) and TEE (*E*) control and monitoring with abolition of RLS (*F*) after implantation no more changes in arterial oxygen saturation were detected and there was subsequent clinical improvement of the patient that was confirmed at the follow-up. Ao, aortic root; LA, left atrium; RA, right atrium.

side, there are 2 rims: the mitral valve rim and right upper pulmonary vein rim.[11] A deficient or absent rim, in particular the IVC rim, is a potential risk factor for embolization of the septal occluder device. Conversely, an oversized occluder, meant to overcome deficiency or inadequacy of the rims, is a risk for erosion because of the increased chance of contact between the device and the atrial wall (high risk of iatrogenic aortic root-to-right atrium fistula).

INTRAOPERATIVE MORPHOLOGIC AND FUNCTIONAL ASSESSMENT

The most accepted and frequently used methods for selection of PFO occluder and its deployment are SB maneuver and TEE monitoring using simultaneous fluoroscopic guidance.[39,40] Fluoroscopy alone seems not sufficient to grant an optimal visualization of the cardiac structures, especially when the anatomy is complex; however, successful closure of simple PFOs without echocardiographic guidance has been reported.[41] Furthermore, some investigators demonstrated that ultrasound imaging modalities considerably lengthen the closure procedure, without adding a concrete benefit in terms of technical success, periprocedural complications, and long-term outcome.[42] The referred population, however, did not present a significant prevalence of anatomic risk factors (only 29% patients with ASA). Although TEE and SB have been shown to represent important requirements for a successful procedure, their positive predictive accuracy and specificity are low.[40] Moreover, both these methods have some drawbacks: in particular, SB can give inaccurate measurements causing possible overestimation or underestimation of the occluder size; it also can cause septum primum membrane damage eventually enlarging the defect.[43] Alternatively, TEE usually requires general anesthesia with/without endotracheal intubation. Furthermore, aspiration, airway obstruction, esophageal perforation, and vocal cord dysfunction have been reported, although infrequently.[44] Finally, when using transesophageal probe, some discomfort is delivered to patients. So far, the intracardiac echocardiographic catheter using both the electronic multielement system[45] and mechanical single element[46,47] (**Table 3**) has been used in the cardiac catheterization laboratory for monitoring and guiding catheter closure of PFO, thus eliminating the cumbersome SB maneuver and the need for general anesthesia or deep sedation during TEE monitoring. Particularly in the authors' on experience,[47,48] the application of rotational IntraCardiac Ecchocardiography (ICE) (Ultra ICE [EP Technologies, Boston Scientific, San Jose, California]) affords monitoring and guiding catheter–based closure of ASD and PFO with or without ASA as well as diagnosing associated atrial septal abnormalities. The pivotal roles of rotational ICE during catheter-based procedures are as follows:

1. It can distinguish between the septum primum (low–echo signal intensity) and the septum secundum (high-signal intensity) (see **Fig. 2**), whereas on transesophageal ultrasound these structures are of similar echogenicity.
2. It is helpful to confirm the presence of additional structural anomalies that could represent contraindications for interventional procedures (ie, partial anomalous drainage of pulmonary veins).
3. It is used to evaluate the spatial relationship of the PFO with other structures, such as the

---

Table 3
Main characteristics of the two ultrasound intracardiac probes

Ultra ICE (Boston Scientific Corporation)	AcuNav (Acuson Corporation)
• FDA approval: June 20, 1997	• FDA approval: December 15, 1999
• Rotational mechanical scanning system	• Electronic scanning system
• Unique siliceous piezoelectric crystal	• Crystal matrix (64 ceramic elements)
• 8.5 over-the-wire catheter	• 10F non–over-the-wire catheter
• 9 MHz frequency	• 5.0–10 MHz frequency agile
• Radial scanning at 360°	• Sector scanning at 90°
• Images on a plane perpendicular to the long axis of the catheter	• Images on a plane parallel to the long axis of the catheter
• Imaging field: 10 cm	• Imaging field: 15 cm
• Platform: ClearView Ultra, Galaxy (EP Technologies, Boston Scientific Corporation, Natick, MA, USA)	• Platform: Sequoia, Aspen, Cypress (Acuson Corporation, Mountain View, CA, USA)
• Single operator use	• Two-operator use
• 3-D reconstruction	• Doppler technique

aorta, superior and inferior caval veins, CS, mitral, and tricuspid valves.

4. It allows morphometric evaluation of PFO directly rather than using indirect measurements of balloon catheter. ICE assessment of the device and its relation to both septum primum and secundum before final release is useful to confirm a stable position and adequate capture of the surrounding septum as well as the alignment of the device with the aortic root and anterior mitral valve leaflet.

Both imaging modalities (TEE and ICE) are used safely and effectively to guide catheter PFO closure. The choice between them depends on patient age, familiarity of the operator with technique, and local cost issues.

DEVICES FOR PFO CLOSURE

Differently from other countries, no devices are approved currently by the US Food and Drug Administration (FDA) for percutaneous PFO closure. For devices that are approved to close other lesions, such as ASDs, closure of PFO is an off-label procedure. Several different occluders have been developed and modified in order to facilitate PFO closure. These differ in their design and technical properties. The basic design and principles behind each of these are similar, although the delivery systems and methods used to deploy them differ. Generally, device occluders are composed of (1) a metallic framework (metal alloy) as a double disk, plate, or anchor with a small connecting central waist, and (2) a biocompatible tissue scaffold attached to the framework (**Table 4**). Blood-compatible tissue scaffolds should promote quick and thorough tissue coverage and elicit a host healing response by rapid encapsulation and complete neoendothelialization. The factors that influence this endothelialization process are

unknown but the PFO occluder must flatten and stabilize the interatrial septum aiding in the process of endothelialization. Factors related to PFO morphology should have some bearing on PFO closure rate and it seems plausible that patients with a larger PFO or a septal aneurysm take longer to obtain full closure. Any of these defects may limit the ability of the occluder to oppose the interatrial septum or prevent good disk apposition and may predispose it to residual shunting. Closure devices are classified based on the different constructive characteristics (**Tables 5** and **6**). Many different devices for PFO closure are currently used in clinical practice (**Fig. 12**).

RECOMMENDATIONS FOR DEVICE SELECTION

As more is understood about the morphology of PFO and the number of occluders increases, then the complexity of PFO closure as an intervention also increases. One of the main challenges that remains is which occluder to use. No single type of occluder is sufficient, and different occluders are required in order to meet the different sizes and morphologies of PFOs. The most important consideration is which occluder best suits the PFO. An attempt should always be made to select the most appropriate occluder for the defect, that is, the choice has to be driven by anatomy (**Tables 7–9**). Although no study has shown a difference in outcome based on device type, device selection for anatomic reasons seems reasonable. Because some devices for PFO closure may better fit specific anatomic conditions,

Table 4
Closure device components

Metallic framework (metal alloy)	316 Stainless stel MP35N Nitinol Phynox or Elgiloy (cobalt-based alloy)
Biocompatible tissue scaffold	Polyester Expanded polytetrafluoroethylene Polyurethane foam Polyvinyl alcohol foam Bioabsorbable polymers

Abbreviation: MP35N, multiphase 35% nickel.

Table 5
PFO closure devices

Double umbrella or double disk devices	CardioSEAL, STARFlex (no more available) Amplatzer IntraSept–AtriaSept Occlutech Figulla Flex Helex Septal Occluder NitOcclud Solysafe Septal Occluder
Bioadsorbable devices	BioSTAR, BioTREK
In-tunnel closure devices	Coherex FlatStent EF SeptRx IPO closure system
Suture-based devices	Sutura SuperStitch EL
Non–device closure (radiofrequency ablation)	Cierra PFX Closure System, Coaptus

Table 6
Overview of currently available and future PFO closure devices

Device's Name	Company	Description	Comment
Amplatzer PFO Occluder	AGA Medical Corporation, Golden Valley, Minnesota, USA	Self-expanding, double disk device made from nitinol wire tightly woven into 2 disks that are covered by Dacron patches	Double disk device The right atrium disk is larger (except on the 18-mm device, on which both disks are of the same size) than the left atrium disk. Connecting waist = 3 mm Currently available sizes: 18, 25, 30, and 35 mm	Largest worldwide experience Randomized trials: PC-trial, RESPECT, PREMIUM
CardioSEAL/ STARFlex	Nitinol Medical Technologies, Boston, Massachussetts, USA	Two square Dacron patches mounted between 4 spring arms made from a cobalt-based alloy (called MP35n) that bend independently. The third-generation STARFlex modification has a self-centering mechanism consisting of flexible nitinol microsprings.	Double umbrella type Currently available sizes: from 17 to 40 mm	CE Mark Europe Randomized trials: CLOSURE I, MIST
BioSTAR		Bioabsorbable collagen heparin-coated, acellular porcine intestinal collagen layer matrix [Organogenesis, Canton, Massachusetts] mounted on the STARFlex double umbrella metallic framework	Double umbrella type	BEST BioSTAR evaluation study Research continuing
Intrasept PFO Occluder	CARDIA, Burnsville, Minnesota, USA	The sails and umbrellas are made from polyvinyl alcohol and are mounted onto the arms made of nitinol.	Double umbrella type Is the evolution of the PFO-Star occluder; the device has articulating center post and end caps, which enable the device to align with the septum. Currently available sizes: 25, 30, and 35 mm	CE Mark Europe Randomized trials: CARDIA PFO Stroke Trial

Helex	W.L. Gore and Associates, Flagstaff, Arizona, USA	Non–self-centering double disk device consisting of a 0.012-in single spiral-shaped nitinol wire frame on which is bonded hydrophilic expanded polytetrafluoroethylene patch attached along its length	Double umbrella type Currently available sizes: 15, 20, 25, 30 and 35 mm	CE Mark Europe Randomized trials: REDUCE Clinical Study
Premere	St. Jude Medical, Maple Grove, Minnesota, USA	Self-expanding dual-anchor arm made of nickel-titanium alloy (nitinol); the right anchor is enveloped between 2 layers of knitted polyester fabric. A flexible polyester braided tether runs through the center of the anchor and holds the 2 anchors together.	Double umbrella type The distance between the 2 anchors is variable. Currently available sizes: 20 and 25 mm	Close-Up study CE Mark Europe
Occlutech Figulla	Occlutech International, Helsingborg, Sweden	Made of a self-expanding nitinol wire mesh. The devices have no hub on the left atrium side	Double disk device Currently available sizes (left atrium/right atrium): 16/18, 23/25, 27/30, and 31/35 mm	CE Mark Europe
Solysafe	Swissimplant AG, Solothurn, Switzerland	It consists of 2 synthetic patches that are attached to wires made of a cobalt-based alloy called Phynox; at each end of the device, the wires are fixed to a wire holder.	Double umbrella type Self-centering device designed for ASD and PFO closure Currently available sizes: 15, 20, 25, 30 and 35 mm	CE Mark Europe Swissimplant stopped the marketing and distribution for all Solysafe products in August 2010.
Coherex FlatStent EF	Coherex Medical, Salt Lake City, UT, USA	Intratunnel nitinol frame with polyurethane foam	In-tunnel device Currently available sizes: 13 and 19 mm	CE Mark Europe
SeptRx Intrapocket PFO Occluder	Intrapocket PFO Occluder, SeptRx	Nitinol in-tunnel closure device. It is advanced into the tunnel of the PFO and stabilized by 2 left atrium anchors that adjust to the tunnel length without changing significantly the configuration of the septum primum.	In-tunnel device Minimal left and right atrial material	InterSEPT (Intunnel SeptRx European PFO Trial) Research continuing

(continued on next page)

Table 5
(continued)

Device's Name	Company	Description	Comment
CoAptus	CoAptus Medical Corporation, Redmond, Washington, USA	Radiofrequency ablation	Research continuing
PFx Cierra	Cierra, Redwood City, California, USA	Monopolar radiofrequency energy to effect closure of a PFO by welding the tissues of the septum primum and septum secundum together	Radiofrequency ablation (nondevice closure) PARADIGM II and III. Research abandoned
HeartStitch	Sutura, Fountain Valley, California, USA	The device consists of polypropylene sutures and individually deployable needles	Suturing device
BioTREK	Nitinol Medical Technologies, Boston, Massachusetts, USA	It consists of 2 synthetic patches made from bioabsorbable polymer. Poly-4-hydroxybutyrate (P4HB) (Tepha, Lexington, Massachusetts) is a novel biosynthetic polymer manufactured using recombinant DNA technology.	Double umbrella type, totally bioabsorbable
Spider PFO/Cera II ASD Closure	Lifetech Scientific, Shenzhen, China	Expanded polytetrafluoroethylene–covered disk on the left atrium side and a nitinol wire mesh frame disk on the right atrial side	Double disk device Currently available sizes: 18, 25, and 30 mm Spider PFO Closure system: results of the EU study
PFM NitOcclud ASD-R Device	Pfm Medical Ag, Köln, Germany	Knitted from a single nitinol wire; double-layer right atrial disk and a single-layer left atrial disk; a polyester membrane facing the left atrium promotes accelerated endothelialization	Double umbrella design Currently available sizes: 20, 26, and 30 mm

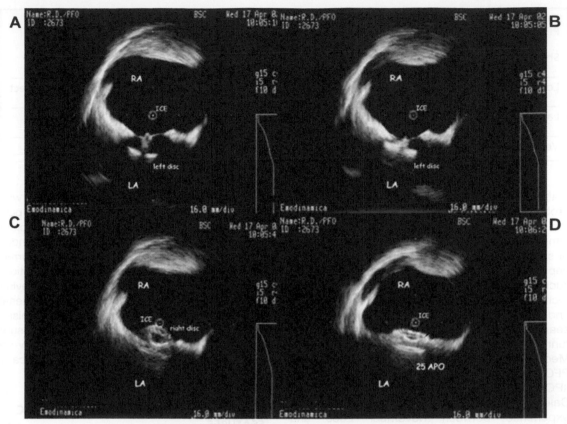

Fig. 12. PFO closure monitoring by rotational ICE (Ultra ICE). In the long-axis 4-chamber parasagittal view: (*A*) left disk opening of the Amplatzer PFO Occluder 25 mm (APO 25); (*B*) APO 25 left disk toward the atrial septum; (*C*) APO 25 right disk opening; (*D*) device correctly implanted (author's data). APO, Amplatzer PFO Occluder; LA, left atrium; RA, right atrium.

in the absence of controlled data it is reasonable to suggest that effort should be put to select the device on an individual basis according to anatomic characteristics. The most appropriate occluder for the morphologic variant of the PFO is selected taking into account the balloon waist size and anatomy of PFO. The atrial size and relation to the mitral valve and aortic root and valve as well as pulmonary and systemic inflows also must considered. Size and type of device selection also may be influenced by other patient factors,

such as clotting disorders and vulnerability to atrial fibrillation. In certain circumstances, a faster seal may be desirable, particularly in patients with multiple thromboembolic events, divers who wish to return to diving as quickly as possible, patients who can only tolerate short periods of antiplatelet treatment, or patients contemplating pregnancy. In these circumstances, it may be appropriate to select an occluder with a lower rate of residual shunt, if the anatomy is suitable (see **Table 9**). Nickel toxicity, thrombus formation, residual shunt,

Table 7
PFO and septal morphology characteristics and suggested closure devices

PFO Anatomy	Amplatzer	STARFlex	Intrasept	Helex	Premere	Occlutech	In-tunnel Devices
Simple	++++	++++	++++	++++	++++	++++	++++
Large ASA	+++	+++	+++	++		+++	
Long-tunnel	++	++	++	++	+++++	++	+++++
Prominent EV	+++	+++	+++	+++	++	+++	+++
LHAS	+++	+++	+++	++	++++	+++	+

Table 8
PFO and septal morphology characteristics and suggested closure devices

Short-tunnel or multiple fenestrations	Double umbrella or double disk devices (Amplatzer PFO Occluder, CardioSEAL device, BioSTAR device, Occlutech device)
Long tunnel	Premere PFO Closure System, Coherex FlatStent EF, SeptRx Intrapockect PFO occluder
Large septal aneurysm	Double umbrella or double disk devices (Amplatzer PFO Occluder, CardioSEAL device, BioSTAR device, Occlutech device)
Very large PFO	Amplatzer ASD Occluder, Occlutech PFO Occluder device

malpositioning, and erosions are active and real problems, whereas the pathophysiology of RLS, the role of coagulation abnormalities, the significance of atrial septal aneurysm, and other sources of shunt remain unresolved issues. Although conceptually highly attractive, newer design concepts, such as suture or radiofrequency-based closure techniques, have failed to demonstrate safety and comparable closure rates. Therefore, the search for the optimal device is ongoing. The in-tunnel closure devices (FlatStent EF [Coherex Medical, Salt Lake City, Utah] and Intrapocket PFO Occluder [SeptRx Intrapocket PFO Occluder (IPO [SeptRx, Inc Freemont, CA, USA], Fremont, California]) are promising. In the authors' early experience between November 2009 and December 2011, 33 patients aged 45 ± 12 years (range 18–70; female/male ratio 3/1) underwent attempted in-tunnel closure of PFO with Coherex FlatStent EF (see **Fig. 12**, **Table 6**). Four 13-mm stents for a tunnel with a balloon-sized diameter less than 8 mm and 29 19-mm stents for a tunnel with a balloon-sized diameter 8 mm to 12 mm were implanted. Device implantation was successful in 30 patients; in 2 patients with less suitable anatomy (septum primum redundancy), a 19-mm FatStent (FS) was implanted, but it was easily retrieved without problems due to a significant residual shunt on the table. One more patient with type II functional tunnel length underwent an uneventful PFO closure (19-mm FS) but, due to problems related with inadvertent release button,

final position was not correct and the device was removed. Clinical follow-up at 12 months was performed in all patients with evidence of complete closure. No device embolization, infective endocarditis, or other serious adverse events occurred (Eustaquio Onorato, MD, personal communication, 2011). The concept of an in-tunnel closure device without significant metallic or other material exposed in both atria is attractive and promises to fulfill most of the requirements of an ideal closure device. Further studies with adequate follow-up results are warranted to confirm long-term efficacy in order to expand its utility.

DEVICE SELECTION BASED ON ANATOMIC FEATURES
Simple PFO

Percutaneous closure of simple PFO is performed with all devices currently available with the aim to seal the patency of the tunnel. Defects with small size may be better suited to a soft flat device (Amplatzer PFO Occluder [AGA Medical Corporation, Golden Valley, Minnesota] [**Fig. 13**] or Helex Septal Occluder [W.L. Gore and Associates, Flagstaff, Arizona]).[5,49] When using the largest PFO closure device ($\geq$30 mm), particular attention must be paid to avoid reaching the free atrial wall or impinging surrounding structures.[4] A tunnel with a wide right or left atrial opening can be challenging to close. The device disk at the broad opening of the tunnel has the tendency to slip

Table 9
PFO and septal morphology characteristics and suggested closure devices

Concerns about nickel	Helex device, in-tunnel closure devices (Coherex FlatStent, SeptRx Intrapocket PFO Occluder), suture-based, radiofrequency-based closure (non–device closure)
Concerns about erosion	Helex device, Premere PFO Closure System, Coherex FlatStent EF, SeptRx Intrapocket PFO Occluder
Risk of thrombus formation	Premere PFO Closure System, Coherex FlatStent EF, Helex device, SeptRx Intrapocket PFO Occluder

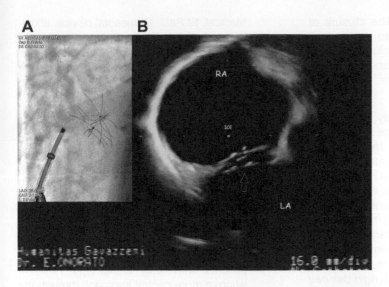

Fig. 13. PFO closure using CARDIA Intrasept PFO occluder (Cardia, Burnsville, Minnesota) under fluoroscopic (*A*) and Ultra ICE (*B*) control and monitoring. Rotational ICE (Ultra ICE) (*B*) shows the septum primum sandwiched between 2 umbrellas of device. Intrasept device (*orange arrow*). LA, left atrium; RA, right atrium.

into the tunnel resulting in unsuccessful closure or even device embolization. Large defects (>10–12 mm) may be better suited to the self-centering ASD occluder.[5] Simple PFO closure procedure is performed according to the usual protocols and with all the devices currently available (including in-tunnel devices) also in the presence of hypermobility of the interatrial septum without ASA (**Fig. 14**).

Complex PFO

Atrial septal aneurysm

The presence of ASA likely contributes to the pathophysiology of paradoxic embolism, and it remains a challenge for PFO treatment. A large ASA may be problematic and needs to be individually considered when selecting the type or size of

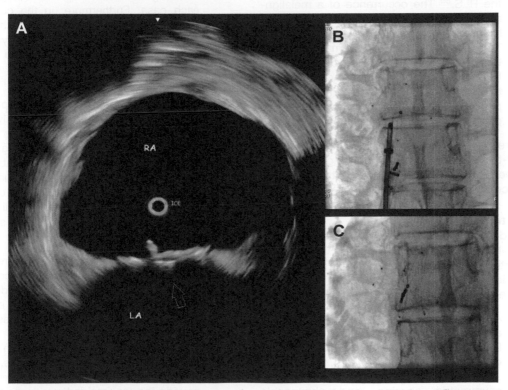

Fig. 14. Long-tunnel PFO closure using Premere PFO Closure System under Ultra ICE (*A*) and fluoroscopic (*B, C*) control and monitoring. Rotational ICE (Ultra ICE) (*A*) shows the device flat and parallel to the septum. Premere device (*orange arrow*). LA, left atrium; RA, right atrium.

the device for adequate closure. The closure of PFO associated with moderate to large ASA usually requires the use of larger occluder devices in order to immobilize the aneurysmatic septum primum between the device disks.[50,51] Procedural strategies are as follows:

- Complete ASA coverage may be accomplished only by a large device or with one approximating the length of the interatrial septum (not exceeding the ratio of 0.8:1), a strategy carrying the inherent risks associated with large-sized devices: arrhythmias, device thrombosis, delayed endothelialization process, residual shunt,[52] and atrial and aortic erosions,[53] particularly in the presence of an aortic septal rim less than 5 mm.[54] Some operators plan to cover a large area of the septum with rigid devices (Amplatzer PFO Occluder and Amplatzer Cribriform Occluder), whereas others prefer to use a soft and malleable device (HELEX Septal Occluder or the BioSTAR device [NMT Medical, Boston, Massachusetts]) that conforms to the existing anatomy.
- Incomplete ASA coverage using a device smaller than the ASA extension may be often sufficient to obtain total abolition of the RLS.[55] The occurrence of a malalignment or dislocation of the device, however, has been reported.[4]
- Transseptal puncture is performed to deploy the device as centrally as possible in the fossa ovalis. This strategy may have potential drawbacks, including aortic puncture, pericardial effusion, tamponade, and the persistence of uncovered fenestration.[56]

Moreover, wear and tear on the sometimes paper-thin septum primum undulating incessantly between the left and the right atrial disks is a concern[57]

Long tunnel
Occluder devices with a short connecting waist are not ideal for the long-tunnel PFO: they end up sitting in the tunnel partially unfolded.[58–62] Techniques advocated to facilitate successful closure include the following:

- A double umbrella–type device with a distensible neck,[61] such as the Amplatzer PFO device, can be used. Very long tunnels, greater than 15 mm to 18 mm, may require a device with a longer connecting waist, asymmetric opening, and changeable distance between the 3 disks, such as the Premere PFO Closure System (St Jude Medical, St Paul, Minnesota) device, allowing a final interdependent positioning of both disks (**Fig. 15**).[5] In the presence of functional tunnel length type I (see **Fig. 4**) and type II (see **Fig. 5**), the implantation of an in-tunnel occluder device (Coherex Flat-Stent PFO Closure System and SeptRx Intrapocket PFO Occluder) is feasible and safe and might represent the treatment of choice in this particular setting of patients (**Fig. 16**).[19,20] The concept of an in-tunnel closure device without significant metallic or other material exposed in both atria is attractive and promises to fulfill most of the requirements of an ideal closure device for this PFO morphology.
- Transseptal puncture may be used in patients with long tunnel–type PFO, in whom a more central approach through the septal flap may result in an improved closure profile of the defect.[63] The experience so far is limited,[60,63,64] residual shunt rate is high,[56] and potential procedure-related risks have been previously described, however.
- Balloon detunnelization technique: the use of a balloon can provide important information about PFO morphology: this may help selecting an individualized strategy for each case. Furthermore, in the case of a long tunnel, the detunnelization technique provides an opportunity to modify PFO anatomy and facilitates standard PFO closure in most patients.[62]

Lipomatous hypertrophy of the atrial septum
In the presence of this anatomic anomaly, the percutaneous PFO closure may be more challenging because the occluder device with a short waist, usually not modifiable, is not able to encroach the thick muscular septum secundum. The procedural difficulties may favor the occurrence of residual shunt or device embolization requiring surgical correction.[65] Procedural strategies are as follows:

- Based on the evidence of literature and author's experience, the classic occluder devices (double disk–type or double umbrella–type) provide a safe and efficacious PFO closure, even in the presence of LHAS.
- When LHAS is not associated with huge ASA, the use of asymmetric devices, such as the Premere PFO Closure System, can provide the maximal independence of the 2 prosthetic components straddling the atrial septum.[66]

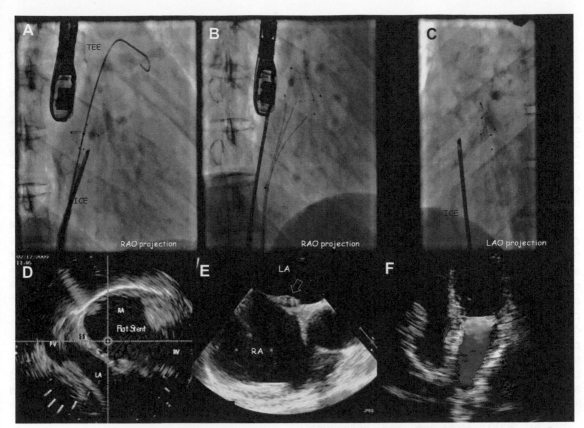

Fig. 15. Long-tunnel–type I PFO closure using Coherex FlatStent EF (19 mm) under simultaneous fluoroscopic, TEE, and ICE guidance. (*A*) FlatStent EF deployed up to the first hard-stop; (*B*) FlatStent EF within the tunnel, final position of the FlatStent EF (*red and orange arrows*) documented by fluoroscopy (*C*); Ultra ICE (*D*) and TEE (*E*); and follow-up TTE color Doppler at 12 months showing optimal device position without residual shunting (*F*) (author's experience). LA, left atrium; RA, right atrium.

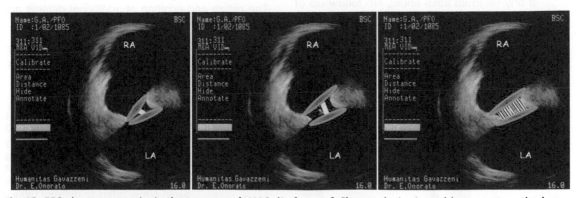

Fig. 16. PFO closure strategies in the presence of LHAS. (*Left panel*) Closure device is unable to capture the hypertrophied septum secundum and slips toward left atrial cavity; (*center panel*) oversplay of the device on the hypertrophied septum secundum with residual shunt and risk of embolization; (*right panel*) device with longer waist capture appropriately both components of atrial septum. LA, left atrium; RA, right atrium. (*Data from* Huie Lin C, Balzer DT, Lasala JM. Defect closure in the lipomatous hypertrophied atrial septum with the Amplatzer muscular ventricular septal defect closure device: a case series. Catheter Cardiovas Interv 2011;78:102–7.)

- A good alternative, as pointed out by Huie Lin and colleagues,[67] is to choose a device with a longer waist (7 mm), such as the Amplatzer Muscular Ventricular Septal Occluder (AGA Medical, Plymouth, Minnesota), that best fits this peculiar anatomy (**Fig. 17**).

In some contexts, LHAS may come to be considered an absolute contraindication to transcatheter closure. For patients with very hypertrophic rims and more than moderate ASA, probably, at the moment, there are no safe and effective devices to be implanted; therefore, alternative medical or surgical therapy should be kept in consideration on an individual basis.

Chiari network and eustachian valve

In the presence of prominent CN/EV, greater attention must be paid during the different phases of the interventional procedure. Most of the cases may be performed with all available devices. As reported by various investigators, the EV in its different degrees may cause complications during percutaneous use of intravascular catheters: hooking[68] and entrapment[69] of catheters has been described. Cooke and colleagues[70] reported a case of CN entanglement and herniation into the left atrium by an atrial septal occluder device.

- In 2000, McMahon and colleagues[71] described 4 patients with ASD and prominent EV, in 3 of whom they used a technique to control the EV using a steerable ablation catheter, avoiding interferences with STAR-Flex (NMT Medical, Boston, Massachusetts) ASD occlusion device placement. In one patient, for whom they did not use this technique, one of the right atrial umbrella legs was entrapped resulting in a tiny residual atrial shunt. No follow-up of this patient was reported. No early complications, however, occurred.
- In 2002, the authors' group[72] demonstrated that the redundant and prominent EV may be wrapped round the delivery cable during

unscrewing (counterclockwise rotation) of the Amplatzer PFO Occluder, interfering with the retrieval of the entire delivery system. The detachment of a piece of the valve is described as similar to an unintentional valve biopsy (**Fig. 18**). To avoid the twisting of a prominent valve round the delivery cable, the long sheath should be gently advanced toward the interatrial septum during device release to be sure that the delivery cable is turning totally freely inside the long sheath.

- In 2006, Butera and colleagues[73] described 3 patients with PFO and prominent EV interfering with the correct placement of right atrial disk of the Amplatzer PFO Occluder. In these cases, using a 6F pigtail catheter to pull down toward the IVC the redundant EV, the correct placement of PFO closure devices was obtained in all patients (pull–push technique).

Multifenestrated ASA and/or PFO associated with a small ASD

Perforated ASAs have been successfully treated by transcatheter device placement, if the interatrial communication is not too large or too close to the mitral valve and there are no more than 2 perforations or small perforations in clusters of 2. The latter may require the placement of 2 devices, whereas aneurysms with multiple perforations may only rarely be treatable with the currently available transcatheter devices and may require lifelong anticoagulation or surgery.[36] The multiple device technique of crossing all the eventual fenestrations, with multiple device implantation, although feasible, does not prevent device/interatrial septal misalignment or aortic impingement. The nature and position of additional defects are important for planning percutaneous closure.

- If 2 defects are close together, they may be effectively closed by a single device (**Fig. 19**)[11,36]

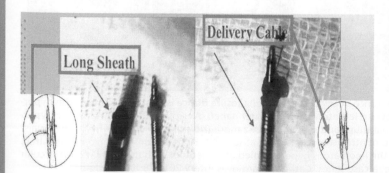

Fig. 17. A piece of the redundant EV interfering with Amplatzer PFO Occluder placement extracted by delivery cable during unscrewing maneuver. left panel *arrow* point at distal portion of the long sheath right panel *arrow* refers to delivery cable.

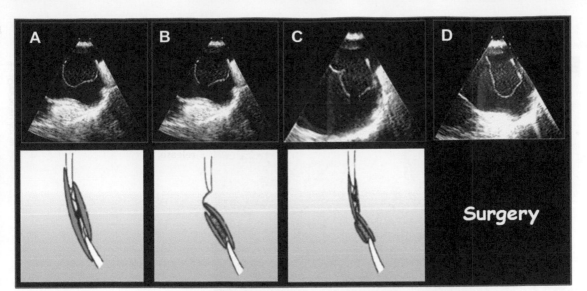

Fig. 18. Multifenestrated ASA treatment options. (*A*) atrial septal aneurysm (*B*) fenestrated atrial septal aneurysm (*C*) multifenestrated atrial septal aneurysm (*D*) huge atrial septal aneurysm. (Schematic drawings and treatment concept *from* Ewert P, Berger F, Vogel M, et al. Morphology of perforated atrial septal aneurysm suitable for closure by transcatheter device placement. Heart 2000;84:328.)

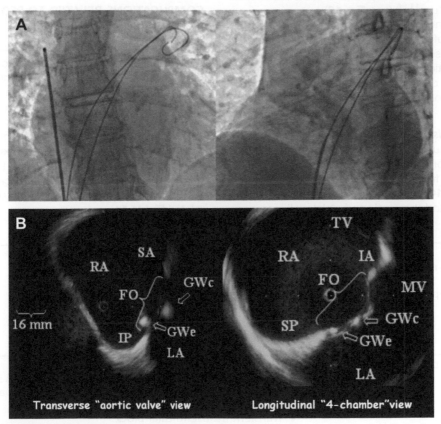

Fig. 19. Double guide wire technique. (*A*) Two 0.035"–260 cm guide wires were introduced via the right femoral vein through a 9F sheath, crossing 2 separate defects by means of 5F Super TorquePlus MP A2 catheter (Johnson & Jonhson Medical Ltd); (*B*) rotational ICE (Ultra ICE) inserted from the contralateral femoral vein, monitoring septal crossing in the 2 orthogonal planes. FO, fossa ovalis; GWc, guide wire central; GWe, guide wire eccentric; IP, inferoposterior rim; LA, left atrium; MV, mitral valve; RA, right atrium; SA, superoanterior rim; SP, superoElse-posterior rim; TV, tricuspid valve.

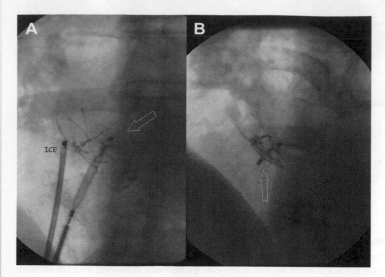

Fig. 20. Previous Intrasept occluder implantation complicated by a late significant residual shunt corrected with an Amplatzer PFO Occluder (18 mm) (*white arrow*) under Ultra ICE and fluoroscopic monitoring. (*A*) Left disk opening; (*B*) second device release.

- Two distant defects usually require 2 separate devices but may be closed by a single device placed equidistant via a transseptal puncture[11,36] (see **Fig. 19**)
- Zanchetta and colleagues[74] described the use of the Amplatzer Cribriform Occluder in cases of multiperforated ASD, keeping attention to cross with the guide wire the most central hole in the fossa ovalis under rotational ICE guidance (**Fig. 20**).

PFO with distorted anatomy

In this particular setting, a deficient rim is a potential risk factor for device embolization (see **Fig. 9**), whereas in the case of aortic root enlargement (see **Fig. 11**C) the chance of contact between the device and the aortic and atrial wall increases the risk for erosion and aortic root-to-right atrium fistula.

COMPLICATIONS RELATED TO PFO CLOSURE PROCEDURE
Procedural Complications

Several different percutaneous devices to close PFOs have been used with overall high success and low complication rates. Since the first report of percutaneous PFO closure,[75] considerable advances in device design let to facilitated delivery and improved occlusion rates. From the meta-analysis of Khairy and colleagues,[76] several complications have been reported in the literature (**Table 10**).[77–79] Furthermore, complications could be also classified as procedure related or device related (**Table 11**).

Table 10
Major and minor procedural complications

Major complications (1.5%)	• Hemorrhage requiring blood transfusion • Cardiac tamponade • Need for surgical intervention • Massive pulmonary embolism • Death
Minor complications (7.9%)	• Bleeding not requiring blood transfusion • Device malpositioning with successful percutaneous reposition • Device embolization with successful catheter retrieval • New-onset atrial arrhythmias (atrial fibrillation) • Transient atrioventricular block • Asymptomatic device thrombosis/device arm fractures • Transient air embolism • Transient ST segment elevation • Femoral arteriovenous fistula • Femoral hematoma

Table 11 Procedure-related and device-related complications	
Procedure-related complications	• Air embolism (1%–3%) • Embolization of thrombus on the device (1%–2%) • Interference with AV valve function (1%–2%) • Systemic or pulmonary venous obstruction (1%) • Atrial flutter or atrial fibrillation • Hematoma (femoral, retroperitoneal)
Device-related complications	• Erosion or perforation of atrial walls or aorta with hemopericardium (1%–2%) • Atrial arrhythmias (1%–3%) • Device arms prolapsing through defects • Device malpositioning or embolization (2%–15%) • Thrombosis on the device

Abbreviation: AV, atrio-ventricular valve function.

Postprocedure Complications

Complications can occur not only in the midterm follow-up but even very late.

Residual shunts after transcatheter closure

Complete PFO closure after percutaneous treatment has been reported in 51% to 100% of patients. Nevertheless, in a minority of patients the initial transcatheter closure attempt may be incomplete and result in persistent residual shunting beyond the expected 8-week to 12-week endothelization period (1%–2% range). Residual shunts are usually the result of a mismatch between the device shape and PFO anatomy. Some of these patients have an additional separate previously unrecognized defect whereas a majority have a residual shunt in the region of the former PFO. Small defects do not seem to have any meaningful clinical significance. In patients with moderate-to-large residual shunts, however, it has been reported a 4-fold increase risk in recurrent paradoxic embolic events compared with patients in whom complete PFO occlusion has been achieved.[80–82] Furthermore, the presence of residual shunting poses a significant clinical dilemma because they can add a higher risk for recurrent neurologic events regardless of antiplatelet or anticoagulant therapy.[3,13] In this situation many cardiologists prefer to re-evaluate patients and use an additional occluder if necessary. Using a further occluder may pose a technical challenge both in its delivery and the choice of device; furthermore, the long-term consequences of multiple occluders within the atrial septum are unknown. These patients represent a current medical challenge and, although it would be intuitive to advise reintervention for shunt closure, the data supporting this or any other alternative strategy are limited and not clearly established.[55,83,84] Treatment options for these patients include medical therapy with antiplatelet or anticoagulation drugs, surgical device removal and patch closure, and percutaneous implantation of a second device. Several investigators reported successful late closure of residual defects by implantation of a second device.[2,10,14] Even in the authors' experience, similar to other reports in the literature, the implantation of a second device has been feasible, safe, and effective (see **Fig. 20**; **Fig. 21**).[4]

Erosions

Erosions of the aortic or atrial wall are a potentially lethal complication of percutaneous closure procedures and can occur at the roof of the right or left atrium or at the atrial junction with the aorta, causing hemopericardium, tamponade, or aortic fistula. The precise frequency of atrial and aortic perforation after percutaneous closure has been estimated to be 0.1%.[85] The reasons for erosion are unknown, but several risk factors have been proposed, all of which increase the chance of contact between the device and the atrial wall: absent or deficient superior–anterior rim[85,86] and device oversizing,[83] both of which predispose toward contact of the device with the aortic root. Erosion of the left or right atrial wall, pressed against the pulsating aorta by the device is a real although rare concern.[57] Oversizing of the device may lead to contact between the edges of the occluder device and the walls of susceptible tissue of the aorta and roof of the atria. Finally, the motion of the device against the tissue can be conceptualized as a repetitive sawing motion.[84,87]

Late cardiac perforations

Late cardiac perforations are considered the most severe complications.[88] Trepels and colleagues[78] described the first case of cardiac perforation using the Amplatzer PFO Occluder device in 2003. This rare complication occurs predominantly in the anterosuperior atrial wall and adjacent to the aorta. The authors believe that a strict long-term follow-up of those patients is mandatory. From an anatomic point of view, this type of

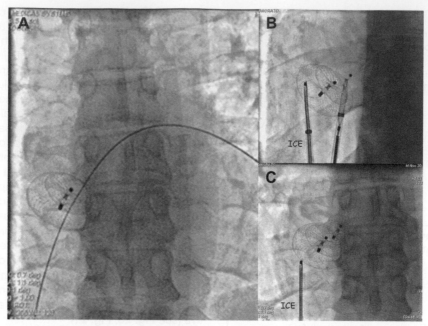

Fig. 21. Significant residual shunt post-PFO closure corrected with a second device Amplatzer PFO Occluder (18 mm) under Ultra ICE and fluoroscopic monitoring. (*A*) Guide wire through the residual defect in the proximity of Amplatzer PFO Occluder (35 mm); (*B*) left disk opening; (*C*) second device implantation.

complication is probably associated with a particular anatomic pattern, that is, when the area of the torus aorticus is bulging within the right atrium and when the plane of PFO is not well aligned with it. Moreover, a diminutive aortic rim may play an important role.[88]

Device embolization

Embolization is among the most common complications reported in the literature[89]: the risk has ranged from 0.5% up to 3%. The causes of device embolization are various: eccentric and large defects, inadequate rims, uncorrect implantation, and/or device choice. Surgery may be needed to explant the occluder devices, but in a majority of cases they are retrieved percutaneously. The most common site of embolization is the left atrium, followed by right ventricle and pulmonary artery.[90] In cases of device embolization toward the left side, it may be argued that the devices placed are undersized or not correctly placed. Embolization usually occurs intraprocedurally or in the first 24 hours, but late embolizations have been reported.[91]

Device explantation

In a recent multicenter survey,[92] a database review has been performed to identify the frequency and causes of PFO device explantation, examining 18 PFO closure centers in Europe and the Unites States. There were 13,736 devices implanted over

the past 3 to 9 years among the 18 centers; 38 devices (0.28% [95% CI, 0.20%–0.37%]) required surgical removal. The most common causes for explantation were chest pain (n = 14), often secondary to nickel allergy; residual shunt (n = 12); thrombus formation on the device (n = 4); pericardial effusion (n = 2); perforation of aortic root or atrial wall (n = 2); recurrent strokes (n = 1); and undocumented reasons (n = 2). Although surgical removal of PFO closure devices is rare, there is a small (0.28%) incidence of severe long-term problems associated with this procedure that might require explantation. Furthermore, the frequency of surgical removal was found device dependent (1 in 126 for CardioSEAL devices [NMT Medical, Boston, Massachussetts], 1 in 480 for Amplatzer devices, and 1 in 600 for the Helex device).

Thrombus formation on the device

Thrombus formation has been reported in large cases series[93,94] and in randomized studies.[95] Overall risk of thrombus formation is low (1%). Thrombi were generally discovered at 6-month follow-up. The incidence varies from 0.2% (Amplatzer PFO Occluder) to 7.1% (CardioSEAL device). Thrombofilic disorders should be routinely searched for because they could be the possible cause of thrombosis in some instances. In most cases, thrombus usually resolved with antiocoagulation therapy (heparin or warfarin), only few required surgical intervention.

Table 12
Overall analysis of retrospective and randomized clinical studies

Authors, Year of Publication	Enrollment Period	Implanted Devices	No of Patients	No of ASA (%)	No of EV/CN/LHAS (%)	Procedural Success	RS	Correlation Between PFO Anatomy, Procedural Success, and Complications
Windecker et al,[80] 2000	1994–1999	BD, PFO Star, APO, AWO, CSSO	80	20 Pts (25%)	NR	78 Pts (98%)	RS was a predictor for recurrent thromboembolic events with a relative risk of 4.2	• No differences in the incidence of intraprocedural complications, RSs, or recurrent thromboembolic events relative to the implanted device • Embolization of an APO into the pulmonary artery 12 h after the procedure in a patient with PFO and a large ASA
Hung, 2000	1989–1994 (Clamshell); 1996–1997 (CSSO)	Clamshell (n = 28), CSSO (n = 13), BD (n = 22)	63	20 Pts (25%)	NR			
Krumsdorf et al,[17] 2001	1997–2000	AWO, CSSF, ASO, APO, PFO Star, Helex	63	63 Pts (100%)			Mild 11%, moderate 3%	
Brockmeier, 2001		APO (n = 4), ASO (n = 45)	48			44 Pts (92%)	5%	
Sievert, 2001	1994–2000	AWO, Sideris, ASDOS, CSSF, APO, Helex	281	64 Pts (22.7%)		281 (100%)		2 Device embolizations (1 Sideris, 1 PFO-Star) in 2 pts

(continued on next page)

Table 12
(continued)

Authors, Year of Publication	Enrollment Period	Implanted Devices	No of Patients	No of ASA (%)	No of EV/CN/LHAS (%)	Procedural Success	RS	Correlation Between PFO Anatomy, Procedural Success, and Complications
Butera, 2001		APO, CSSF, PFO Star	35		NR			
La Rosée, 2001		ASDOS, PFO Star, ASO, APO	102		NR	99 Pts (97%)		PFO (n = 60), ASD (n = 41), ASD + PFO (n = 1)
Du, 2002	1995–2000	AWO, ASO, APO	18	NR	NR		0%	
Braun et al,[64] 2002	1998–2001	PFO Star	276	62 Pts (22%)		276 Pts (100%)		• Transseptal puncture in 1 patient (short distance of the PFO channel to the anterior mitral valve leaflet) • 1 Device embolization (30-mm generation II device) • 1 Dislodgement into the proximal orifice of the PFO channel (long PFO channel), surgical removal effective.
Martin, 2002	1995–2001	Sideris, CSSO	110	16 Pts (14%)		110 Pts (100%)		• 4 Reinterventions for significant RS or malalignment: surgically (n = 3) and percutaneously (n = 1) treated • Second device (n = 8) to accomplish effective PFO closure

Bruch, 2002	1997–2001	ASO, APO, PFO Star, CSSF	66	33 Pts (61.1%)	NR	66 Pts (100%)	0%	PFO (n = 54), ASD (n = 12)
Silverman, 2003	2002	CSSO	16	15 Pts (93.7%)				
Hong, 2003		US multicenter clinical trial	50	17 Pts (34%)		49 Pts (98%)	6.25%	
Onorato, 2003	1999–2002	APO, PFO Star, Helex	256	86 Pts (34%)	EV 43 pts (17%),	49 Pts (98%)	6.25%	
Schrader, 2003	1994–2003	Rashkind occluder (n = 2), BD (n = 2), ASDOS (n = 20), AWO (n = 2), CSSF (n = 13), PFO Star (n = 379), APO (n = 23)	457	169 Pts (37%)				
Kay, 2004	1995–1998	AWO	3		NR		18.8% at 2 y	
Windecker, 2004	1994–2000		150		NR			
Schwerzmann et al,[55] 2004	1998–2001	PFO Star, APO	100	50 Pts (50%)		100 Pts (100%)	6% (APO), 34% (PFO Star) 16% Severe shunt only with PFO Star	
Anzola, 2004	2001–2004	APO, PFO Star, HELEX	140	66 Pts (47%)		140 Pts (100%)	ASA tended to be over-represented in pts who failed to attain a full closure	
Alameddine, 2004	Forecast registry	CSSF	272					

(continued on next page)

Table 12
(continued)

Authors, Year of Publication	Enrollment Period	Implanted Devices	No of Patients	No of ASA (%)	No of EV/ CN/LHAS (%)	Procedural Success	RS	Correlation Between PFO Anatomy, Procedural Success, and Complications
Braun, 2004	1998–2002	PFO Star, APO, CSSF	307	70 Pts (23%)	NR	307 Pts (100%)	• 6% at 1 Y • The risk of stroke recurrence was not associated with the presence of an ASA or a small RS • No major differences in the rate of RS between the 3 types of implanted devices	• Transseptal puncture in 1 patient (short distance of the PFO channel to the anterior mitral valve leaflet) • 3 Device dislodgements (2 surgical removal; 1 conservative management)
Post, 2005	1999–2003	CSSF, APO, PFO Star, Helex	112		NR			No significant differences in outcome or occurrence of any type of complication between the different types of devices
Wahl et al,[51] 2005	1999–2003	Sideris, AWO, ASO/APO, CSSF, PFO Star, Helex	141	141 pts (100%)	NR	99.3%	Minimal 8%, moderate 4%, large 2%	• 1 Device embolization • Device size categorized as small (<30 mm; n = 83 pts) or large (>30 mm; n = 58 pts) had no impact on the incidence of procedural complications (small 1.2% vs large 0%; $P = .40$) and RS rate (small 15% vs large 14%; $P = .89$) in pts with ASA + PFO
Chatterje, 2005	2001–2003	APO	55	8 (15%)	NR	55 Pts (100%)	4%	

El Said et al,[9] 2005	1997–2002	CSSO	47	14 Pts	NR	45 Pts (95%)	5%	• Trans-septal puncture in 5 pts (long-tunnel) • Complex PFO did not increase risk of RS or recurrent neurologic symptoms after device closure
Errmann, 2005			100		NR			
Spies, 2006	1998–2004	Cardia PFO Occluder (first 3 generations: I–III)	403	154 Pts (38.2%)	NR	403 Pts (100%)	10.8% (Equal frequencies among 3 PFO occluder generations)	
Billinger, 2006		Helex	128	38 (29.7%)	NR	127 (99.2%)	10%	
Büscheck et al,[58] 2006	Close Up Trial	Premere	67	18 Pts (26.9%)	NR	67 Pts (100%)	14%	• 73 Pts enrolled: unsuitable anatomy (ASD or large PFO) in 6 pts
Egred, 2007	2003–2005	Amplatzer (n = 166), CSSF (n = 13)	185			179 Pts (96.8%)		PFO (n = 109) + ASD (n = 76)
Fischer, 2008	1999–2005	Starflex	154	57 Pts (37.5%)		153 Pts (99%).		Unsuccessful implantation during the early experience (n = 1)
Krizanic, 2008	2006	Occlutech Figulla	37	NR		36 Pts (97.3%)	12% at 180 d	A defect size of over 13 mm was an exclusion criterion
Ruiz, 2008	SUPERSTITCH F-I-M tiral							
Wahl, 2009	1998–2006	APO	620	207 Pts (33%)		620 (100%)	9% at 6 Mo (moderate 2%, large 1%)	Fluoroscopic monitoring without echocardiography
Ford, 2009	2001–2006	ASO (n = 348), CardioSEAL (n = 4)	352	83 Pts (23.6%)		352 Pts (100%)		
Rigatelli et al,[54,66] 2010	2006–2009	ASO/Cribriform, Premere	10				Hypertrophy (n = 8) and LHAS (n = 2)	Misalignment of the 25/25 Cribriform in 2 pts

(continued on next page)

Table 12
(continued)

Authors, Year of Publication	Enrollment Period	Implanted Devices	No of Patients	No of ASA (%)	No of EV/CN/LHAS (%)	Procedural Success	RS	Correlation Between PFO Anatomy, Procedural Success, and Complications
Zimmermann, 2010	2006–2007	SeptRx Device F-I-M trial	13	4 Pts	EV 4 Pts	11 Pts	0%	Anatomic exclusion criteria: tunnel shorter than 5 mm (n = 1), tunnel longer than 12 mm (n = 1)
Diaz, 2010	1995–2007		424				5% Moderate-to-large RS at 6 mo	The variations in baseline interatrial septal anatomy, PFO characteristics, and type and size of closure device used failed to predict RS at 6 mo
Thaman, 2011	2006–2008	APO, Helex, Premere	166	45 Pts (27%)		166 Pts (100%)	Large RS at 12 mo: 7.5% (APO), 31.2% (Helex), 10.5% (Premere)	• Long tunnel in 29 pts (17%) • Predictors of RS: septal aneurysm and type of occluder device
Rigatelli, 2011	2005–2009	Premere	70			70 Pts (100%)		Long tunnel (>10 mm) = 70 pts
Fischer, 2011	2005–2008	APO	114	55 Pts (48%)	NR	114 Pts (100%)	8% (Small shunt)	
Bissessor, 2011			70					
Van Den Branden 2011	2008–2009	Occlutech Figulla	82	PFO 22 pts (46%)				PFO (48 pts) + ASD (34 pts)

Scacciatella et al,[96] 2011		APO, Cribriform, Premere (n = 1) e Cardia Intrasept (n = 3)	95	71 pts (74.5%)	EV 22 pts (23.2%)	95 pts (100%)	3.2% moderate-to-severe RS	• Severe RS in 2 pts: second percutaneous repair (n = 1), surgical repair (n = 1) • Septal erosion (n = 1) 8 mo after PFO closure; successful surgical repair
Siddiqui, 2011	2006–2010	APO, Helex	132	29%		132 Pts (100%)	At 6 mo: 7% (Helex), 5% (APO)	• Monitoring tool: TEE (n = 117), ICE (n = 15) • Immediate embolization of a 30-mm Amplatzer Cribriform (fluoroscopic guidance alone) in patient with highly mobile ASA (total septal excursion of 2.5 cm). A larger 35-mm Cribriform occluder was successfully placed
Rigatelli, 2012	2005–2009	Cribriform	160	160 (100%)		160 Pts (100%)		
CLOSURE I, 2012	2003–2008	CSSF	405	362 pts (89.4%)		315 Pts with effective closure at 6 mo (86.1%)		• Thrombus in left atrium in 4 pts • Degree of RS not related to the presence or absence of ASA

Abbreviations: APO, Amplatzer PFO Occluder; ASDOS, Atrial Septal Defect Occlusion System; ASO, Amplatzer Septal Occluder; AWO, Angel-wings Occluder; BD, buttoned device; CN, Chiari network; CSSF, CardioSEAL/Starflex; CSSO, CardioSEAL septal occlude; n°, number; NR, not reported; PFO-STAR, Cardia PFO-STAR Occluder (Cardia, Inc, Burnsville, Minnesota); pts, patients; RS, residual shunt.

REVIEW OF OBSERVATIONAL AND RANDOMIZED STUDIES ABOUT THE INFLUENCE OF PFO ANATOMY ON SUCCESSFUL TRANSCATHETER CLOSURE

Several studies have been conducted to find which anatomic and clinical features can predict the outcome of patients with their PFO closed, but results are often contradictory and controversial. There is still no consensus about how to stratify the PFO anatomy to determine the risk to develop major adverse events or residual shunt after catheter PFO closure. In addition, univariate and multivariate analysis performed in numerous published studies (Table 12) based on single or multicentric experiences did not identify any correlation between the different anatomic features of PFO, even those considered most difficult and complex, and the incidence of major adverse events. Even taking into consideration study limitations (small patient sample), El Said and colleagues[9] also confirmed that the presence of a complex PFO morphology does not increase the risk of residual shunt or recurrent neurologic symptoms after device closure, thus not altering the successful outcome. More recently Scacciatella and colleagues[96] described a high-risk population in which only patients with anatomic risk factors, such as ASA or EV, developed complications, or had a severe residual shunt, suggesting a possible correlation between anatomic features and functional outcome. Moreover, in this population the presence of high-risk characteristics seems more likely to be correlated to the persistence of residual shunt than to the occurrence of complications, which are probably influenced by a more complex set of factors. In a retrospective study, Shafi and colleagues[97] analyzed 51 patients undergoing PFO closure. Univariate analysis was used to determine which preprocedure variables predicted increased risk of inadequate PFO closure or recurrent clinical events. Variables examined included age, gender, left ventricular ejection fraction, tunnel length, aneurysm base length, degree of aneurysmal phasic excursion, degree of protrusion, and PFO size. Univariate analysis revealed larger PFO size ($F = 4.72$, $P = .036$) as the only independent predictor of residual shunting after PFO closure.

SUMMARY AND FINAL RECOMMENDATIONS

Percutaneous closure of PFO is increasingly considered the preferred treatment of young patients who have had a cryptogenic stroke via paradoxic embolism. Patients with PFO have a large variety of anatomic features: mild to moderate ASA, large and huge ASA, multiperforated fossa ovalis, hypertrophic or lipomatosus rims, and long-tunnel PFO. These different anatomic characteristics, often combined with each other may have an impact on immediate procedural results and outcomes. The ability to assess the associations of the different features by TEE or better by ICE have been suggested as the key for lowering potential failures or complications and to increase the long-term occlusion rate. The characteristics of an ideal device have been pointed out but are unclear in many cases (Table 13): new-generation devices, such as the biodegradable BioSTAR, the in-tunnel closure devices, or nothing-behind techniques (radiofrequency ablation and suture-mediated device) for different reasons do not seem the best options for complex anatomies.

In conclusion

- Percutaneous PFO closure is a simple, minimally invasive, safe, and effective procedure in experienced centers and skilled hands but not totally risk free.
- Lower profile and less foreign material could reduce risk of thrombus formation.
- Softer devices and in-tunnel devices could reduce septal distortion and risk of atrial fibrillation.
- Bioresorbable devices and nothing-behind techniques could prevent long-term device-related complications.
- New devices need to be rigorously tested for not only efficacy but also for durability.

A tailored approach is based on certain PFO devices fitting better to certain anatomic conditions

Table 13 Properties of an ideal PFO closure device	
Clinical	Nonarrhythmogenic Nonthrombotic Nonallergenic No increased chance of endocarditis Minimal requirement for postprocedural medication
Technical	Complete closure Low procedural risk of complications No risk of embolization Minimal impact on surrounding structures (no erosion)
Staff	Simple to implant Short time required for training Short procedural time Short hospital stay–day case procedure
Financial	Cost effective

and other devices fitting better to certain patient conditions: clotting disorder, atrial fibrillation, and nickel allergy.

ACKNOWLEDGMENTS

The authors greatly appreciate Gian Paolo Anzola, MD, for technical help and valuable suggestions.

REFERENCES

1. Hagen PT, Scholz DG, Edwards WD. Incidence and size of patent foramen ovale during the first 10 decades of life: an autopsy study of 965 normal hearts. Mayo Clin Proc 1984;59:17–20.

2. Mas JL, Arquizan C, Lamy C, et al. Recurrent cerebrovascular events associated with patent foramen ovale, atrial septal aneurysm, or both. N Engl J Med 2001;345:1740–6.

3. Cabanes L, Mas J, Cohen A, et al. Atrial septal aneurysm and patent foramen ovale as risk factors for cryptogenic stroke in patients less than 55 years of age: a study using transesophageal echocardiography. Stroke 1993;24:1865–73.

4. Muench A, Boccalandro F, Ellis K, et al. Approaches to correct device malposition in percutaneous PFO closure: anatomical and technical implications. Catheter Cardiovasc Interv 2005;64:338–44.

5. McKenzie JA, Edwards W, Hagler DJ. Anatomy of the patent foramen ovale for the interventionalist. Catheter Cardiovasc Interv 2009;73:821–6.

6. Calvert PA, Rana BS, Kydd AC, et al. Patent foramen ovale: anatomy, outcomes and closure. Nat Rev Cardiol 2011;8:148–60.

7. Schuchklenz HW, Weihs W, Horner S, et al. The association between the diameter of a patent foramen ovale and the risk of cerebrovascular evetns. Am J Med 2000;109:456–62.

8. Ho SY, McCarthy KP, Rigby ML. Morphological features pertinent to interventional closure of patent oval foramen. J Interv Cardiol 2003;16:33–8.

9. El Said HG, McMahon CJ, Mullins CE, et al. Patent foramen ovale morphology and impact on percutaneous device closure. Pediatr Cardiol 2005;26:62–5.

10. Marshall AC, Lock JE. Structural and compliant anatomy of the patent foramen ovale in patients undergoing transcatheter closure. Am Heart J 2000; 140:303–7.

11. Rana BS, Thomas MR, Calvert PA, et al. Echocardiographic evaluation of patent foramen ovale prior to device closure. JACC Cardiovasc Imaging 2010;3: 749–60.

12. Silver MD, Dorsey JS. Aneurysms of septum primum in adults. Arch Pathol Lab Med 1978;102:62–5.

13. Pearson AC, Nagelhout D, Castello R, et al. Atrial septal aneurysm and stroke: a transesophageal echocardiographic study. J Am Coll Cardiol 1991; 18:1223–9.

14. Agmon Y, Khanderia BK, Meissner I, et al. Frequency of atrial septal aneurysms in patients with cerebral ischemic events. Circulation 1999;99: 1942–4.

15. Marazano M, Roudaut R, Cohen A, et al. Atrial septal aneurysm. Morphological characteristics in a large population: pathological associations. A French multicenter study on 259 patients investigated by transoesophageal echocardiography. Int J Cardiol 1995;52:59–65.

16. Hanley PC, Tajik AJ, Hynes JK, et al. Diagnosis and classification of atrial septal aneurysm by two-dimensional echocardiography: report of 80 consecutive cases. J Am Coll Cardiol 1985;6:1370–82.

17. Krumsdorf U, Keppeler P, Horvath K, et al. Catheter closure of atrial septal defects and patent foramen ovale in patients with an atrial septal aneurysm using different devices. J Interv Cardiol 2001;14:49–55.

18. Lucas JF, Radtke WAK, Bandisode VM, et al. Characteristics of interatrial communication in patients undergoing transcatheter device closure of atrial septal defects for cryptogenic stroke. Echocardiography 2005;22:814–7.

19. Ruygrok PN. The Coherex FlatStent: an advance in patent foramen ovale closure. Expert Rev Med Devices 2010;7(2):193–9.

20. Onorato E, Ambrosini V, Rubino P, et al. Coherex FlatStent™ EF closure system: a novel concept of in-tunnel PFO closure device. Early Italian Experience. Abstract presentation at Annual SCAI Meeting, San Diego May 5-8, 2010. Catheter Cardiovasc Interv 2010;75:S151.

21. O'Connor S, Recavarren R, Nichols LC, et al. Lipomatous hypertrophy of the interatrial septum: an overview. Arch Pathol Lab Med 2006;130:397–9.

22. Prior JT. Lipomatous hypertrophy of cardiac interatrial septum: a lesion resembling hibernoma, lipoblastomatosis and infiltrating lipoma. Arch Pathol 1964;78:11–5.

23. Heyer CM, Kagel T, Lemburg SP, et al. Lipomatous hypertrophy of the interatrial septum: a prospective study of incidence, imaging findings, and clinical symptoms. Chest 2003;124:2068–73.

24. Augoustides JG, Weiss SJ, Ochroch AE, et al. Analysis of the interatrial septum by transesophageal echocardiography in adult cardiac surgical patients: anatomic variants and correlation with patent foramen ovale. J Cardiothorac Vasc Anesth 2005;19:146–9.

25. Shirani J, Roberts WC. Clinical, electrocardiographic and morphologic features of massive fatty deposits ("lipomatous hypertrophy") in the atrial septum. J Am Coll Cardiol 1993;22:226–38.

26. Ayan K, De Boeck B, Velthuis BK, et al. Lipomatous hypertrophy of the interatrial septum. Int J Cardiovasc Imaging 2005;21:659–61.

27. Tatli S, O'Gara PT, Lambert J, et al. MRI of atypical lipomatous hypertrophy of the interatrial septum. Am J Roentgenol 2004;182:598–600.

28. Calè R, Andrade MJ, Canada M, et al. Lipomatous hypertrophy of the interatrial septum: report of two cases where histological examination and surgical intervention were unavoidable. Eur J Echocardiogr 2009;10:876–9.

29. Chiari H. Uber netzbildungen im rechten vorhof des herzens. Beitr Pathol Anat 1897;22:1–10.

30. Corliss CE. Patten's human embryology: elements of clinical development. New York: McGraw-Hill; 1976.

31. De Dominicis E, Ometto R, Frigiola A, et al. Echocardiographic patterns of persistence of the right sinus venosus valve. G Ital Cardiol 1985;15:80–3.

32. Limacher MC, Gutgesell HP, Vick GW, et al. Echocardiographic anatomy of the Eustachian valve. Am J Cardiol 1986;57:363–5.

33. Okamoto M, Beppu S, Nagata S, et al. Echocardiographic features of the Eustachian valve and its clinical significance. J Cardiogr 1981;11:271–6.

34. Battle-Diaz J, Stanley P, Kratz C, et al. Echocardiographic manifestation of persistent of the right sinus venosus valve. Am J Cardiol 1979;43:850–3.

35. Maeno YV, Boutin C, Benson LN, et al. Three-dimensional transesophageal echocardiography for secundum atrial septal defects with a large Eustachian valve. Circulation 1999;99:E11.

36. Ewert P, Berger F, Vogel M, et al. Morphology of perforated atrial septal aneurysm suitable for closure by transcatheter device placement. Heart 2000;84:327–31.

37. Bertaux G, Eicher JC, Petit A, et al. Anatomic interaction between the aortic root and the atrial septum: a prospective echocardiographic study. J Am Soc Echocardiogr 2007;20(4):409–14.

38. Caputi L, Carriero MR, Parati EA, et al. Postural dependency of right to left shunt: role of contrast-enhanced transcranial Doppler and its potential clinical implications. Stroke 2008;39:2380–1.

39. Hellenbrand WE, Fahey JT, McGowan FX, et al. Transesophageal echocardiographic guidance of transcatheter closure of atrial septal defect. Am J Cardiol 1990;66:207–13.

40. Godart F, Rey C, Francart C, et al. Two-dimensional echocardiographic and color Doppler measurements of atrial septal defect, and comparison with the balloon-stretched diameter. Am J Cardiol 1993;72:1095–7.

41. Hildick-Smith D, Behan M, Haworth P, et al. Patent foramen ovale closure without echocardiographic control: use of "standby" intracardiac ultrasound. JACC Cardiovasc Interv 2008;1:387–91.

42. Wahl A, Praz F, Stirnimann J, et al. Safely and feasibility of percutaneous closure of patent foramen ovale without intraprocedural echocardiography in 825 patients. Swiss Med Wkly 2008;138(39–40):567–72.

43. King TD, Thompson SL, Mills NL. Measurements of the atrial septal defect during cardiac catheterization. Experimental and clinical results. Am J Cardiol 1978;41:41–2.

44. Urbanowicz JH, Kernoff RS, Oppenheim G, et al. Transesophageal echocardiography and its potential for esophageal damage. Anesthesiology 1990;72:40–3.

45. Hijazi Z, Wang Z, Cao Q, et al. Transcatheter closure of atrial septal defects and patent foramen ovale under intracardiac echocardiographic guidance: feasibility and comparison with transesophageal echocardiography. Catheter Cardiovasc Interv 2001;52:194–9.

46. Jan SL, Hwang B, Lee PC, et al. Intracardiac ultrasound assessment of atrial septal defect: comparison with transthoracic echocardiographic, angiocardiographic and balloon-sizing measurements. Cardiovasc Intervent Radiol 2001;24:884–96.

47. Zanchetta M, Onorato E, Rigatelli G, et al. Intracardiac echocardiography-guided transcatheter closure of secundum atrial septal defect. A new efficient device selection method. J Am Coll Cardiol 2003;42:1677–82.

48. Onorato E, Casilli F, Zanchetta M. Intracardiac echocardiography by Ultra ICE in "Percutaneous interventions in congenital heart disease." London: Informa Healthcare; 2007. p. 49.

49. Meier B. Pacman sign during device closure of the patent foramen ovale. Catheter Cardiovasc Interv 2003;60:221–3.

50. Rigatelli G, Cardaioli P, Braggion G, et al. Transesophageal echocardiography and intracardiac echocardiography differently predict potential technical challenges or failures of interatrial shunts catheter-based closure. J Interv Cardiol 2007;20:77–81.

51. Wahl A, Krumsdorf U, Meier B, et al. Transcatheter treatment of atrial septal aneurysm associated with patent foramen ovale for prevention of recurrent paradoxical embolism in high-risk patients. J Am Coll Cardiol 2005;45(3):377–80.

52. Greutmann M, Greutmann-Yantiri M, Kretschmar O, et al. Percutaneous PFO closure with Amplatzer PFO: predictors of residual shunt at 6 months follow-up. Congenit Heart Dis 2009;4:252–7.

53. Schoen SP, Wiedeman S, Block M, et al. Interatrial septal closure devices and aortic perforation: a note of caution. J Invasive Cardiol 2009;21:E39–41.

54. Rigatelli G, Ronco F, Cardaioli P, et al. Incomplete aneurysm coverage after patent foranem ovale closure in patients with huge atrial septal aneurysm: effect on left atrial functional remodeling. J Interv Cardiol 2010;23:362–7.

55. Schwerzmann M, Windecker S, Wahl A, et al. Implantation of a second closure device in patients

with residual shunt after percutaneous closure of patent foramen ovale. Catheter Cardiovasc Interv 2004;63:490–5.

56. Tande AJ, Knickelbine T, Chavez I, et al. Transseptal technique of percutaneous PFO closure results in persistent interatrial shunting. Catheter Cardiovasc Interv 2005;65:295–300.

57. Meier B. Iatrogenic atrial septal defect, erosion of the septum primum after device closure of a patent foramen ovale as a new medical entity. Catheter Cardiovasc Interv 2006;68:165–8.

58. Büscheck F, Sievert H, Kleber F, et al. Patent foramen ovale using the Premere device: the results of the CLOSEUP trial. J Interv Cardiol 2006;19: 328–33.

59. Chintala K, Turner DR, Leaman S, et al. Use of balloon pull-through technique to assist in Cardio-SEAL device closure of patent foramen ovale. Catheter Cardiovasc Interv 2003;60:101–6.

60. Ruiz CE, Alboliras ET, Pophal SG. The puncture technique: a new method for transcatheter closure of patent foramen ovale. Catheter Cardiovasc Interv 2001;53:369–72.

61. Meier B. Closure of patent foramen ovale: technique, pitfalls, complications, and follow up. Heart 2005;91: 444–8.

62. Spence MS, Khan AA, Mullen MJ. Balloon assessment of patent foramen ovale morphology and the modification of tunnels using a balloon detunnelisation technique. Catheter Cardiovasc Interv 2008;71: 222–8.

63. McMahon CJ, El Said HG, Mullins CE. Use of the transseptal puncture in transcatheter closure of long tunnel-type patent foramen ovale. Heart 2002; 88:E3, 22.

64. Braun MU, Ehrhard K, Strasser RH, et al. Occlusion by catheter intervention in patent foramen ovale via additional transseptal puncture. Z Kardiol 2002;91: 659–62.

65. Al-Faleh H, Marquis JF, Chan KL. Device closure of a patent foramen ovale in a patient with lipomatous hypertrophy of the atrial septum. Can J Cardiol 2005;21:789–90.

66. Rigatelli G, Dell'Avvocata F, Giordan M, et al. Transcatheter patent foramen ovale closure in spite of interatrial septum hypertrophy or lipomatosis: a case series. J Cardiovasc Med (Hagerstown) 2010;11: 91–5.

67. Huie Lin C, Balzer DT, Lasala JM. Defect Closure in the lipomatous hypertrophied atrial septum with the Amplatzer muscular ventricular septal defect closure device: a case series. Catheter Cardiovasc Interv 2011;78:102–7.

68. Salmeron O, Rarco P, Nunez L. A unusual complication of right catheterization: hooking of the catheter in Chiari network. Arch Inst Cardiol Mex 1966;36: 387–90.

69. Sopher SM, Grace AA, Spencer CH, et al. Entrapment of an ablation catheter in the cardiac venous system: a case report. Pacing Clin Electrophysiol 1998;21:1306–8.

70. Cooke JC, Gelman JS, Herper RW. Chiari network entanglement and herniation into the left atrium by an atrial septal defect occluder device. J Am Soc Echocardiogr 1999;12:601–3.

71. McMahon CJ, Pignatelli RH, Rutledge JM, et al. Steerable control of the Eustachian valve during transcatheter closure of secundum atrial septal defects. Catheter Cardiovasc Interv 2000;51:455–9.

72. Onorato E, Pera IG, Melzi G, et al. Persistent redundant Eustachian valve interfering with Amplatzer PFO occluder placement: anatomico-clinical and technical implications. Catheter Cardiovasc Interv 2002;55:521–4.

73. Butera G, Montinaro A, Carminati M. The "pull-push" technique to deal with a redundant Eustachian valve interfering with placement of a PFO Occluder. Catheter Cardiovasc Interv 2006;68:961–4.

74. Zanchetta M, Rigatelli G, Pedon L, et al. Catheter closure of perforated secundum atrial septal defect under intracardiac echocardiographic guidance using a single Amplatzer device: feasibility of a new method. J Invasive Cardiol 2005;17:262–5.

75. Bridges ND, Hellenbrand W, Latson L, et al. Transcatheter closure of patent foramen ovale after presumed paradoxical embolism. Circulation 1992; 86:1902–8.

76. Khairy P, O'Donnell CP, Landzberg MJ. Transcatheter closure versus medical therapy of patent foramen ovale and presumed paradoxical thromboemboli: a systematic review. Ann Intern Med 2003;139: 753–60.

77. Vanderheyden M, Willaert W, Claessens P, et al. Thrombosis of a patent foramen ovale closure device: thrombolytic management. Catheter Cardiovasc Interv 2002;56:522–6.

78. Trepels T, Zeplin H, Sievert H, et al. Cardiac perforation following transcatheter PFO closure. Catheter Cardiovasc Interv 2003;58:111–3.

79. Ischinger TA, Kemkes B, Boosfeld C. Partial malposition of PFO closure device: indication for elective surgical removal? discussion of indications, procedural and anatomical aspects. Z Kardiol 2003;92:188–92.

80. Windecker S, Wahl A, Chatterjee T, et al. Percutaneous closure of patent foramen ovale in patients with paradoxical embolism: long-term risk of recurrent thromboembolic events. Circulation 2000;101:893–8.

81. Dearani JA, Ugurlu BS, Danielson GK, et al. Surgical patent foramen ovale closure for prevention of paradoxical embolism related cerebrovascular ischemic events. Circulation 1999;100:II171–5.

82. Homma S, Di Tullio MR, Sacco RL, et al. Surgical closure of patent foramen ovale in cryptogenic stroke patients. Stroke 1997;28:2376–81.

83. El-Said HG, Moore JW. Erosion by the Amplatzer septal occluder: experienced operator opinions at odds with manufacturer recommendations? Catheter Cardiovasc Interv 2009;73:925–30.

84. Crawford GB, Brindis RG, Krucoff MW, et al. Percutaneous atrial septal occluder devices and cardiac erosion: a review of the literature. Catheter Cardiovasc Interv 2012;80(2):157–67.

85. Amin Z, Hijazi ZM, Bass JL, et al. Erosion of amplatzer septal occluder device after closure of secundum atrial septal defects: review of registry of complications and recommendations to minimize future risk. Catheter Cardiovasc Interv 2004;63: 496–502.

86. Grayburn PA, Schwartz B, Anwar A, et al. Migration of an Amplatzer Septal Occluder device for closure of atrial septal defect into the ascending aorta with formation of an aorta-to-right atrial fistula. Am J Cardiol 2005;96:1607–9.

87. Murphy JC, Walsh SJ, Spence MS. Late aortic perforation with an Atriasept device resulting in life-threatening tamponade. Catheter Cardiovasc Interv 2010;76:132–4.

88. Raffa GM, Pellegrini C, Lentini S, et al. Minimally invasive video-assisted surgery for iatrogenic aortic root-to-right atrium fistula after incomplete percutaneous occlusion of patent foramen ovale: case report and review of the literature. J Card Surg 2008;23(1):75–8.

89. Chessa M, Carminati M, Butera G, et al. Early and late complications associated with transcatheter occlusion of secundum atrial septal defect. J Am Coll Cardiol 2002;39:1061–5.

90. Dibardino DJ, McElhinney DB, Kaza AK, et al. Analysis of the IS food and drug administration manufacturer and user faciliity device experience database for adverse events involving AMPLATZER septal occluder devices and comparison with the society of thoracic congenital cardiac surgery database. J Thorac Cardiovasc Surg 2009;137:1334–41.

91. Mashman WE, King SB, Jacobs C, et al. Two cases of device embolization of Amplatzer septal occluder devices to the pulmonary artery following closure of secundum atrial septal defect. Catheter Cardiovasc Interv 2005;65:588–92.

92. Verma SK, Tobis JM. Explantation of patent foramen ovale closure devices. A multicenter survey. JACC Cardiovasc Interv 2011;4:579–85.

93. Krumsdorf U, Ostermayer S, Billinger K, et al. Incidence and clinical course of thrombus formation on atrial septal defect and patient foramen ovale closure devices in 1,000 consecutive patients. J Am Coll Cardiol 2004;43:302–9.

94. Baronowski A, Skowasch M, Hofmann I, et al. Thrombus formation of ASD and PFO devices: frequency and clinical importance. Circulation 2006; 114:785.

95. Taafe M, Fischer E, Baronowski A, et al. Comparison of the three patent foramen ovale closure devices in a randomized trial (AMPLATZER versus Cardio-SEAL and HELEX Occluder). Am J Cardiol 2008; 101:1353–8.

96. Scacciatella P, Butera G, Meynet I, et al. Percutaneous closure of patent foramen ovale in patients with anatomical and clinical high-risk characteristics: long-term efficacy and safety. J Interv Cardiol 2011;24:477–84.

97. Shafi NA, McKay RG, Kiernan FJ, et al. Determinants and clinical significance of persistent residual shunting in patients with percutaneous patent foramen ovale closure devices. Int J Cardiol 2009;137(3): 314–6.

Transcatheter Closure of Membranous Ventricular Septal Defects—Old Problems and New Solutions

Gianfranco Butera, MD, PhD*, Luciane Piazza, MD,
Antonio Saracino, MD, Massimo Chessa, MD, PhD,
Mario Carminati, MD

KEYWORDS

- Ventricular septal defect • Closure • Membranous • Conduction system • Arrhthmias
- Transcatheter

KEY POINTS

- Perimembranous defects are the most common type of ventricular septal defect.
- Transcatheter closure has been attempted with a number of devices with variable success rates.
- High closure rates have been achieved with the Amplatzer Membranous Occluder; however, concerns have been raised regarding the incidence of device-induced complete heart block.
- A newer Amplatzer device has been designed with modifications to target the possible pressure points on the conduction tissue.

INTRODUCTION

Ventricular septal defects (VSDs) are the most common congenital cardiac malformation, accounting for over one-fifth of all defects.[1] Seventy percent are located in the area of the membranous septum, with various extensions toward the inlet, outlet, or apical components of the right ventricle. These are called perimembranous defects. Defects opening directly beneath both the aortic and pulmonary valves are defined as doubly committed and juxta-arterial, or supracristal. These defects are rare in western countries, but are more frequent in Asian countries. VSDs can also be located entirely within the muscular portion of the septum, and these account for around 15% of patients seen in postnatal life. The defects can be multiple as in the Swiss cheese septum.

Surgical closure of a congenital VSD was performed for the first time by Lillehei and associates in 1954.[2] Since that time, surgical closure has come to be regarded as the gold standard for treatment; however, it remains associated with morbidity and mortality,[3–11] with associated postoperative discomfort, the need for sternotomy, and residual scar. Complications due to significant residual leaks are reported in up to 2% of patients,[3–7] while iatrogenic atrioventricular block can occur in around 1% to 8% of cases.[3–11] Reoperations due to indications other than residual leakage are needed in a further 2% of subjects.[3–7] The occurrence of postpericardiotomy syndrome, arrhythmias, infections, and respiratory or neurologic complications has been also reported.[3–7] Mortality occurs rarely in the current era.[3–7] The risk for all these events is increased in small

Pediatric Cardiology and GUCH Unit, Policlinico San Donato IRCCS, Via Morandi 30, San Donato Milanese 20097, Italy
* Corresponding author.
E-mail address: gianfranco.butera@grupposandonato.it

Intervent Cardiol Clin 2 (2013) 85–91
http://dx.doi.org/10.1016/j.iccl.2012.09.003
2211-7458/13/$ – see front matter © 2013 Elsevier Inc. All rights reserved.

interventional.theclinics.com

infants, patients with multiple defects or apical defects, those with associated lesions, or when additional surgery is required in patients with residual defects.[3–5] It has been reported that negative long-term effects on developmental and neurocognitive function may occur in children who undergo cardiopulmonary bypass surgery.[10] Therefore, various attempts have been made to develop less invasive techniques to reduce morbidity, mortality, and psychological stress associated with surgery.

HISTORY

In 1988, Lock and colleagues[12] reported the first human experience of transcatheter closure of muscular VSDs. They closed defects in 7 patients using the Rashkind double umbrella device. Since then, various devices have been used, such as the Clamshell or CardioSeal-Starflex device,[13,14] the Sideris buttoned device,[15] and Gianturco coils.[16] The rate of success of such procedures has been reported between 77% and 100% of cases, while residual shunting was reported in between 35% and 100% of cases.[12–20] Furthermore, the procedure was technically difficult when using these devices, and complications were encountered with some frequency.[12–20]

Introduction of the Amplatzer family of devices has markedly widened the application of transcatheter techniques for closure of these defects.[21,22] This is particularly true for perimembranous defects. Due to the proximity of these defects to the aortic and the atrioventricular valves, devices designed for other applications did not fit perfectly when used in this setting.[13,14] With the introduction of the specially designed eccentric Amplatzer device, general closure of these defects become feasible.[22,23]

INDICATIONS AND PATIENT SELECTION

Indications for closure are symptoms of heart failure, or signs of left heart volume overload. In patients, and in particular in children with left atrial and ventricular overload, closure may be needed in order to prevent pulmonary arterial hypertension, ventricular dilation, arrhythmias, aortic regurgitation, and development of double-chambered right ventricle. Even subjects with small defects without symptoms of cardiac failure or overload may need closure if they experience endocarditis. Soufflet and colleagues[24] showed that midterm outcome of small and unclosed perimembranous VSDs in young adults is not uneventful. In fact, during a median follow-up of 6 years (range 4–38 years), 4% of subjects experienced endocarditis. Nine percent of patients had pulmonary hypertension, and 1% died suddenly.

Large defects are associated with signs and symptoms of cardiac failure in early infancy, and they have to be treated surgically in the first months of life. Defects of moderate size may also be responsible for failure to thrive, respiratory infections, and diastolic left heart overload. Surgical repair is currently the only option for doubly committed or supracristal defects, for perimembranous defects associated with prolapse of aortic valve and aortic regurgitation, and for any defect associated with malalignment of the muscular outlet septum, or straddling and overriding atrioventricular valves.

ECHOCARDIOGRAPHIC PREPROCEDURAL EVALUATION

Transthoracic echocardiography is mandatory to assess the size, number, and location of the defect. The presence of a rim of tissue of 2 mm or more between the aortic valve and the defect is considered a prerequisite for device closure. The left parasternal long-axis view will demonstrate the defect. In short-axis view, at the level of the aortic valve, it is possible to locate exactly the perimembranous VSD (supracristal defects between 12 and 1 o'clock, membranous defects between 9 and 12 o'clock, and perimembranous defects between 7 and 9 o'clock). Four-chamber and 5-chamber views may demonstrate perimembranous defects and their extension.

TECHNIQUE AND EQUIPMENT
Device

The original Amplatzer membranous occluder (St. Jude Medical, Golden Valley, Minnesota) has 2 discs of unequal size (**Fig. 1**). The aortic rim of the asymmetric left ventricular disc exceeds the dimensions of the connecting waist by only 0.5 mm, so as to avoid impingement on the aortic valve, whereas the apical end is 5.5 mm larger than the waist. This apical end of the left ventricular disc contains a platinum marker to facilitate

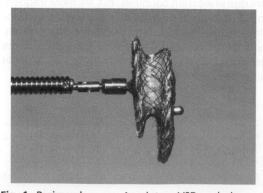

Fig. 1. Perimembranous Amplatzer VSD occluder.

correct orientation during implantation. The right ventricular disk is symmetrical, and it exceeds the diameter of the connecting waist by 2 mm throughout its circumference. The device is available in sizes from 4 to 18 mm, and requires delivery sheaths from 7 to 9 French. The delivery system consists of a delivery cable and a pusher catheter having a sharp curvature of 180° inferiorly. This allows correct orientation of the left ventricular disc during implantation. It has a flattened part of the socket that matches the flat portion of the microscrew, in order to force the larger part of the left ventricular disc to be oriented downwards so that it points to the left ventricular apex.[23,25–35]

Procedure and Technique of Implantation

All procedures are performed under general anesthesia, with fluoroscopic and transoesophageal echocardiographic control. Full heparinization, using 100 IU/kg, is given routinely. Patients receive a dose of cephalosporin during catheterization, and 2 further doses at 8-hour intervals.

Vascular access is via the right femoral artery and vein. Angiography is performed using 60° left anterior oblique plus 20° cranial view (**Fig. 2**, top left). An angiogram of the ascending aorta is also performed in 50° left atrial oblique view to check for aortic insufficiency. The size of the defect and its relationship to the aorta are confirmed. The defect is crossed from the left ventricle by using a Right Judkins or a Right Amplatzer catheter (Cordis Corp, Miami, Florida) and a Terumo wire (Terumo, Tokyo, Japan). The catheter is advanced to the pulmonary arteries or the superior or inferior caval vein. The Terumo wire is then replaced by the soft exchange noodle wire (St. Jude Medical, Golden Valley, Minnesota). The noodle wire is snared with a gooseneck snare, exteriorized from the femoral vein, and an arteriovenous circuit is created (see **Fig. 2**, top middle). The St. Jude Medical braided sheath is advanced over the wire up to ascending aorta. Sometimes this maneuver is quite difficult. A kissing technique may be needed, using the tip of the sheath and the arterial catheter over the wire. Another technique consists in holding the guide wire circuit taut and pushing the sheath and the dilator over this quite rigid system. The dilator is withdrawn approximately 10 cm; the sheath is slowly withdrawn, and the arterial catheter advanced, making a loop of the wire that is then pushed into the left ventricular apex. The sheath is advanced over the wire until it reaches the apex of the left ventricle, and the wire

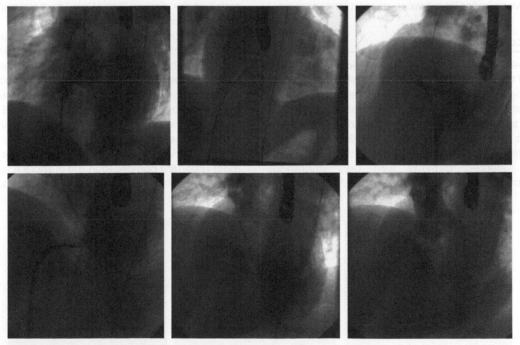

Fig. 2. Perimembranous VSD percutaneous closure. Cine angiograms in the hepatoclavicular projection. *Top left*: angiogram demonstrates a single perimembranous VSD. *Top middle*: arterovenous circuit through the VSD. *Top right*: cine image showing the position of the delivery sheath towards the apex of the left ventricle. *Bottom left*: opening of the left ventricular disc. *Bottom middle*: left ventricular angiogram after device release, showing good device position and trivial residual shunt. *Bottom right*: ascending aortogram showing relationship between aortic valve and device and no aortic regurgitation.

is gently removed (see **Fig. 2**, top right). The device, having been sized at equal to or 1 mm larger than the size of the defect, is secured on the delivery cable, and the flat part of the microscrew is aligned with the flat part of the capsule of the pusher catheter. The device is advanced up to the tip of the sheath, and the entire system is withdrawn to the left ventricular outflow tract. The left disc is deployed (see **Fig. 2**, bottom left), echocardiographic monitoring being of paramount importance at this stage to confirm normal function of both mitral and aortic valves. The platinum marker of the distal disc should point downwards. The proximal disc is then deployed on the right side of the septum, and angiographic testing is done before releasing the device (see **Fig. 2**, bottom middle and right).

When it is difficult to achieve the position of the braided sheath toward the left ventricular apex; the sheath can be left in the ascending aorta and the left ventricular disc opened under the aortic valve while coming with the sheath from the aorta. Then the right ventricular disc is opened by advancing the delivery cable. After 10–15 minutes, left ventricular angiogram and aortogram are repeated to assess possible residual shunting or aortic regurgitation. Throughout the procedure, the electrocardiogram is carefully screened in order to assess the occurrence of abnormalities of atrioventricular conduction or tachyarrhythmias.

Outcomes

At the beginning of their experience, the authors used the muscular occluder in 10 selected patients, having at least 5 mm distance between the superior rim of the defect and the aortic valve. The device was successfully deployed by using a retrograde or an anterograde approach (**Fig. 3**). Similar good results with the use of a muscular device for properly selected patients with perimembranous defects have been already reported.[36,37]

When the membranous occluder became available, indications were expanded also to patients having only 1 to 2 mm distance between the defect and the aortic valve.[23,25]

Pooling data from the literature, the authors calculate the mean rate of successful closure at 98.5%, with 95% confidence interval from 95% to 100%. In their series[32] among the 104 patients who had the device successfully implanted, complete closure was 97% at 6 months, as in previous reports.[25–35]

The most common morphologic variation is the presence of an aneurysm of the ventricular septum. The authors found this feature in one-third of their patients. Usually, the authors tried to close the true anatomic hole with the more appropriate device, as judged from case to case. Sometimes, when the redundant tissue of the aneurysm was relatively small, the device could cover the hole along with the aneurysm. In cases of very large aneurysms, the device was implanted within the aneurysm itself, with the aim of closing the true anatomic hole, and not to place the device at the entrance on the left ventricular side, in order to avoid insertion of a dangerously oversized device. Studies reported in the literature show that major acute complications occur in 1.3% of cases, with 95% CI from 0 to 3%.

The most important complications are embolization of the device, hemolysis, aortic regurgitation, and disturbances of conduction. In their series, embolization occurred in 2 cases, but the authors could retrieve the device and successfully implant a second device in both. Transient hemolysis occurred in 2 out of 35 cases in the phase 1 clinical trial carried out in the United States,[31] and in 2 out of 104 of the authors' patients.[32] Trivial aortic and tricuspid regurgitation related to insertion of the device occurred in only 3 cases in the authors' series. Complete heart block was the most important complication the authors encountered. It occurred acutely, albeit transiently, during

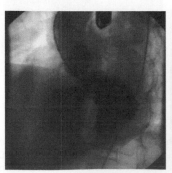 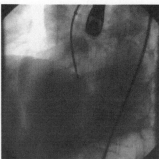 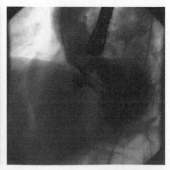

Fig. 3. High muscular VSD. Left anterior oblique with cranial angulation angiographic views. *Left*: left ventricular angiography showing left-to-right shunting. *Middle*: retrograde transaortic closure by using a muscular Amplatzer VSD occlude. *Right*: left ventricular angiography showing the device in place with trivial residual shunting.

the procedure in 1 patient, within 48 hours after the procedure in 2 patients, 1 of occurrences was permanent. In another patient, permanent heart block was noted 4 months afterward, and then after more than 6 months, but again permanently, in a final patient. Implantation of a pacemaker was required in 6 of 104 patients (5.7%). No instances of complete heart block were reported by Thanoupoulos and colleagues[26] in 10 children, or by Bass and colleagues[25] in 25 cases. Complete atrioventricular block, however, was reported in 2 out of 35 patients (5.7%) by Fu and colleagues,[29] in 2 out of 100 subjects by Holzer and colleagues,[31] and in 1 out of 12 patients (8%) during catheter manipulation leading to abandonment of the procedure by Pedra and colleagues.[30] Also in the authors' experience, the procedure was aborted in 2 patients after the occurrence of transient complete atrioventricular block during catheter maneuvers. From data published in the literature, the authors calculate the incidence of complete atrioventricular block needing implantation of a pacemaker to be 2.6%, with 95% CI from 0% to 4%.

The occurrence of complete heart block is the major issue in percutaneous closure of perimembranous defects. The proximity of the conduction tissues to the rims of the perimembranous defect explains how sometimes a simple catheter or wire manipulation across the defect may cause heart block. If heart block occurs after placement of the device, this is related to the expansion of the device against the conducting tissue. Therefore, the use of oversized devices should be avoided. Complete heart block may also occur, however, when the discs appear nicely flat on both sides. In the authors' patients, an oversized device could have been possibly used in 1 patient, but not in the 2 others. Other mechanisms should be considered. The device may give a chronic inflammatory reaction or scar formation in the conduction tissue. Furthermore, nitinol is a memory shape alloy, whose progressive expansion and flattening against the conduction tissue and its vascular supply may play a major role.

Steroid therapy in high doses with aspirin may be useful,[38] as was observed previously in some cases of complete atrioventricular block occurring subsequent to surgery. However, results in complete atrioventricular block (cAVB) after device implantation are not always predictable and stable.[39]

NEW SOLUTIONS

A new Amplatzer Membranous VSD Occluder 2 device and delivery system has been developed and presents major changes compared to the first version (**Fig. 4**). First, the device's left disc has an elliptical and concave shape that adapts to the left ventricular outflow and provides improved retention and stability. It is available in 2 configurations: eccentric, with a 1 mm superior rim and a 2 mm inferior rim; and concentric, with a 3 mm superior rim, to adapt to the variations in available subaortic tissue superior to the defect. The nitinol wire is considerably thinner to decrease the rigidity of the device, and it is arranged in a dual layer configuration.

The external layer is especially thin, to impact with minimal radial pressure while the inner part provides stability. In order to reduce clamp force against the ventricular septum, the waist length was also increased from 1.5 to 3 mm. This change evolved from the experience of muscular VSD occluder use in subjects with high muscular VSD where no cAVB occurred.[36,37]

Polyester patches are sewn into the disks, to ensure rapid occlusion. Both versions of the device (eccentric and concentric) are available in 9 waist diameters (from 4 to 10 mm in 1 mm increments plus 12 and 14 mm). Second, the new TorqVue 4 delivery system has been redesigned to assure better positioning of the device in the left ventricular outflow tract. The novel pusher catheter facilitates easier rotation outside the sheath to assure proper orientation of the occluder while the delivery system remains stable.

Recently 2 reports[40,41] have been published on the use of this new occluder. Bass and Gruenstein[40] studied this new device in vitro and in

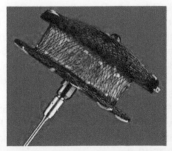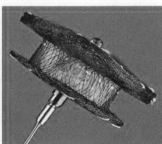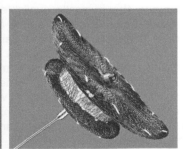

Fig. 4. Perimembranous II Amplatzer VSD occluder. *Left*: 1 mm rim device. *Middle*: 3 mm rim device. *Right*: device profile.

a swine model. They showed that the device had 75% reduction in radial force, 45% reduction in clamping force, and increased stability as compared to the previous version. The device was implanted in 6 swine with naturally occurring perimembranous VSDs with immediate, 1-, 7-, 30-, and 90-day follow-up by echocardiography, angiography, and final pathologic examination. The device was successfully implanted in all animals and was retrievable and repositionable. There was complete occlusion of the VSD in 5 of 6 cases without embolization. There was no thrombus formation on the device or occurrence of complete heart block. A single instance of a tiny residual shunt was attributed to capture of tricuspid valve apparatus. Velasco-Sanchez and colleagues[40] reported the first human cases showing the feasibility and safety of percutanous perimembranous VSD closure with the new device in a pediatric and adult patient. Short-term follow-up of both patients showed no atrioventricular conduction disturbances, no valve interference and, in the case of the first patient, progressive decrease of the residual shunt, until disappearance. The implantation technique did not vary significantly from the previous version of the device, except that perfect positioning of the device is now even more important, due to the elliptic shape of the left ventricular disk.

It is too early to anticipate a reduction of cAVB, and follow-up has been too short; however, the special design and the softness of the outer nitinol layer are expected to decrease the incidence of AV block in comparison to the previous version of the device. Nevertheless, patient selection, defect assessment, and adequate device size are still necessary. The current device design has allowed successful closure of a large perimembranous VSD with no aortic rim in an 18 kg child. However, in smaller children and infants, the radius of curvature of the left disk might not be adapted to the anatomy of the left ventricular outflow tract of an infant, resulting in subaortic stenosis.

SUMMARY

In summary, the currently available data show that percutanous closure is a safe and effective procedure in highly specialized centers and in children aged more than 6 years. Appropriate patient selection is of paramount importance to the success of the procedure. A new device is now available. Its characteristics will probably reduce the risk of complications, including cAVB. However, more data in a large series of patients with long-term follow-up are needed to demonstrate the safety and efficacy of this

new device, and in particular a decrease in AV block occurrence.

REFERENCES

1. Rudolph AM. Ventricular septal defect. In: Rudolph AM, editor. Congenital diseases of the heart: clinical–physiological considerations. 2nd edition. Armonk (NY): Futura Publishing Company; 2001. p. 197–244.
2. Lillehei CW, Cohen M, Warden HE, et al. The results of direct vision closure of ventricular septal defects in eight patients by means of controlled cross circulation. Surg Gynecol Obstet 1955;101:446–66.
3. Kouchoukos NT, Blackstone EH, Doty DB, et al. Ventricular septal defect. In: Kouchoukos NT, Blackstone EH, Doty DB, editors. Kirklin/barratt-boyes. 3rd edition. Philadelphia: Elsevier Science; 2003. p. 850–910.
4. Roos-Hesselink JW, Meijboom FJ, Spitaels SE, et al. Outcome of patients after surgical closure of ventricular septal defect at a young age: longitudinal follow-up of 22-34 years. Eur Heart J 2004;25:1057–62.
5. Mavroudis C, Backer CL, Jacobs JP. Ventricular septal defect. In: Mavroudis C, Backer CL, editors. Pediatric cardiac surgery. 3rd edition. St Louis (MO): Mosby Inc; 2003. p. 298–320.
6. Nygren A, Sunnegard J, Berggren H. Preoperative evaluation and surgery in isolated ventricular septal defects: a 21 years perspective. Heart 2005;83: 198–204.
7. Monro JL, Alexiou C, Salmon AP, et al. Follow-up and survival after primary repair if congenital heart defects in children. J Thorac Cardiovasc Surg 2003;126:511–20.
8. Hobbins SM, Izukawa T, Radford DJ, et al. Conduction disturbances after surgical correction of ventricular septal defect by the atrial approach. Br Heart J 1979;41:289–93.
9. Bol-Raap G, Weerheim J, Kappetein AP, et al. Follow-up after surgical closure of congenital ventricular septal defect. Eur J Cardiothorac Surg 2003;24:511–5.
10. Visconti KJ, Bichell DP, Jonas RA, et al. Developmental outcome after surgical versus interventional closure of secundum atrial septal defect in children. Circulation 1999;100(Suppl 19):II145–50.
11. Tucker EM, Pyles LA, Bass JL, et al. Permanent pacemaker for atrioventricular conduction block after operative repair of perimembranous ventricular septal defect. J Am Coll Cardiol 2007;50:1196–200.
12. Lock JE, Block PC, McKay RG, et al. Transcatheter closure of ventricular septal defects. Circulation 1988;78:361–8.
13. Janorkar S, Goh T, Wilkinson J. Transcatheter closure of ventricular septal defects using the Rashkind device: initial experience. Catheter Cardiovasc Interv 1999;46:43–8.

14. Kalra GS, Verma PK, Dhall A, et al. Transcatheter device closure of ventricular septal defects: immediate results and intermediate follow-up. Am Heart J 1999;138:339–44.

15. Sideris EB, Walsh KP, Haddad JL, et al. Occlusion of congenital ventricular septal defects by the buttoned device. "Buttoned device" Clinical Trials International Register. Heart 1997;77:276–9.

16. Kalra GS, Verma PK, Singh S, et al. Transcatheter device closure of ventricular septal defects using detachable steel coil. Heart 1999;82:395–6.

17. Bridges ND, Perry SB, Keane JF, et al. Preoperative transcatheter closure of congenital muscular ventricular septal defects. N Engl J Med 1991;324:1312–7.

18. Latiff HA, Alwi M, Kandhavel G, et al. Transcatheter closure of multiple muscular ventricular septal defects using Gianturco coils. Ann Thorac Surg 1999; 68:1400–1.

19. Chaudari M, Chessa M, Stumper O, et al. Transcatheter coils closure of muscular ventricular septal defects. J Invasive Cardiol 2001;14:165–8.

20. Knauth AL, Lock JE, Perry SB, et al. Transcatheter device closure of congenital and post-operative residual ventricular septal defect. Circulation 2004; 110:501–7.

21. Amin Z, Gu X, Berry JM, et al. New device for closure of muscular ventricular septal defects in a canine model. Circulation 1999;100:320–8.

22. Gu X, Han YM, Titus JL, et al. Transcatheter closure of membranous ventricular septal defects with a new nitinol prosthesis in a natural swine model. Catheter Cardiovasc Interv 2000;50:502–9.

23. Hijazi ZM, Hakim F, Hawaleh AA, et al. Catheter closure of perimembranous ventricular septal defects using the new Amplatzer membranous ventricular septal defect occluder: initial clinical experience. Catheter Cardiovasc Interv 2002;56:508–15.

24. Soufflet V, Van de Bruaene A, Troost E, et al. Behavior of unrepaired perimembranous ventricular septal defect in young adults. Am J Cardiol 2010; 105(3):404–7.

25. Bass JL, Kalra GS, Arora R, et al. Initial human experience with the Amplatzer perimembranous ventricular septal occluder device. Catheter Cardiovasc Interv 2003;58:238–45.

26. Thanopoulos BD, Tsaousis GS, Karanasios E, et al. Transcatheterer closure of a perimembranous ventricular septal defects with the Amplatzer asymmetric ventricular septal defect occluder: preliminary experience in children. Heart 2003;89:918–22.

27. Hijazi ZM. Device closure of ventricular septal defects. Catheter Cardiovasc Interv 2003;60:107–14.

28. Arora R, Trehan V, Kumar A, et al. Transcatheter closure of congenital ventricular septal defects. Experience with various devices. J Interv Cardiol 2003;16:83–91.

29. Fu YC, Hijazi ZM, Amin Z, et al. Transcatheter closure of perimembranous ventricular septal defects using the new Amplatzer membranous ventricular septal defect occluder: result of the U.S. phase I trial. J Am Coll Cardiol 2006;47:319–25.

30. Pedra CA, Pedra SR, Esteves CA, et al. Percutaneous closure of perimebranous ventricular septal defects with the Amplatzer device: technical and morphological considerations. Catheter Cardiovasc Interv 2004;61:403–10.

31. Holzer R, de Giovanni J, Walsh K, et al. Transcatheter closure of perimembranous ventricular septal defects using the Amplatzer membranous ventricular septal defect device occluder: immediate and midterm results of an international registry. Catheter Cardiovasc Interv 2006;68:620–8.

32. Butera G, Carminati M, Chessa M, et al. Transcatheter closure of perimembranous ventricular septal defects. J Am Coll Cardiol 2007;50:1189–95.

33. Zuo J, Xie J, Yi W, et al. Results of transcatheter closure of perimembranous ventricular septal defect. Am J Cardiol 2010;106:1034–7.

34. Carminati M, Butera G, Chessa M, et al. Transcatheter closure of congenital ventricular septal defects: results of the European Registry. Eur Heart J 2007; 28:2361–8.

35. Predescu D, Chaturvedi RR, Friedberg MK, et al. Complete heart block associated with device closure of perimembranous ventricular septal defects. J Thorac Cardiovasc Surg 2008;136(5):1223–8.

36. Arora R, Trehan V, Thakur AK, et al. Transcatheter closure of congenital muscular ventricular septal defect. J Interv Cardiol 2004;17:109–15.

37. Szkutnik M, Qureshi SA, Kusa J, et al. Use of the Amplatzer muscular ventricular septal defect occluder for closure of perimembranous ventricular septal defects. Heart 2007;93:355–8.

38. Yip WC, Zimmerman F, Hijazi ZM. Heart block and empirical therapy after transcatheter closure of perimembranous ventricular septal defect. Catheter Cardiovasc Interv 2005;66:436–9.

39. Butera G, Gaio G, Carminati M. Is steroid therapy enough to reverse complete atrioventricular block after percutaneous perimembranous ventricular septal defect closure? J Cardiovasc Med (Hagerstown) 2009;10:412–4.

40. Velasco-Sanchez D, Tzikas A, Ibrahim R, et al. Transcatheter closure of perimembranous ventricular septal defects: initial human experience with the Amplatzer® membranous VSD occluder 2. Catheter Cardiovasc Interv 2012. http://dx.doi.org/10.1002/ccd.24361. [Epub ahead of print].

41. Bass JL, Gruenstein D. Transcatheter closure of the perimembranous ventricular septal defect—preclinical trial of a new Amplatzer device. Catheter Cardiovasc Interv 2012;79:1153–60.

Stenting of Lesions in Patent Ductus Arteriosus with Duct-Dependent Pulmonary Blood Flow

Focus on Case Selection, Techniques and Outcome

Mazeni Alwi, MBBS, MRCP*, Marhisham Che Mood, MD

KEYWORDS

- PDA stenting • Branch pulmonary artery stenosis • Cyanotic heart disease • In-stent thrombosis

KEY POINTS

- Patent ductus arteriosus (PDA) in cyanotic heart disease has a diverse morphology that encompasses its shape, origin in the aorta, and site of insertion onto the pulmonary artery.
- The main indications for PDA stenting are bridging palliation whereby the PDA is the sole source of pulmonary blood flow, and to augment pulmonary blood flow following right ventricular outflow tract intervention in some patients with pulmonary atresia with intact ventricular septum.
- The major complications of PDA stenting are PDA spasm, migration of stent, stent thrombosis, pulmonary hypertension, and accelerated branch pulmonary stenosis in vulnerable patients.
- Further studies are necessary to define the role and limitations of PDA stenting in cyanotic congenital heart disease.

 Videos of patent ductus arteriosus stenting via the femoral artery route in a severely hypoxic newborn with Ebstein anomaly, severe tricuspid regurgitation, and "functional" pulmonary atresia accompany this article at http://www.interventional.theclinics.com/

INTRODUCTION

With advances in surgical techniques and perioperative care, important milestones have been achieved in the primary repair of major congenital heart lesions in the neonatal period or early infancy.[1,2] Despite this tendency and desirability for primary repair, palliative systemic pulmonary shunt in the form of modified Blalock-Taussig (mBT) shunt remains a commonly performed procedure as technical feasibility precludes neonatal primary repair in certain cyanotic lesions such as those requiring complex conduit surgery. On the other hand, in hearts with a single-ventricle, transitional postnatal physiology precludes definitive repair, hence palliative mBT continues to be relevant in the modern era.

Despite being performed without cardiopulmonary bypass and its palliative nature, it is recognized that the neonatal mBT shunt, unlike that

The authors have no financial disclosures to make in relation to the subject matter of this article.

Department of Paediatric Cardiology, Institut Jantung Negara (National Heart Institute), 145, Jalan Tun Razak, Kuala Lumpur 50400, Malaysia

* Corresponding author.

E-mail address: mazeni@ijn.com.my

interventional.theclinics.com

performed in older children carries a significant risk of morbidity and mortality. Extensive data from the Society of Thoracic Surgery database over an 8-year period reported a mortality of 7.2%. Pulmonary atresia intact ventricular septum (PAIVS) was an independent risk factor for death, with a mortality of 15.6%.[3] Weight less than 2.5 kg was another independent risk factor for increased mortality.

Maintaining ductal patency for the longer term seems the logical, more physiologic alternative to a surgical shunt. Santoro and colleagues[4] have demonstrated that stenting the patent ductus arteriosus (PDA) is as effective as the mBT shunt in promoting a global pulmonary artery growth and, in addition, ensures an even distribution of pulmonary blood flow. However, keeping the ductus arteriosus reliably patent until the time of definitive repair, generally at 6 to 12 months of age for conduit surgery or first-stage cavopulmonary anastomosis, has remained a challenge until recently. Advances in coronary intervention in adult cardiology have led to the availability of stents that are highly flexible, have excellent radial strength and low thrombogenicity, with sizes, lengths, guide wires, and catheters that are well suited for stenting the neonatal PDA.[5–8] However, despite its technical feasibility in general, PDA stenting cannot be universally recommended because in a significant proportion of cyanotic congenital heart disease (CHD), this may have a negative impact on the branch pulmonary arteries and may undermine long-term survival.

ANATOMY: PDA IN CYANOTIC CHD

When the PDA occurs as an isolated lesion it is usually a short conical-shaped structure that arises from the proximal descending aorta, running anterosuperiorly and slightly leftward to insert onto the dome of the main pulmonary artery (MPA), slightly towards the origin of the left pulmonary artery (LPA). The pulmonary end of the PDA is the narrowest part, and the aortic end forms the ampulla. In the setting of cyanotic CHD, PDA morphology is remarkably diverse, ranging from one that resembles PDA as an isolated lesion to the bizarre.[9,10] It is crucial that a detailed assessment of the PDA and related anatomy is performed. Apart from case selection, the PDA morphology and its relationship to the aorta and pulmonary artery affects the feasibility and technical aspects of the procedure.

Origin in the Aorta

The PDA in conditions such as PAIVS, tricuspid atresia, Ebstein anomaly, and simple transposition of the great artery (TGA) commonly arises from the proximal descending aorta, resembling an isolated lesion. In the majority of patients, however, the PDA arises more proximally from the underside of the arch opposite the origin of the left subclavian artery or left common carotid artery (in the setting of a left aortic arch and vice versa). The PDA runs inferiorly toward the pulmonary artery, giving it a vertical orientation, often with a curve as it inserts onto the pulmonary artery. In tetralogy of Fallot with pulmonary atresia (TOF-PA) its origin may be even more proximal, opposite the brachiocephalic trunk.[11] In a small number of patients, generally not seen outside TOF-PA, the PDA arises from the left subclavian artery as a long tubular structure resembling a surgically constructed shunt on angiography (**Fig. 1D**).

Pulmonary End of PDA: Site of Insertion

In CHD with left aortic arch, the PDA tends to insert onto the pulmonary end at the origin of the LPA or even more distally, although in some lesions there is a tendency for insertion onto the dome of the MPA as in isolated PDA. In those that insert onto the LPA, appearance of LPA stenosis may be readily seen even at presentation in the newborn period. The phenomenon of "pulmonary coarctation" in cyanotic CHD is well recognized.[12–14] In this clinical setting, ductal tissue smooth muscle has a tendency to extend into the walls of the LPA, and causes stenosis as the ductus constricts. In lesions where the MPA is absent or severely attenuated, the PDA may cause bilateral branch pulmonary artery (PA) stenosis (**Fig. 2**). TOF-PA, transposition of great artery–ventricular septal defect–pulmonary atresia (TGA-VSD-PA), congenitally corrected TGA-VSD-PA (ccTGA-VSD-PA), and complex single ventricle with heterotaxy have a propensity for this. On the other hand, PDA in PAIVS, tricuspid atresia, Ebstein anomaly, and simple TGA tends to insert normally onto the MPA, leading to a lesser propensity for LPA stenosis (**Box 1**).

Disconnected Pulmonary Arteries

The branch pulmonary arteries may uncommonly be disconnected in conditions such as TOF, TGA-VSD-PS, and ccTGA-VSD-PS, whereby the PDA supplies the LPA (when the aortic arch is left sided), whereas flow to the right PA is from the morphologic right or pulmonary ventricle. In this setting, constriction of ductal tissues around the LPA may cause luminal discontinuity, although occasionally there may be anatomic disconnection. It is important to recognize this early before ductal closure occurs to salvage the LPA, failing which the left lung will

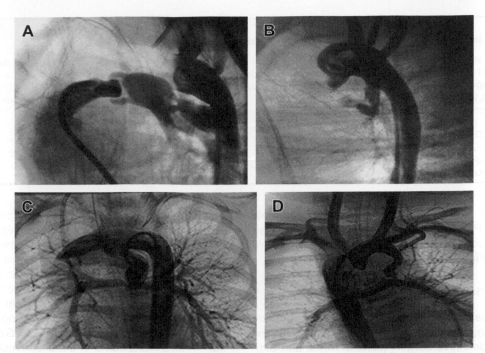

Fig. 1. Various origins of patent ductus arteriosus (PDA) arising from the aorta. (*A*) PDA arising from the proximal descending aorta in a patient with pulmonary atresia with intact ventricular septum (PAIVS). It has the configuration of an isolated PDA (ie, relatively short and straight with a conical shape). (*B*) More proximal origin of PDA, opposite the origin of the left subclavian artery in another patient with PAIVS. (*C*) Very proximal origin of PDA, opposite the origin of the brachiocephalic trunk in a patient with tetralogy of Fallot with pulmonary atresia (TOF-PA), left aortic arch. There is also bilateral branch pulmonary artery stenosis in this patient, whose main pulmonary artery (MPA) is absent. (*D*) PDA originating from the left subclavian artery/brachiocephalic trunk in a patient with TOF-PA, right aortic arch.

not be perfused ("absent" LPA). Far less commonly, anatomic discontinuity (adventitial and luminal) of the pulmonary arteries are seen, particularly in TOF-PA whereby bilateral PDAs supply the respective disconnected branch (**Fig. 3**).[15,16]

Shape of the PDA

The PDA in cyanotic CHD tends to be an elongated, tubular structure, with some having more than 1 curve. There is remarkable variation in the

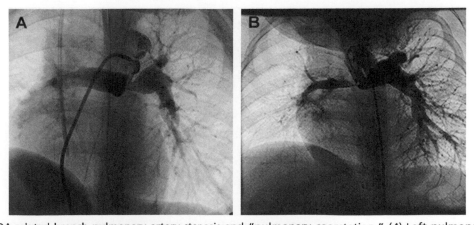

Fig. 2. PDA-related branch pulmonary artery stenosis and "pulmonary coarctation." (*A*) Left pulmonary artery (LPA) stenosis in a patient with TOF-PA. (*B*) Very severe, bilateral branch pulmonary artery stenoses in another patient with TOF-PA. The MPA is absent. (*From* Alwi M, Choo KK, Latiff HA, et al. Initial results and medium-term follow up of stent implantation of patent ductus arteriosus in duct-dependent pulmonary circulation. J Am Coll Cardiol 2004;44:438–45; with permission.)

shape of these PDAs, from those that resemble isolated PDA to one that is bizarre, characterized by marked tortuosity with acute bends in multiple planes (**Fig. 4**).

INDICATIONS FOR PDA STENTING

The most common indication is to provide a bridging palliation in cyanotic CHD until the time of definitive surgery (conduit repair and bidirectional Glenn shunt) whereby the PDA becomes the sole source of pulmonary blood flow. The second indication is in PAIVS (and occasional cases of critical PS) whereby the patient may remain hypoxic even following successful abolition of right ventricular (RV) outflow obstruction, often due to significant RV hypoplasia. PDA stenting in this setting provides additional pulmonary blood flow. It is well recognized in PAIVS that following successful interventions to the RV outflow tract (RVOT) there may be a need for unplanned mBT shunt or PDA stenting within days of the procedure.[17–19] The authors have adopted the approach of electively stenting the PDA at the time of RVOT intervention in selected patients, to help stabilize patients after the procedure and avoid unplanned additional procedures (**Fig. 5**).[19] The American Heart Association Scientific Statement categorized the first indication (as temporary bridging palliation) as class IIb, and an additional source of pulmonary blood flow following RV outflow intervention in PAIVS as class IIa.[20] A third indication is in the uncommon situation of Ebstein anomaly with severe tricuspid regurgitation leading to the phenomenon of functional pulmonary atresia during the transitional postnatal physiology. PDA stenting avoids the need for prolonged prostaglandin E_1 (PGE_1) infusion and hospital stay, as these patients tend to become unstable following mBT shunt. With establishment of forward flow from the right ventricle, the PDA stent tends to become self-limiting. The fourth indication, rarely encountered in the Western world, is neonates with simple TGA whose left ventricle has involuted. PDA stenting is alternative to preparing the left ventricle for

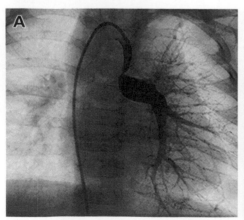
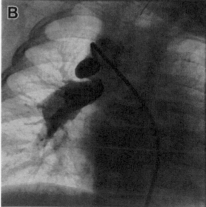

Fig. 3. Disconnected pulmonary arteries and bilateral PDA in a patient with TOF-PA. (*A*) Left PDA supplying the left pulmonary artery (LPA). There is severe constriction at the site of PDA insertion. (*B*) Right PDA supplying the right pulmonary artery, with a less severe constriction at the site of insertion. Both PDAs were stented. (*From* Alwi M. Stenting of ductus arteriosus: case selection, technique and possible complications. Ann Pediatr Cardiol 2008;1(1):38–45; with permission.)

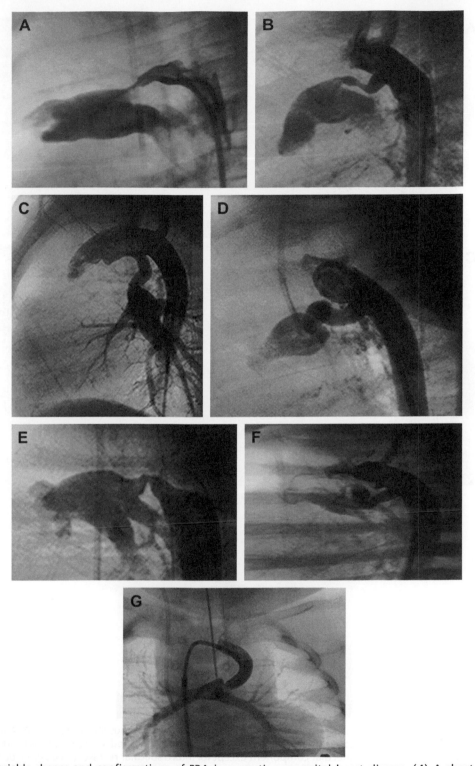

Fig. 4. Variable shapes and configurations of PDA in cyanotic congenital heart disease. (*A*) A short, straight conical PDA that resembles isolated PDA in a patient with tricuspid atresia. (*B–D*) PDAs in cyanotic heart disease tend to be elongated with 1 or more curves. (*E*) Constriction in the mid-segment of PDA instead of at the distal end. (*F*) PDA with bizarre configuration: long and tortuous with very severe constriction at its pulmonary end. (*G*) PDA arising from the left subclavian artery, resembling a surgically constructed Blalock-Taussig shunt. (*A, B, F From* Alwi M. Stenting of ductus arteriosus: case selection, technique and possible complications. Ann Pediatr Card 2008;1(1):38–45.)

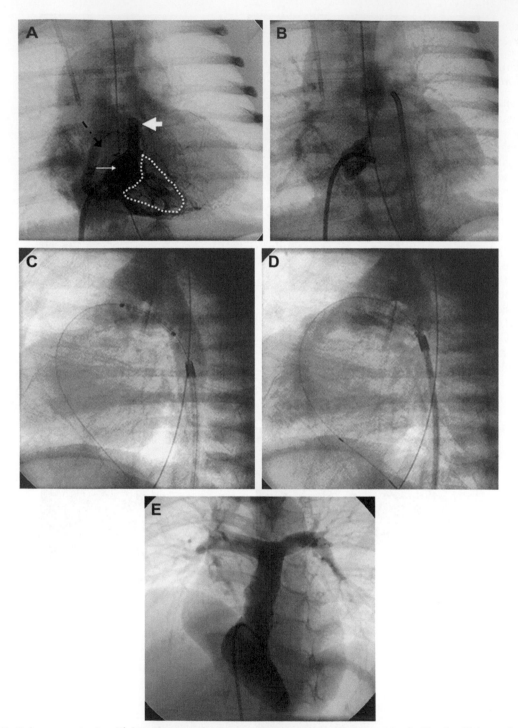

Fig. 5. Pulmonary atresia with intact ventricular septum (PAIVS) with membranous atresia. Elective PDA stenting at the time of radiofrequency valvotomy and balloon dilatation. (*A*) Well-developed inlet (*thin arrow*) and infundibulum (*thick arrow*), but absent trabecular component except for intertrabecular recesses (*area within dotted line*). A large right ventricle to right coronary connection with no stenosis is seen (*broken arrow*). (*B*) Right ventricular (RV) angiogram following pulmonary valvotomy. Transient reactive spasm reduces cavity of RV inlet and infundibulum. (*C, D*) Stent implantation via the femoral artery route. (*E*) 4 years after the procedure. There is excellent overall growth of the right ventricle, especially the trabecular component. The PDA stent has closed and is hardly visible. (*From* Alwi M, Choo KK, Radzi NA, et al. Concomitant stenting of the patent ductus arteriosus and radiofrequency valvotomy in pulmonary atresia with intact ventricular septum and intermediate right ventricle: early in-hospital and medium-term outcomes. J Thorac Cardiovasc Surg 2011;141:1355–61; with permission.)

anatomic repair by PA banding and mBT shunt (**Box 2**).[21]

Patient Selection: Which Patients Should be Excluded?

Branch PA stenosis (usually the left), as already discussed, poses an additional challenge at the time of repair of complex congenital cardiac lesions, and often leaves significant residual stenosis which requires reinterventions and may undermine late survival. Hence it is important to delineate this at the time of presentation. Because of its pathogenesis (infiltration of ductal smooth muscles into the walls of branch PA that later constrict and cause fibrosis), PDA stenting is likely to accelerate and worsen this particular problem. In the authors' view its presence is a contraindication to PDA stenting, especially in patients destined for single-ventricle repair. A metallic stent embedded in dense fibrotic tissues would pose difficulty during surgical reconstruction. Vida and colleagues[22] reported that operations after PDA stenting are safe. However, the presence of PDA stents requires additional surgical maneuvers on the pulmonary arteries in nearly half of the patients, and above all on the LPA. Furthermore, repeated postoperative interventions are still required on the PA branches. Thus conditions such as TOF-PA, TGA-VSD-PA, ccTGA-VSD-PA, and single

ventricle in the setting of heterotaxy are generally not suitable unless LPA stenosis has been firmly excluded. Suitability for PDA stenting is more favorable in PAIVS, tricuspid atresia, Ebstein anomaly, and simple TGA with involuted left ventricle. It is generally possible to detect this and exclude patients by echocardiography. Detailed angiographic evaluation will further exclude patients in whom this was not detected at the initial noninvasive assessment.

As the stent relies on the constricting ductal tissue to keep it in position, another exclusion factor is when the PDA is insufficiently constricted. There is a risk of stent migration if the pulmonary end of the PDA is larger than 2.0 mm (for a 4.0-mm stent). This can be gauged by the presence of a loud murmur coupled with mild cyanosis, and confirmed by 2-dimensional echo, although occasionally this can only be decided on subsequent angiography. For this reason the authors practice stopping PGE$_1$ infusion 6 hours before the procedure (see later discussion). It is also unlikely to be technically feasible to stent an overly tortuous, long PDA, another factor for exclusion.

Finally, if the femoral artery route is used, patients weighing less than 2.5 kg should be excluded because of the risk of damage to the vessel by the 4F-long sheath. For the femoral venous route the weight limit is also 2.5 kg, as the branch pulmonary arteries would be too small relative to the desired stent size for patients below this weight. The authors' practice is to maintain patients on PGE$_1$ infusion until the minimum weight is attained (**Box 3**).

Preprocedure Planning

Detailed echocardiography should be performed before the procedure to evaluate the intracardiac anatomy, and with particular emphasis on the pulmonary arteries, the PDA, and the aortic arch, as discussed in the preceding section on anatomy. Although angiographic details will be required, the initial echocardiographic data provide an idea on how the procedure is to be approached, the likely complexity of the procedure, and whether PDA stenting should be delayed on account of insufficient ductal constriction, or excluded because of the presence of obvious branch pulmonary stenosis (PS). Where PDA stenting is contemplated as an adjunct to RV outflow intervention in PAIVS or critical PS with a seemingly small right ventricle, echocardiographic evaluation of the RV size is essential.

As mentioned earlier, unless this is poorly tolerated, PGE$_1$ infusion should be stopped 6 hours before the procedure. The authors strongly

---

Box 2
Indications for PDA stenting

- To maintain the PDA as the sole source of pulmonary blood flow in cyanotic heart disease until the time of definitive surgery: conduit repair in TOF-PA and lesions with similar physiology, and bidirectional Glenn shunt in hearts with single-ventricle physiology.

- To augment the pulmonary blood flow in PAIVS and critical PS with moderate RV hypoplasia following interventions to abolish RVOT obstruction. Elective PDA stenting at the time of valvotomy in selected patients avoids the need for unplanned PDA stenting or mBT shunt following RVOT interventions.

- Severe Ebstein anomaly with functional pulmonary atresia: avoids prolonged PGE$_1$ infusion during the transitional postnatal physiology.

- Simple TGA with involuted left ventricle to prepare the left ventricle for the arterial switch operation as alternative to PA banding and mBT shunt.

recommend that all procedures should be done under general anesthesia and that the patient be returned to the intensive care unit (ICU) for immediate postprocedure management.

In view of the uncommon but very serious problem of acute in-stent thrombosis, there may be merit in commencing low-dose aspirin, 5 mg/kg, at least 1 day before the procedure as

an extrapolation of adult cardiology practice in coronary intervention. However, this is open to debate because theoretically aspirin may promote ductal closure, particularly in preterm infants.[23,24]

Vascular Access and Hemodynamic Monitoring

The femoral vein is cannulated with a 5F sheath if this is likely to be required for stent delivery, as in TOF-PA with proximal origin of PDA, or if a prior RVOT intervention is to be performed in PAIVS and critical PS. Otherwise, internal jugular access is obtained for drugs and fluids.

The femoral artery is cannulated with a 4F sheath for angiography and stent delivery. In addition, either of the axillary arteries may be cannulated if this route is likely to be required for stent delivery. Another arterial access should be obtained for postprocedure hemodynamic monitoring.

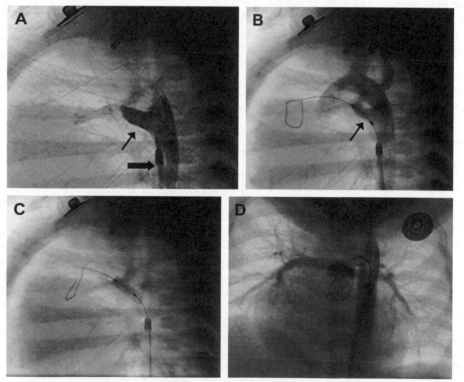

Fig. 6. Patent ductus arteriosus stenting via the femoral artery route in a severely hypoxic newborn with Ebstein anomaly, severe tricuspid regurgitation, and "functional" pulmonary atresia. A step-by-step description of the procedure is also available in video form (Videos 1–4). (*A*) Lateral aortic angiogram showing a short straight PDA arising from the proximal descending aorta. Very severe constriction at the pulmonary end. Large arrow indicates tip of a 4F long sheath. The tip of a 4F Judkins Right (JR) catheter is in the PDA ampulla (*small arrow*). (*B*) Tip of a Choice PT Extra Support guide wire looped in the MPA. Balloon and stent are positioned along the length of the PDA (*arrow*). (*C*) Expansion of balloon and stent. (*D*) Aortic angiogram after stent expansion in left anterior oblique (LAO)-cranial projection well opacifies the pulmonary arteries. The pulmonary end of the stent is at the dome of the MPA, away from the LPA.

Aortic angiography is then performed to evaluate the PDA, the pulmonary arteries, and the aortic arch. The emphasis is on the morphology, size and length, origin from the aorta and insertion onto the PA, and the presence or otherwise of PDA-related branch PA stenosis. The authors start with the anteroposterior and lateral projections, and for examination of the pulmonary bifurcation the left anterior oblique (LAO)-cranial projection (in levocardia patients) is usually valuable. Other projections may be required to obtain a good evaluation of the PDA and anatomy of the PA.

PROCEDURE

Once baseline angiography has established that the PDA is sufficiently constricted (usually at the pulmonary end), that it is not extremely tortuous, and that there is no PDA-related branch PA stenosis, PDA stenting may be approached by the femoral artery, the femoral vein, or the axillary route, depending on the aortic origin of the PDA and the intracardiac anatomy.

Femoral Artery Route

As this is the most commonly used route, a full description of the entire procedure including choice of stent size and length is given in this subsection. For the following subsections, only the relevant discussion on delivery route is given. **Fig. 6** provides a step-by-step description of this technique. Videos 1–4 (available at http://www.interventional.theclinics.com/) show the same procedure.

- This approach is used when the PDA originates from the proximal descending aorta resembling an isolated PDA, or those that arise slightly more proximally, opposite the left subclavian artery or toward the left common carotid artery. This is more commonly seen in tricuspid atresia (TA), PAIVS, Ebstein anomaly, and simple TGA, and much less so in TOF-PA and related lesions.
- Following angiography the femoral artery sheath is replaced with a 4F long sheath (Cook Inc, Bloomington, IN, USA) with its tip near the PDA ampulla.
- For a PDA with near normal aortic origin or opposite the left subclavian artery, a 4F Judkins Right (JR) catheter is engaged in the PDA ampulla. A 0.014-inch (0.356 mm) diameter coronary guide wire is gently steered across the PDA and anchored in a distal PA

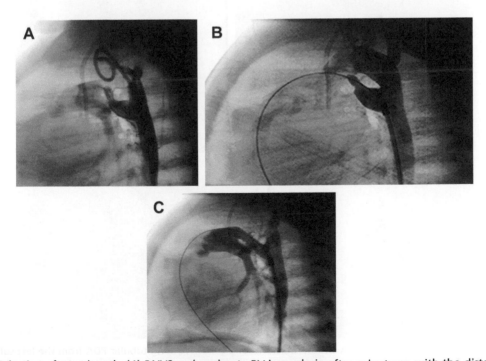

Fig. 7. Selection of stent length. (A) PAIVS and moderate RV hypoplasia after valvotomy, with the distal half of the PDA nearly at right angle to the ampulla. (B) With the guide wire across, the PDA becomes straighter and slightly shorter. The stent length chosen is based on PDA length measured with this maneuver. (C) The stented PDA has become completely straight.

branch (a Tuohy-Borst Y-connector is needed to prevent back-bleeding as the catheter lumen is 0.035 inches [0.889 mm] in diameter). A guide wire of moderate stiffness such as the Choice PT Extra Support (Boston Scientific, Miami, FL, USA), which has a tip-load of 3 g, generally provides adequate support for delivery of the balloon-stent assembly, especially during passage across a constricted PDA. Occasionally when the PDA is severely constricted or tortuous, a softer wire such as the BMW (Abbott Vascular, Santa Clara, CA, USA) may be used for ease of steering across the PDA.

- Once the body of the guide wire is across the PDA and its tip is securely anchored in a distal pulmonary branch, the JR catheter is removed and the angiogram is repeated with contrast injection via the side port of the long sheath. The guide wire tends to straighten the PDA, and choice of stent

length is based on measurement after placement of the guide wire (**Fig. 7**).

Choice of stent size and length

- As a general rule, a 4.0-mm diameter stent is selected for a body weight of 3.0 to 3.5 kg, and 4.5-mm diameter for infants weighing more than 3.5 kg. The stent length is selected according to the measurement with the guide wire across the PDA (current coronary stents do not shorten significantly with full expansion). The entire length of the PDA should be stented as much as possible to prevent accelerated closure of the unstented part. It is preferable to use only one stent, although occasionally errors in measurement require a second stent to be implanted. The exception is for the PDA that arises from the subclavian artery, which tends to be longer, as a single long stent

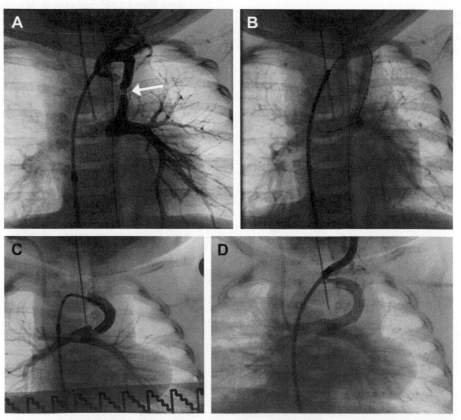

Fig. 8. The entire length of the PDA should be stented. (*A*) TOF-PA, long tubular PDA from the left subclavian artery (LSA). Two months after the procedure, there is severe stenosis at the junction of the stented and unstented part of the PDA (*arrow*). (*B*) Second stent implanted to cover unstented part. (*C*) Another TOF-PA patient with a long, curving PDA from the LSA. Three stents cover the entire PDA and maintain its configuration. A single long stent may distort the pulmonary arteries.

that straightens out the PDA may distort the pulmonary arteries (**Fig. 8**).

Balloon-stent assembly

- To prevent slippage of stent off the balloon by the rubber valve of the long sheath during insertion, a short piece of a 4F regular sheath is cut off and used as stent protector. The balloon-stent assembly is pushed gently over the guide wire, usually without much difficulty even across a severely constricted PDA, owing to its very low profile. Repeat angiograms via the side port of the long sheath are performed to ensure precise positioning of the stent. It is critical that the constricted part of the PDA is stented, without too much protrusion into the MPA or aorta. Once correct stent position is obtained, the stent is expanded according to the pressure required. Once the balloon is deflated and removed, an angiogram is repeated to assess the stent position and to determine whether additional stents are

required if the length selected is inadequate. At the end of the procedure, the authors recommend keeping the wire across the stented PDA for 10 to 15 minutes. In the rare event of acute stent thrombosis (see later discussion on complications), this measure allows a quick passage of balloon for dilations to mechanically break up the thrombus. A rapid, major drop in oxygen saturation after a remarkable increase following stent expansion is an ominous sign for this complication.

- For PDA with a more proximal origin (ie, opposite the left subclavian or left common carotid artery), the tip of the JR catheter may not be able to engage well the PDA ampulla for passage of the guide wire. A cut pigtail that leaves a U-shaped tip is more suited for this type of PDA. It may be very difficult to steer the Choice PT Extra Support guide wire beyond its floppy tip in this situation, particularly if the PDA is severely constricted and has a distal curve. A useful technique is to gently steer a soft

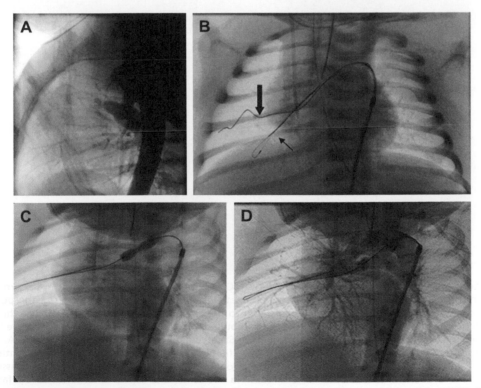

Fig. 9. Buddy-wire technique. (*A*) PDA arising proximally opposite the LSA in a patient with PAIVS. The acute angle between the PDA and descending aorta did not permit passage of the Choice PT Extra Support guide wire from the femoral artery route. (*B*) Passage of BMW wire (*thick arrow*) reduced the acute angle, allowing passage of Choice PT wire (*thin arrow*) across the PDA to be anchored in a distal branch. The BMW wire was then removed. (*C*) Balloon and stent tracked over the wire and positioned across the PDA, and inflated. (*D*) Fully expanded stent. The pulmonary arteries are well opacified, with no stenosis of the LPA in the LAO-cranial view.

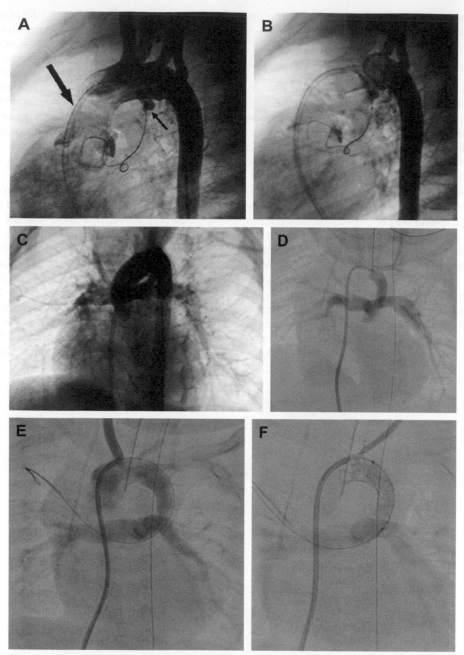

Fig. 10. Stent implantation by femoral-vein route in TOF-PA. (*A*) A short PDA arising from underneath the aortic arch opposite the origin of the brachiocephalic trunk. There is severe constriction at the pulmonary end (*thin arrow*). A 5F JR guide catheter was passed into the aortic arch from the femoral vein via the ventricular septal defect (VSD), with its tip facing the PDA ampulla. A Choice PT wire was steered across the PDA and was well anchored in a distal branch (*thick arrow*). (*B*) Stent and balloon positioned across the PDA. (*C*) Fully expanded stent. Both pulmonary arteries are well opacified in this LAO-cranial view. (*D*) Another patient with TOF-PA and left aortic arch with a long tubular PDA from the LSA. (*E*) A JR guide catheter was passed antegradely into the aortic arch from the femoral vein via the ventricular septal defect with its tip facing the PDA orifice. The guide wire was anchored in the right upper lobe branch. (*F*) Fully expanded stent.

guide wire such as the BMW wire well across the PDA. This wire tends to straighten the PDA and allows passage of the Choice PT Extra Support (buddy-wire technique, **Fig. 9**). The BMW wire is then removed and stent delivery may proceed as already described.

Femoral Vein Route

- If the PDA arises proximal to the left common carotid artery, as may commonly occur in TOF-PA and lesions with similar physiology, it is unlikely that a guide wire could be steered well across the PDA by the femoral artery route.
- The presence of a VSD allows balloon-stent delivery via the femoral vein with the use of 5F coronary guiding catheters (0.058-inch [1.47 mm] lumen), either with a JR shape or, if it is unable to engage the PDA ampulla, an XB (extra back up) guide catheter with its tip cut off to give an inverted-U shape. As the guide catheter is stiff, it is advisable to first maneuver a diagnostic 5F JR catheter into the ascending aorta and arch via the VSD, and replace this with the guide catheter over an exchange wire. A coronary guide wire can then be anchored in a distal PA branch for balloon and stent delivery (**Fig. 10**).
- The same technique and coronary guide catheter is well suited for the PDA originating from the left subclavian artery.
- A note of caution: complete heart block may occur with this technique, as the stiff coronary guide catheter presses against the atrioventricular node.
- The femoral vein route may also be used in PAIVS (and critical PS) once the pulmonary valve has been opened with balloon dilatation. However, the guide wire often requires to be introduced from the aortic end when the PDA is severely constricted, hence the need for snaring and exteriorizing the guide wire from the femoral vein to get the guide catheter across the PDA. Alternatively, the femoral artery route may used as described.

Axillary Artery Route

- This route may be used as alternative to the femoral vein route in TOF-PA or similar lesions whereby a PDA with very proximal origin precludes that of the femoral artery. Less commonly, in single-ventricle lesions with a PDA of proximal origin, this may be the only feasible route. This technique provides direct access to the PDA and does not require a long introducer sheath for balloon-stent delivery. In fact this technique was used in the first human experience of PDA stenting, but via a cut-down.[25] However, few cardiologists are familiar with axillary artery cut-down, and a follow-up study does raise concerns about the long-term effect on upper limb circulation.[26]
- Recently, Schranz and Michel-Behnke[27] have demonstrated percutaneous access of the axillary artery for neonatal interventions including PDA stenting as a feasible and reliable technique, obviating a cut-down.

Immediate Postprocedure Care and Follow-Up

Following the procedure, the patient is returned to the ICU for continued ventilation, hemodynamic monitoring, and supportive care for at least 24 hours. Patients who require minimal support are extubated the following day. Heparin infusion is continued at 10 to 20 units/kg/h for 72 hours while aspirin is commenced on return to the ICU. It is common for the oxygen saturation to be at least 90% following PDA stenting, but this

---

Box 4
Complications of patent ductus arteriosus (PDA) stenting

Acute, Procedure Related
- Spasm of PDA, sudden severe hypoxia with guide-wire or catheter manipulation
- Slippage of unexpanded stent
- Migration of expanded stent
- Transient complete heart block with the femoral vein route (stiff guide catheter pressing on the atrioventricular node at VSD rim)

Acute, Stent Related
- Acute in-stent thrombosis
- Overshunting and heart failure ± pulmonary edema in cases of a relatively large stent to a single lung
- Myocardial dysfunction in PAIVS with RV-coronary connections

Late Problems
- Accelerated branch PA stenosis in susceptible patients
- Pulmonary hypertension from chronic over-shunting

is expected to decrease and stabilize to 80% to 90% over a few days.[7] Some patients may exhibit overt signs of overshunting and may benefit from diuretics, usually for a few weeks. A rapid, major drop in oxygen saturation strongly suggests in-stent thrombosis, which can be readily confirmed by echocardiography and should be managed promptly (see later discussion). Patients with PAIVS and those with RV-coronary connections in particular may develop hemodynamic instability and may require longer supportive treatment.[19]

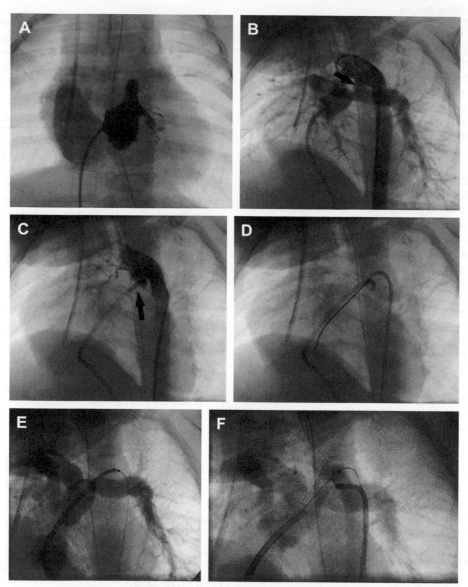

Fig. 11. PDA spasm in a patient with PAIVS soon after valvotomy and balloon dilatation. (*A*) Preliminary angiogram showing bipartite right ventricle with good inlet and infundibulum but no apical trabecular component. (*B*) Aortography in LAO-cranial projection showing good opacification of the pulmonary arteries via the PDA (*arrow*). A 5F JR catheter was placed beneath the valve plate ready for perforation. (*C*) Rapid, sudden hypoxia caused by PDA spasm. Arrow shows a 5F JR catheter in the main pulmonary artery with its tip at the PDA insertion. Aortography shows no opacification of the pulmonary arteries attributable to PDA spasm. (*D*) Prostaglandin infusion was recommenced and the BMW wire steered across the PDA from the aortic side. This wire was snared and exteriorized out of the femoral vein to allow placement of the 5F JR guide catheter for stent-balloon delivery. (*E*) Stent and balloon positioned across the PDA. (*F*) Fully expanded stent. Pulmonary arteries are well opacified in this LAO-cranial view.

Following discharge, the patient should be reviewed every 6 to 12 weeks until the time of definitive surgery. In the majority, this would be bidirectional Glenn anastomosis or conduit repair, whereas for PAIVS patients with borderline right ventricle, longer follow-up may be required before the next intervention is decided, or satisfactory RV growth with biventricular circulation has been attained and the PDA stent is deemed no longer necessary.[19]

Potential Complications and Management

Complications fall into 2 categories, those related to the procedure and those that result from having a stent in the PDA itself (**Box 4**).

As the procedure is performed in fragile hypoxic neonates, several serious complications may potentially occur. Passage of a guide wire across the PDA may induce spasm, resulting in sudden, severe hypoxemia (**Fig. 11**). However, this is a surprisingly uncommon occurrence. PGE_1 infusion should be on standby for readministration during the procedure, should this occur.

Slippage of stent off the balloon, and migration or embolization of expanded or unexpanded stent may occur, especially when the guide wire is not securely anchored in a distal pulmonary branch. This complication generally requires surgical removal, as percutaneous retrieval of a rigid metallic stent in a neonate is likely to be difficult and may cause major injury. Alternatively this may be pushed and expanded in a truly distal peripheral branch (**Fig. 12**). Bearing in mind that the coronary stent can only undergo limited redilatation, it should not be expanded in a major lobar artery.

In TOF-PA and similar conditions whereby access to the PDA is from the venous side and the through the VSD, the stiff coronary guiding catheter may press on the atrioventricular node and cause transient complete heart block. The procedure should be expedited to avoid permanent damage, and if this is not possible the axillary artery approach may be an alternative.

Once the PDA has been successfully stented a marked increase in oxygen saturation will be observed, often accompanied by a significant drop in aortic diastolic pressure. Frank heart failure from overshunting is rare, but a relatively large stent to a single lung may cause pulmonary edema. In PAIVS patients with significant RV-coronary connections, this may result in myocardial ischemia and left ventricular

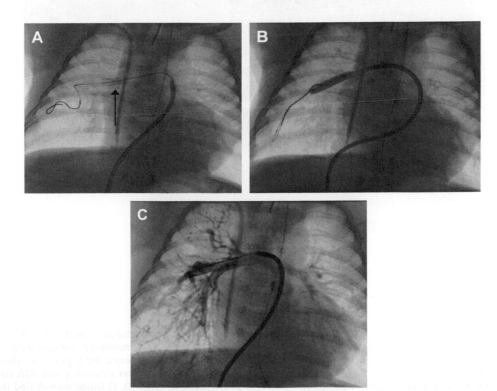

Fig. 12. Migration of expanded stent in a patient with PAIVS after valvotomy and balloon dilatation. (*A*) The expanded stent migrated to the right pulmonary artery and the guide wire was passed through the stent lumen (*arrow*). (*B, C*) With an inflated balloon the stent was pushed to a middle lobar branch and dilated further.

dysfunction, even though RV-dependent coronary circulation has been excluded at initial assessment. It is likely that the unusually high mortality and morbidity following mBT shunt in neonates with this disease is related to this.[3]

Acute in-stent thrombosis is by far the most serious complication of this procedure, although fortunately it is an uncommon occurrence. It manifests dramatically with a rapidly progressive hypoxemia, occurring during the procedure itself

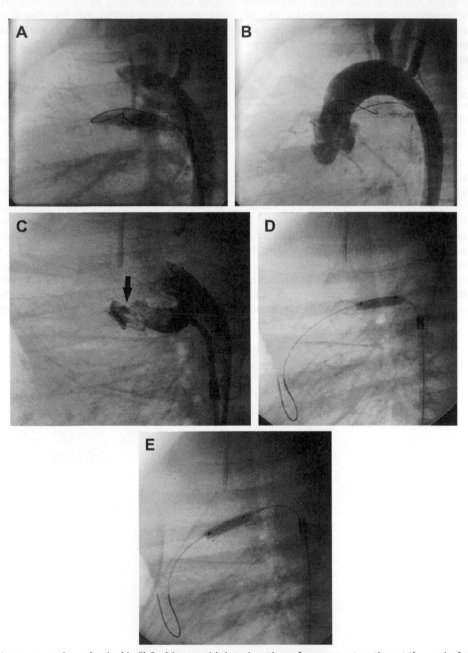

Fig. 13. Acute stent thrombosis. (*A, B*) Sudden, rapid deterioration of oxygen saturation at the end of the stenting procedure in a patient with PAIVS. The guide wire is still across the PDA. Thrombolytic therapy with streptokinase resulted in major bleeding. (*C*) Another patient with PAIVS and moderate RV hypoplasia. There was sudden deterioration of oxygen saturation in the intensive care unit 1 hour after valvotomy and PDA stenting. Angiogram shows thrombus within the pulmonary end of the stent (*arrow*). (*D, E*) Guide wire drilled through the thrombus and repeated balloon dilatations recanalized the stent. The heparin dose was increased, and no recurrence occurred. (*From* Alwi M. Stenting of ductus arteriosus: case selection, technique and possible complications. Ann Pediatr Cardiol 2008;1(1):38–45; with permission.)

or hours later. The authors instituted thrombolytic therapy in 2 cases, but this led to severe bleeding and death in 1 of the patients. One patient received emergent mBT shunt. In another patient, mechanically disrupting the thrombus by drilling a guide wire through followed by repeated balloon dilatations was effective (**Fig. 13**). The correct management of this uncommon problem is yet to be established, but this technique avoided the real risk of severe bleeding that may complicate pharmacologic thrombolysis. For this reason, the authors recommend leaving the guide wire across the expanded stent for 10 to 15 minutes at the end of the procedure.

Late Complications and Problems

A problem that significantly limits the role of PDA stenting is the propensity for accelerated and more severe branch PA stenosis in a significant number of patients, especially those with TOF-PA and related lesions, as discussed earlier. This complication will likely lead to the need for future rehabilitation of the affected PA by surgery, stent implantation, and redilatation (**Fig. 14**B and C). Hence, the importance of case selection with detailed angiographic evaluation cannot be overemphasized.

Mild heart failure from overshunting is not uncommon in the weeks following the procedure.

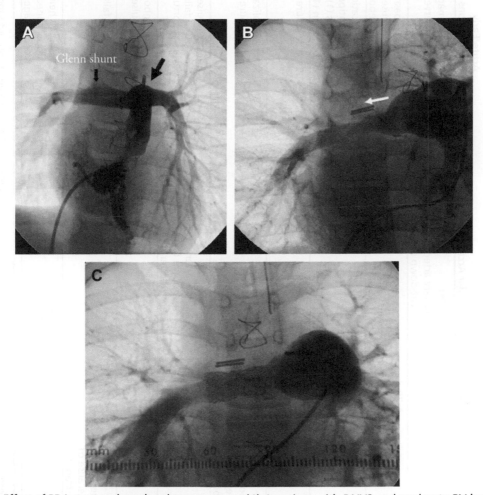

Fig. 14. Effect of PDA stent on branch pulmonary artery. (*A*) A patient with PAIVS and moderate RV hypoplasia, 2 years after valvotomy and PDA stenting. At 1½ ventricle repair (bidirectional Glenn shunt [*small arrow*], closure of atrial septal defect). The PDA stent was divided and clipped (*large arrow*). There was no LPA stenosis as the PDA inserted onto the dome of main pulmonary artery. (*B*) A patient with congenitally corrected transposition of great artery with ventricular septal defect and pulmonary atresia, right aortic arch, PDA insertion onto right pulmonary artery (RPA). The patient developed progressive RPA stenosis after PDA stenting. The PDA stent was divided and clipped at the time of conduit repair and RPA arterioplasty was performed. The stent remnant is hardly visible (*arrow*). (*C*) Stent implantation in RPA for persistent stenosis. (*B* and *C From* Alwi M. Stenting of ductus arteriosus: case selection, technique and possible complications. Ann Pediatr Cardiol 2008;1(1):38–45; with permission.)

Table 1
Experience of PDA stenting for duct-dependent pulmonary circulation from published studies

Trial Authors,[Ref.] Year	Total Patients (N) Total Stents (N)	Age	Vascular Access	CHD Pathology	Acute/Early Complications (n)	Late Problems (n)
Schneider et al,[5] 1998	21 32	13.3 d (median)	FA (8) Axillary artery cut-down (13)	Diverse	Arterial damage (2) Early reintervention (2)	Stent stenosis requiring redilatation (5) Occlusion of LSCA (1)
Gibbs et al,[29] 1999	19	4–78 d	—	Diverse (11) HLHS (8)	2 died of spasm Failed because of tortuosity (2) Stent thrombosis	
Michel-Behnke et al,[#] 2004	21	10.5 d (median)	—	Diverse	Stent dislocation/stent embolization (3) Thrombosis (1) FA occlusion (1)	Stent stenosis <6 mo (3) LPA stenosis (3)
Gewilling et al,[6] 2004	10 13	6 d (median)	FA (2) FV (8)	Mainly PAIVS Critical PS with short straight ducts	Cardiac failure (3)	Stent occlusion
Alwi et al,[7] 2004	56 (5 not done because of tortuosity)	2.3 mo (median)	FA (43) FV (8)	Diverse	Stent embolization (1) Cardiac failure (1)	Blocked stent <3 mo (1) Stent stenosis <6 mo (8) Worsening preexisting branch PA stenosis (7)
Santoro et a,[30] 2008	26	9 d (median)	FA (24) Axillary artery cut-down (1) Carotid arteriotomy (1)	Diverse	Transient pulse loss (1) Procedural failure due to tortuosity (2)	Stent thrombosis (1) Stent redilatation (4)
Alwi et al,[19] 2011	37	10 d (median)	FA FV	PAIVS with moderate RV hypoplasia LCOS (2)	Stent thrombosis (1) Transient pulse loss (5)	1 died after RVOT surgery
Hussain et al,[28] 2008	21 (5 not done because of tortuosity)	24 d (mean)	—	Diverse	Procedural failure (2)	Stent stenosis 2 died of PAH post Glenn surgery
Odemis et al,[31] 2012	13	10.5 d (median)	FA (12) FV(1)	Diverse	Pulmonary hemorrhage (1) Retroperitoneal hemorrhage (1)	Stent stenosis

Abbreviations: FA, femoral artery; FV, femoral vein; HLHS, hypoplastic left heart syndrome; LCOS, low cardiac output syndrome; LPA, left pulmonary artery; LSCA, left subclavian artery; PA, pulmonary artery; PAH, pulmonary arterial hypertension; PAIVS, pulmonary atresia with intact ventricular septum; PS, pulmonary stenosis; RV, right ventricular; RVOT, right ventricular outflow tract.

Occasionally this persists and causes elevated PA pressure, especially if the stented PDA is to a single lung. Hence, a stent of smaller diameter should be implanted when the PDA supplies a single lung. In patients destined for the single-ventricle pathway, the first stage of cavopulmonary anastomosis may have to be planned early if persistent overshunting raises concern for elevated pulmonary resistance.[28]

In general, a stented PDA affords a less durable palliation compared with the mBT shunt. Because definitive surgery is often planned at 6 to 12 months of age, or earlier if necessary, durability of palliation is generally not an issue.

CLINICAL RESULTS IN THE LITERATURE

Gibbs and colleagues[25] first reported on the human application of PDA stenting in 2 neonates with complex cyanotic heart disease. Although the procedures were successful, the technical difficulties and complications may have discouraged many. It was also the early era of stents in coronary interventions, and applying this to small neonates was truly challenging. Gibbs concluded later that PDA stenting in duct-dependent pulmonary blood flow carried a high risk and that the duration of palliation was poor.[29] Schneider and others later reported more favorable results in a more sizable series of patients with diverse CHD.[5–8,30,31] These results are summarized in **Table 1**.

The small number of published clinical studies and the relatively small number of patients in each demonstrate that PDA stenting has yet to gain wide acceptance as an alternative to the mBT shunt. Procedural failure is significant because of severe tortuosity in some of these PDAs. The acute or early complications were also significant, and these included stent migration and thrombosis, cardiac failure, spasm and vascular injury, and hemorrhage. At short-term to medium-term follow-up, early failure of palliation owing to stent stenosis requiring redilatation was also significant. In the current era of pediatric cardiac surgery, earlier definitive repair should be able to mitigate this problem to a large degree.

Early in their experience, the authors overlooked the problem of accelerated branch PA stenosis in susceptible patients.[7]

Given the generally limited durability of palliation, the development of pulmonary hypertension that led to death in 2 patients after bidirectional Glenn shunt is surprising.[28] No details are available, but this result flags for caution in not oversizing the stent in patients destined for the single-ventricle pathway.

Overall, the results appear to compare less favorably with the surgical shunt but, from the authors' experience, in well-selected patients and in certain clinical settings such as PAIVS with questionable RV size, PDA stenting has its merits. This procedure merits further evaluation through well-conducted collaborative studies.

SUMMARY

Maintaining ductal patency is an attractive, less invasive alternative to surgical aortopulmonary shunt. Applying coronary stent technology and modifying its techniques for the PDA has made this objective feasible. However, PDA in cyanotic heart disease has a remarkably diverse morphology that encompasses its shape, origin in the aorta, and site of pulmonary insertion. In a significant proportion, these features limit the technical feasibility of PDA stenting or make it an unsuitable alternative to surgical shunt. The main indications for PDA stenting are to provide bridging palliation in cyanotic heart disease whereby the PDA is the sole source of pulmonary blood flow until the time of definitive repair, and to provide additional source of pulmonary blood flow after RVOT interventions in PAIVS and critical PS with moderate RV hypoplasia. Less common indications are to provide palliation in severe Ebstein anomaly during the transitional postnatal physiology, and in simple TGA with involuted left ventricle, to prepare the left ventricle for anatomic repair. The aortic origin of the PDA and the intracardiac anatomy dictate the approach for the procedure, chiefly the femoral artery route, femoral venous route, or axillary artery route. Major complications are those related to the procedure such as PDA spasm, transient complete heart block, stent migration, or those related to the stent, which include acute stent thrombosis, pulmonary hypertension, and accelerated branch PA stenosis.

A review of the literature indicates that PDA stenting has not gained wide acceptance among pediatric cardiologists worldwide. Published studies involve relatively small numbers of patients. Although most demonstrated feasibility and safety of the procedure, more studies are required to evaluate its advantages, limitations, and potential complications, and to define its role in the management of cyanotic CHD. The durability of palliation from PDA stenting tends to be inferior to surgical shunt, but this is not a major issue given the current practice of definitive repairs in the first year of life.

SUPPLEMENTARY DATA

Supplementary data related to this article can be found online at http://dx.doi.org/10.1016/j.iccl. 2012.09.011.

REFERENCES

1. Di Donato RM, Jonas RA, Lang P, et al. Neonatal repair of tetralogy of Fallot with and without pulmonary atresia. J Thorac Cardiovasc Surg 1991;101: 126–37.

2. Reddy VM, Liddicoat JR, McElhinney DB, et al. Routine primary repair of tetralogy of Fallot in neonates and infants less than three months of age. Ann Thorac Surg 1995;60:S592–6.

3. Petrucci O, O'Brien SM, Jacobs ML, et al. Risk factors for mortality and morbidity after the neonatal Blalock-Taussig shunt procedure. Ann Thorac Surg 2011;92(2):642–52.

4. Santoro G, Capozzi G, Caianiello G, et al. Pulmonary artery growth after palliation of congenital heart disease with duct-dependent pulmonary circulation: arterial duct stenting versus surgical shunt. J Am Coll Cardiol 2009;54(23):2180–6.

5. Schneider M, Zartner P, Sidiropoulos A, et al. Stent implantation of the arterial duct in newborns with duct-dependent circulation. Eur Heart J 1998;19: 1401–9.

6. Gewillig M, Boshoff DE, Dens J, et al. Stenting the neonatal arterial duct in duct-dependent pulmonary circulation: new techniques, better results. J Am Coll Cardiol 2004;43:107–12.

7. Alwi M, Choo KK, Latiff HA, et al. Initial results and medium-term follow up of stent implantation of patent ductus arteriosus in duct-dependent pulmonary circulation. J Am Coll Cardiol 2004;44: 438–45.

8. Michel-Behnke I, Akintuerk H, Thul J, et al. Stent implantation in the ductus arteriosus for pulmonary blood supply in congenital heart disease. Catheter Cardiovasc Interv 2004;61:242–52.

9. Alwi M. Stenting the patent ductus arteriosus in duct-dependent pulmonary circulation: techniques, complications and follow-up issues. Future Cardiol 2012;8(2):237–50.

10. Alwi M. Stenting of ductus arteriosus: case selection, technique and possible complications. Ann Pediatr Card 2008;1(1):38–45.

11. Abrams SE, Walsh KP. Arterial duct morphology with reference to angioplasty and stenting. Int J Cardiol 1993;40:27–33.

12. Elzenga NJ, Gittenberger-de Groot AC. The ductus arteriosus and stenoses of the pulmonary arteries in pulmonary atresia. Int J Cardiol 1986; 11:195–208.

13. Elzenga NJ, von Suylen RJ, Frohn-Mulder I, et al. Juxtaductal pulmonary artery coarctation. An under-estimated cause of branch pulmonary artery stenosis in patients with pulmonary atresia or stenosis and a ventricular septal defect. J Thorac Cardiovasc Surg 1990;100:416–24.

14. Moon-Grady AJ, Teitel DF, Haley FL, et al. Ductus-associated proximal pulmonary artery stenosis in patients with right heart obstruction. Int J Cardiol 2007;114:41–5.

15. Barbero-Marcial M, Atik E, Baucia JA, et al. Reconstruction of stenotic or nonconfluent pulmonary arteries simultaneously with a Blalock Taussig shunt. J Thorac Cardiovasc Surg 1988;95:82–9.

16. Murphy DN, Winlaw DS, Cooper SG, et al. Successful early surgical recruitment of the congenitally disconnected pulmonary artery. Ann Thorac Surg 2004;77:29–35.

17. Agnoletti G, Piechaud JF, Bonhoeffer P, et al. Perforation of the atretic pulmonary valve: long-term follow up. J Am Coll Cardiol 2003;41:1399–403.

18. Humpl T, Söderberg B, McCrindle BW, et al. Percutaneous balloon valvotomy in pulmonary atresia with intact ventricular septum: impact on patient care. Circulation 2003;108:826–32.

19. Alwi M, Choo KK, Radzi NA, et al. Concomitant stenting of the patent ductus arteriosus and radiofrequency valvotomy in pulmonary atresia with intact ventricular septum and intermediate right ventricle: early in-hospital and medium-term outcomes. J Thorac Cardiovasc Surg 2011;141:1355–61.

20. Feltes TF, Bach E, Beekman RH, et al. Indications for cardiac catheterization and intervention in pediatric cardiac disease: a scientific statement from the American Heart Association. Circulation 2011;123: 2607–52.

21. Sivakumar K, Francis E, Krishnan P, et al. Ductal stenting retrains the left ventricle in transposition of great arteries with intact ventricular septum. J Thorac Cardiovasc Surg 2006;132(5):1081–6.

22. Vida VL, Speggiorin S, Maschietto N, et al. Cardiac operations after patent ductus arteriosus stenting in duct-dependent pulmonary circulation. Ann Thorac Surg 2010;90(2):605–9.

23. Narayanan-Sankar M, Clyman RI. Pharmacology review: pharmacologic closure of patent ductus arteriosus in the neonate. Neoreviews 2003;4: e215–21.

24. Momma K, Hagiwara H, Konishi T. Constriction of fetal ductus arteriosus by non-steroidal anti-inflammatory drugs: study of additional 34 drugs. Prostaglandins 1994;28(4):527–36.

25. Gibbs JL, Rothmann MT, Rees MR, et al. Stenting of the arterial duct: a new approach to palliation for pulmonary atresia. Br Heart J 1992;67:240–5.

26. Viswanathan S, Arthur R, Evans JA, et al. The early and mid-term fate of the axillary artery following

axillary artery cut-down and cardiac catheterization in infants and young children. Catheter Cardiovasc Interv 2012. [Epub ahead of print].

27. Schranz D, Michel-Behnke I. Axillary artery access for cardiac interventions in newborns. Ann Pediatr Card 2008;1(2):126–30.

28. Hussain A, Al-Zharani S, Muhammed AA, et al. Midterm outcome of stent dilatation of patent ductus arteriosus in ductal-dependent pulmonary circulation. Congenit Heart Dis 2008;3(4):241–9.

29. Gibbs JL, Uzun O, Blackburn ME, et al. Fate of the stented arterial duct. Circulation 1999;99:2621–5.

30. Santoro G, Giao G, Palladino MT, et al. Stenting of the arterial duct in newborns with duct-dependent pulmonary circulation. Heart 2008;94:925–9.

31. Odemis E, Haydin S, Guzeltas A, et al. Stent implantation in the arterial duct of the newborn with duct-dependent pulmonary circulation: single centre experience from Turkey. Eur J Cardiothorac Surg 2012;42(1):57–60.

Stenting Options for Coarctation of the Aorta

Elchanan Bruckheimer, MBBS[a],*,
Carlos Augusto Cardoso Pedra, MD, PhD[b,c]

KEYWORDS

- Coarctation • Angioplasty • Stent • Covered stent

KEY POINTS

- Surgery is the preferred intervention in neonatal period and infancy.
- Recoarctation or aneurysm formation may be encountered during follow up. Complications include paradoxical hypertension, pleural effusion and spinal cord damage [in older patients].
- Balloon dilation for coarctation was the initial technique for transcatheter intervention. The use is controversial due to relatively high incidence of recoarctation and aneurysm formation. Complications include aneurysm formation, dissection and aortic rupture.
- Bare metal stent implantation for coarctation may result in less aortic wall injury than balloon angioplasty alone. Use is relatively safe and highly effective. Complications include aneurysm formation, stent malposition, stent fracture and vascular access injury.
- Covered stent implantation has a decreased incidence of aortic wall injury.
- Use is relatively safe and highly effective. It is the treatment of choice with coexistence of PDA or aneurysm, circumferential fracture of previously implanted stent, atretic/sub-atretic coarctation and older patients. Complications include stent malposition and potential side branch closure, vascular access injury.
- Technical considerations for stent implantation include: Implantation technique is challenging and demanding; Redilation over time is feasible; Long term follow up imaging is essential.

INTRODUCTION: NATURE OF THE PROBLEM

Coarctation of the aorta is a narrowing of the aortic lumen, usually of the thoracic descending aorta in the region just distal to the left subclavian artery. Although there are many variants of the anatomic position and length of the narrowing and associated lesions, such as a bicuspid aortic valve, hypoplastic transverse aortic arch, and aberrancies of the head vessels, the effect of the narrowing has the commonly shared features of increased afterload on the left ventricle, exposure of the upper body to hypertension, flow disturbance in the thoracic aorta, and decreased perfusion to the lower body.[1,2] Overall coarctation accounts for approximately 7% of live births with congenital heart disease and can present in infancy, adolescence, or adulthood depending on the balance between the degree of flow disturbance and the compensatory mechanisms available to overcome it. Untreated coarctation has a poor prognosis with most patients suffering from significant morbidities associated with hypertension, including premature death due to heart failure, endocarditis, cerebral

Conflict of Interest: Elchanan Bruckheimer, MBBS, is a paid consultant for Atrium Medical who manufactures the Advanta V12 LD covered stent.
[a] Pediatric Cardiac Catheterization, Schneider Children's Medical Center Israel, Kaplan 14, Petach Tikva, Israel;
[b] Catheterization Laboratory for Congenital Heart Disease, Instituto Dante Pazzanese de Cardiologia, Avenida Doutor Dante Pazzanese, 500 CEP 04012-180, Sao Paulo, Brazil; [c] Catheterization Laboratory for Congenital Heart Disease, Hospital do Coração, Sao Paulo, Brazil
* Corresponding author.
E-mail address: elchananb@bezeqint.net

Intervent Cardiol Clin 2 (2013) 115–129
http://dx.doi.org/10.1016/j.iccl.2012.08.002
2211-7458/13/$ – see front matter © 2013 Elsevier Inc. All rights reserved.

vascular accidents, and premature coronary artery disease.[3] Despite successful treatment by surgery, balloon angioplasty, or stent implantation, the coarctation can recur from a variety of causes, including scarring, failure to match somatic growth, and tissue ingrowth.[4–7]

Surgical repair of coarctation was first described in 1944[8] and since then many techniques have been developed depending on the anatomy. These include resection and end-to-end anastomosis, patch repair, arch augmentation, and, less commonly, insertion of a bypass graft.[9] Surgery is the preferred treatment of infants with coarctation and is successful; however, in older patients, complications are more common and can be severe, particularly when an adequate collateral circulation has not developed and spinal cord damage can ensue.[9] Balloon angioplasty has been an acceptable technique for 3 decades for the relief of coarctation.[10–12] It is successful in cases of recoarctation[13] after surgical repair in infants but the use of this technique in native coarctations at all ages remains controversial due to the disruption of the intima and media of the aortic wall predisposing to a high incidence for future aneurysm formation.[10–12] The aortic wall in coarctation is primarily abnormal and this is compounded by the flow disturbance over time so that in adult patients, tortuousity, thinning, cystic medial necrosis, and calcification may be present, further increasing the predisposition to dissection, aneurysm formation or even rupture.[14]

Stent implantation for coarctation of the aorta has gained popularity since its initiation in 1991 with the rationale that overdilation, dissection, and elastic recoil of the aorta are avoided with this technique and the pinning of the intimal flaps to the aortic wall after tearing of the intima and media promote healing.[15–20] The stent can reinforce weakened areas within the aortic wall and provide a framework for neointima formation to cover the tear. These features of stenting result in less aortic injury than balloon angioplasty[20] but dissection and aneurysm formation remain an important issue. Other complications of stent implantation include malposition, stent fracture, and femoral artery damage[5–7] and their use is restricted to patients with vascular access of adequate size for the large delivery system, which is typically greater than 8F for stents that can achieve an adult size of at least 18 mm. The implantation of stents of narrower maximal diameters may allow for smaller delivery systems and the treatment of infants and young children; however, the need for repeated reintervention to further dilate the stent to match somatic growth and the limited maximal diameter restrict the use of stents in this group of patients.[17–19]

Covered stent implantation was initially introduced for the treatment of coarctation associated with aneurysms or a patent ductus arteriosus (PDA) and for tight or atretic native lesions.[21–23] More recently, with the reasoning that the material cover supplements the advantages of bare stent implantation, providing additional protection to the acutely disrupted aortic wall and the downstream area of poststenotic dilation, the use of covered stents has broadened as the primary treatment of coarctation in some centers.[24] The literature on the use of covered stents is encouraging but has been limited to small clinical series and case reports.[21–27] These stents require larger delivery systems than bare metal stents and an additional limitation to use is the potential to jail important side branches, typically the left subclavian artery.

This article reviews the currently available options for stenting coarctation of the aorta, the equipment and techniques, and reported outcomes. This review is not intended to be comprehensive but to provide a practical framework for interventionalists to approach the straightforward but challenging lesion of coarctation of the aorta.

INDICATIONS FOR TREATMENT

Coarctation of the aorta, native or recurrent, is diagnosed[23,28,29] when the following are present:

- There is a difference in systolic blood pressure of 20 mm Hg between the upper and lower limbs.
- There are echocardiographic findings of coarctation, including 2-D imaging of narrowing in the descending aorta, a Doppler gradient with turbulence of color Doppler and persistence of the gradient into diastole, and an abnormal Doppler tracing with damping of the signal in the abdominal descending aorta.
- Hemodynamic evaluation demonstrates a peak-to peak pressure gradient greater than 20 mm Hg.
- Imaging (aortography, CT, or MRI) demonstrates a significant narrowing in the descending thoracic aorta.

Although it is generally accepted that coarctation should be treated when a pressure gradient greater than 20 mm Hg[17–19,30,31] is recorded, it has been suggested that milder obstructions and gradients may benefit from stent implantation by decreasing left ventricular diastolic pressure and preserving systolic and diastolic left ventricular function in the long term.[32,33] Mild obstructions should be relieved when associated with hypertension at rest, abnormal blood pressure response during exercise, progressive left ventricular hypertrophy, and in cases of complex heart disease, in particular Fontan palliations. The pressure gradient may be less than 20 mm Hg when a large collateral circulation is present or ventricular function is depressed.[28]

Stenting reduces the gradient at the coarctation site more effectively than balloon dilation,[7,34,35] and, therefore, the authors consider this technique in all patients in whom vascular access appropriate for the required delivery system is available. Exception is made in small children due to the need for repeated reinterventions to match somatic growth. The authors routinely stent patients with coarctation and who weigh more than 20 kg.

Covered stent implantation is indicated in patients with coarctation[21–27]:

- Associated with aneurysm or degenerative changes of the aortic wall suggested by the presence of an aneurysmal ascending aorta or significant aortic tortuosity
- Associated with a PDA

- Critical or atretic obstructions
- Age over 18 years
- Aortitis, Turner syndrome, Williams syndrome
- Aortic wall injury (aneurysm, dissection, or rupture) after balloon dilation, bare stent implantation, or surgery
- Presence of circumferential fractures within a previously implanted stent in the aorta with malalignment or protrusion of the stent struts into the aortic wall on repeat angiography, MRI, or CT (**Figs. 1–5**).

Due to improvements in balloon and stent technologies, which afford lower profile systems and the encouraging results from recent reports, the authors now use covered stents as the first choice for treatment of coarctation of the aorta in suitable patients.

STENTS

A variety of types of stents are available for treatment of coarctation and can be divided into

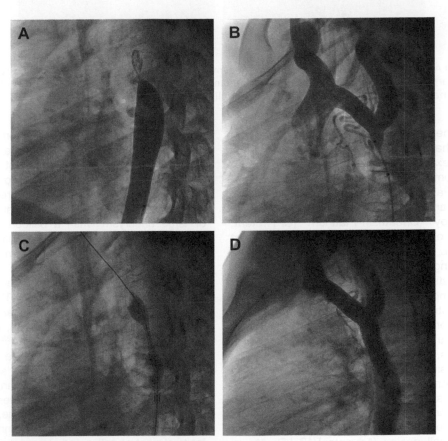

Fig. 1. (*A, B*) Lateral projection shows subatretic coarctation in 24-year-old adult with power injection of contrast below and above the coarctation. (*C*) Implantation of Advanta V12 LD covered stent on a 12-mm balloon. The delivery sheath is placed behind the partially inflated balloon to prevent movement during inflation. (*D*) Lateral view angiogram after further dilation to 16 mm 3 months after initial implantation.

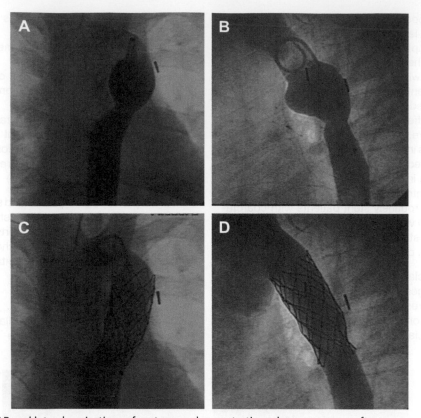

Fig. 2. (*A, B*) AP and lateral projections of aortogram demonstrating a large aneurysm after surgery with a Dacron patch 18 years previously. (*C, D*) CP covered stent implanted and dilated to cover the aneurysm with edges well apposed to native aortic wall above and below suture lines.

groups depending on stent design, material, and size, each having advantages and disadvantages.

Balloon-expandable bare metal stents[5,6,17] are the most commonly used and are made from stainless steel (Palmaz Genesis, Johnson and Johnson; Mega LD and Maxi LD series, ev3), platinum-iridium alloy (Cheatham-Platinum [CP] stent, NuMED),[18] or chromium-cobalt alloy (AndraStent XL and XXL, Andramed).[36] The chromium-cobalt alloy is stronger than stainless steel and, therefore, thinner struts allow for a lower crimped profile without compromising radial strength. Closed cell stents are strong and rigid (Palmaz Genesis) and markedly foreshorten whereas open cell stents (Mega LD and Maxi LD), although weaker, foreshorten less, conform to the anatomy, and allow access to side branches. A hybrid open-closed cell stent (AndraStent) combines the advantages of these designs. Balloon-expandable expanded polytetrafluoroethylene (ePTFE)-covered stents are available in a closed cell design (CP stent) and open cell design (Advanta V12 LD, Atrium Medical) **(Fig. 6)**.

Self-expanding bare nitinol stents have been reported in the treatment of coarctation of the aorta although their use is uncommon.[27,37] Self-expandable stent grafts, which are commonly used for the endovascular treatment of thoracic aortic aneurysms, have been used in special circumstances usually when the degree of coarctation is mild and there is an aortic-bronchial fistula or large aneurysm when a balloon-expandable covered stent is inadequate. A self-expanding covered stent for aneurysm exclusion is probably safer than the balloon-expandable because it avoids an additional local vascular trauma caused by the radial forces of the balloon. These stents typically require a large delivery system of greater than 18F, have lower radial strength, and do not allow further expansion in the future.[23,27]

The choice of stent depends on the coarctation anatomy and associated lesions, size of the patient, the experience and preferences of the operator, and availability. In the literature, and the authors' personal experience, balloon-expandable stents are the most commonly used for treatment of native and recurrent coarctation, and the interventionalist treating coarctation should be familiar with the properties of these stents.[38,39]

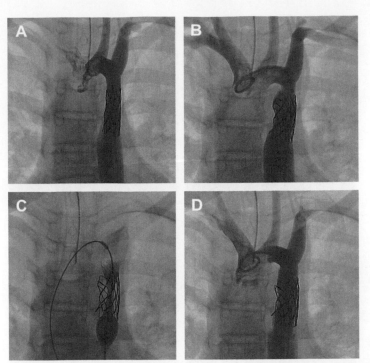

Fig. 3. (*A*) AP aortogram after covered CP stent implantation for native coarctation. (*B*) AP aortogram after further dilation on follow-up with 14-mm balloon. There is an aneurysm on the medial aspect at the top of the stent and the stent is flared in to the aneurysm. (*C*) An Advanta V12 LD covered stent is dilated in the stent up to 14-mm to reach the base of the left subclavian artery. (*D*) The coarctation is dilated to 16 mm and the aneurysm is closed.

The Palmaz XL 14-series stents can be dilated up 25 mm, and are available in 30-mm to 50-mm lengths. They are laser-cut from a rigid stainless steel tube and shorten significantly during expansion and by almost 50% when expanded to their full diameter. Palmaz stents, with their closed-cell design, have little to no flexibility and do not conform to the contour of the aortic arch. The Palmaz Genesis XD stent is also laser-cut from stainless steel and the closed-cell design is modified by a sigma hinge interposed between the cells, which affords some flexibility around curves and also reduces the degree of shortening on expansion. The Genesis stents are available in multiple lengths but cannot be expanded further than 18 mm. This limitation makes the use of this stent inappropriate for larger aortas and patients. Unless the aorta is expected to reach a diameter significantly greater than 18 mm, the radial strength and flexibility of the Genesis stent make it a good option for treatment of lesions that lie across the curve between the transverse arch and the descending aorta. Concerns have been raised, however, with regard to fracturing when expanded to large diameters.[38,39]

The CP stent is composed of a 90% platinum and 10% iridium alloy, with the metal wires arranged in a zig pattern.[18] Earlier versions of the stent were prone to fracture and refinements in the welding process using gold have been successfully used to minimize this problem.[18] CP stents with 8 zigs can be expanded up to 25 mm and shorten less than the Palmaz stents, with the 39-mm and 45-mm lengths usually appropriate.[23,25]

The Maxi LD stent is made from stainless steel with an open cell design affording flexibility and reduces the risk of jailing side branches, making it especially useful in dilations of the transverse arch. In addition, when expanded in a staged fashion with progressively larger diameter balloons, it displays minimal foreshortening. The long-term resistance to fracturing, however, when expanded to 20 mm to 25 mm, is not known.[38]

The AndraStent XL and XXL stents are hybrid open-closed cell cobalt-chromium stents that can be dilated up to 25 mm and 32 mm, respectively, and are available in a variety of lengths. This combination of high radial strength with a lower profile, conformability, and minimized shortening make it a good candidate for the

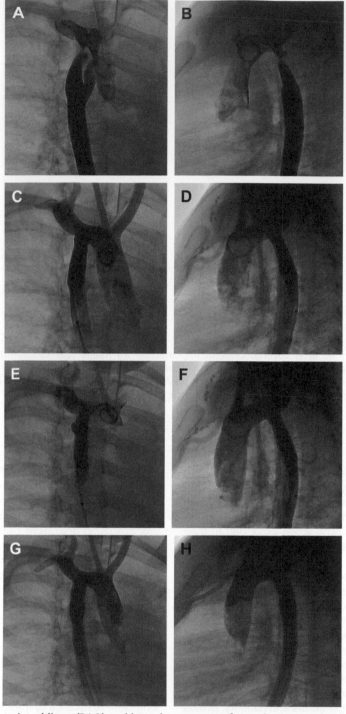

Fig. 4. (*A, B*) Right anterior oblique (RAO) and lateral aortogram of complex coarctation in 6-year-old girl with a right aortic arch, tight coarctation, and aberrant left subclavian artery. The right subclavian artery is enlarged because it is the major supply of collateral flow. (*C, D*) RAO and lateral aortogram after Genesis 1990 bare stent implanted and dilated to 9 mm. (*E, F*) RAO and lateral aortogram at 2-year follow-up demonstrating a small aneurysm on the RAO view. (*G, H*) RAO and lateral aortogram after Advanta V12 LD covered stent implantation on 12-mm balloon. The aneurysm is excluded and the stent dilated appropriately to the diameter of the transverse arch.

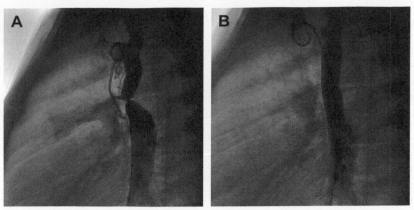

Fig. 5. (*A*) Lateral projection shows severe coarctation and a small PDA in a 10-year-old boy. There is a small bronchial collateral. (*B*) Implantation of Advanta V12 LD covered stent on a 12-mm balloon with further dilation to 14 mm. The stent dilates the coarctation appropriate to the size of the transverse arch and closes the PDA.

treatment of coarctation of the aorta, particularly in curved anatomy. Because this stent is new, the reported experience is encouraging but limited.[36]

There are 2 ePTFE balloon-expandable covered stents currently available. The covered CP stent is the standard CP stent covered with an ultrathin stretchable ePTFE membrane applied to a stent using biodegradable adhesives[18,23] and is also available crimped and premounted on a BIB balloon (NuMed).

The Advanta V12 LD stent is a stainless steel open cell stent encapsulated by a covering of

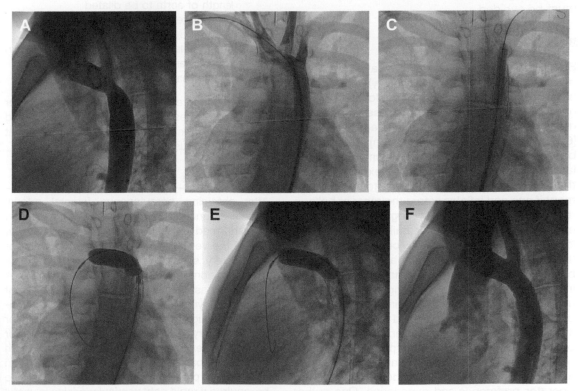

Fig. 6. (*A*) Lateral projection shows mild coarctation at isthmus. (*B*) AP view—Rosen guide wire in right subclavian artery for stent implantation. (*C*) Guide wire in left subclavian artery with 6-mm balloon to align stent to wall of artery. (*D, E*) AP and lateral views with guide wire in ascending aorta so that the back end of the 14-mm balloon lays the stent down on the arch. (*F*) Stent dilates arch appropriately and flush with the native vessel walls.

ePTFE on the interior and exterior aspects. It is available in 3 lengths (29 mm, 41 mm, and 61 mm) and is premounted on high-pressure balloons of 12-mm, 14-mm, and 16-mm diameters. The stent can be incrementally dilated, by 4 mm at a time, to avoid tearing of the ePTFE, up to a maximal diameter of 22 mm.[26]

In countries, such as the United States, where the availability of covered stents is limited, interventionalists have reported on the use of self-fabricated covered stents[40,41] for high-risk patients or during acute aortic wall complications.

The major concern with the implantation of covered stents in the aorta is the risk of side branch occlusion, particularly of the left subclavian artery or the spinal artery, resulting in paraplegia. The major concern with the implantation of covered stents in the aorta is the risk of side branch occlusion, particularly of the left subclavian artery or the spinal artery resulting in paraplegia.[42,43] The latter complication is usually avoided by not implanting a covered stent below the ninth thoracic vertebra. An additional concern with the use of covered stents is when distal migration occurs because the stent cannot be easily parked without occluding side branches and the origins of the renal and mesenteric arteries must be avoided.

BALLOONS

Balloon-expandable stents are available premounted (as described previously) or need to be crimped on to a balloon for deployment. There are 2 types of balloon commonly used for deployment, single-balloon catheters (eg, Powerflex [6–12 mm] and Maxi LD [14–25 mm]) and the BIB balloon (balloon-in-balloon) (Numed). Single large-diameter balloons tend to expand first at their ends, which may predispose to stent movement if one end inflates before the other or balloon rupture if the stent has sharp edges. The BIB catheter is made from an inner balloon and a 1-cm longer outer balloon that is twice the diameter of the inner balloon and they are available in outer-balloon sizes of 8 mm to 24 mm. They offer the important advantage of opening the stent more uniformly along its length, resulting in more control over its precise placement and preventing stent flaring and migration; however, they are more bulky than their single counterparts. The choice of balloon depends on the coarctation anatomy and dimensions, the stent to be implanted, and operator preference and experience. One author (EB) always uses single balloons whereas the other (CACP) uses the BIB for special cases. Single-balloon catheters are preferable in smaller

patients to reduce risk to the femoral artery at the access site, whereas the BIB balloon is helpful in precise positioning in transverse arch stenting. On occasions, high-pressure balloons, such as the Mullins balloons (NuMed) and Atlas balloons (Bard), may be needed to dilate up a residual waist, particularly in postsurgical coarctations. Generally, a balloon that is slightly longer (approximately 1 cm) than the stent is used for implantation.

TECHNIQUE

The implantation techniques for bare and covered stents in coarctation of the aorta vary among institutions and depend on the anatomy of the coarctation and materials used.[15–41] Despite this variation, there are several steps that are common to all coarctation stent procedures:

- Vascular access
- Crossing the lesion
- Hemodynamic assessment
- Definition of anatomy by aortography
- Measurement of diameters of transverse arch, isthmus, coarctation, and descending aorta at the level of the diaphragm and length of aorta to be dilated
- Guide wire positioning
- Sheath advancement
- Stent implantation, positioning, and dilation
- Assessment and postdilation
- Sheath removal

The procedure is generally performed under general anesthesia because it is painful and patient movement at the time of stent deployment can be hazardous.

Vascular Access

After obtaining percutaneous femoral arterial access, a hand injection of contrast media should be performed through the sheath to assess the size of the vessel and, if of appropriate size, for the delivery sheath. A second vascular access may occasionally be used for serial angiograms in order to assist proper positioning of the stent during deployment and this may be achieved transeptally through a femoral vein or using a radial or brachial artery. A second access is indicated for more complex cases, such as transverse arch stenting, subatretic coarctation, and when an aneurysm is present.[17] Venous access may also be required if rapid right ventricular pacing is useful for stent positioning. This is of importance when stenting the aortic arch or using covered stents in proximity to head vessels or when significant aortic regurgitation, creating large pressure swings, is present.[30] After vascular access is obtained, heparin sulfate (100–150 IU/kg; maximum 10,000 IU total) is given intravenously and the activated clotting time (ACT) should be maintained at greater than 200 seconds. The authors administer intravenous antibiotics prior to stent implantation.

Crossing the Lesion

The lesion is typically crossed from the descending aorta with the aid of a shaped (Berenstein or Cobra) end-hole catheter and a hydrophilic guide wire. Subatretic lesions are often more easily crossed from above, with the anatomy creating a funnel, which guides the tip, and this can then be snared and exteriorized through a femoral sheath below. In patients with atretic coarctation, a discrete atretic segment may be perforated from above or below using a transseptal needle, stiff end of a coronary wire, or a radiofrequency catheter.[23,44]

Hemodynamic Assessment

The peak pressure gradient is assessed via simultaneous measurements above and below the lesion or by pullback across the lesion if it was easy to cross. The pressure gradient may be less than that measured by arm-leg cuff blood pressure due to the use of general anesthesia lowering the systemic vascular resistance and this can be rectified with fluids and medications to create a stable state. Extensive collateral flow may also reduce the peak gradient. In these situations, the indication for intervention should be based on the clinical, echocardiographic and angiographic findings.

Aortography and Measurement

Aortic angiograms are typically obtained in the anteroposterior (AP) and lateral projections or using shallow left anterior oblique or shallow right anterior oblique projections with caudal angulation. A high-volume, rapid injection in the region of the coarcted segment using a 5F marker pigtail (eg, Merrit Medical) catheter usually suffices to define the anatomy and enable accurate measurements of the diameters of the transverse arch, aortic isthmus, coarctation, poststenotic dilatation, and descending aorta at the level of the diaphragm. The recent introduction of 3-D rotational angiography in to the pediatric cardiac catheterization laboratory provides an additional tool to understand complex coarctation anatomies. The rotation provides multiple individual frames of the aorta, each from a different angle, which affords a more detailed assessment of the spatial anatomic

relationship between a coarcted segment and the implanted stent or associated aneurysm than that obtained from a standard biplane view.

The initial stent diameter chosen should at least match the diameter of the aorta adjacent to the coarctation for it to anchor well. The final stent diameter should be similar to that of the isthmus or distal transverse arch. In coarctations in which there is a large degree of mismatch, initial relief should be provided at a diameter that the stent is well opposed and stable. Further dilation to the final diameter can be performed some months later. The use of covered stents in this setting adds extra protection to the aortic wall.[17,18,23–26] The length of the aorta to be stented should be measured from above the region of tapering proximal to the coarctation to well in to the poststenotic dilation. This is important to avoid the distal edge of the stent touching the aortic wall here to avoid dissection. In long lesions requiring 2 or more stents, it is important to telescope the stents with sufficient overlap so they can be dilated together and not come apart because the stent edge is forced in to the aortic wall and the risk of dissection is increased. With covered stents, the length is decided on with the above considerations and taking in to account the position of side branches. In the poststenotic dilation area, the covered stent deflects the flow away from the wall toward the center. The anatomy needs to be carefully assessed for the presence of aneurysms/dissections, especially in patients with recoarctation after previous intervention.

Guide Wire Positioning

Prior to intervention, a long support wire with a soft tip, such as a 260-cm 0.035" Rosen wire or Amplatz Super Stiff Guide Wire, is parked in the ascending aorta or right or left subclavian artery, depending on the straightest wire course and angulation of the lesion. The softer Rosen wire does not distort the anatomy and usually provides sufficient support for advancing of the sheath and stent implantation. The distal position of the tip of the wire is changed during the procedure if the stent needs to be shaped to match the aortic contour (see **Fig. 6**). It is important not to place the wire in the left subclavian artery if the balloon for stent implantation enters the artery because the oversizing of the artery by the tip of the balloon can damage the artery or, alternatively, the balloon milks downwards and changes the position of the stent.

Sheath Advancement

A popular sheath for stent delivery is the 75-cm long Cook RB-Mullins sheath (Cook Cardiology), which has a radiopaque tip and a sidearm for contrast injections and pressure measurements. The French size of the long sheath required for stent implantation depends on the profile of the balloon and generally needs to be 1F to 2F larger. When using a covered CP stent, the sheath may need to be 2F to 3F larger than the implanting balloon. The Brite Tip 55-cm sheath (Cordis) is a useful sheath, especially in the smaller patients when a delivery system of up to 9F is required. The sheath is advanced over the wire through the lesion and the dilator removed. A hand injection of contrast through the sideport is useful for establishing the site for implantation with relationship to anatomic bony landmarks.

Stent Implantation, Positioning, and Dilation

If the selected stent is not premounted, it is manually crimped on to the chosen balloon. A piece of umbilical tape looped around the stent and pulled at both ends to help tighten the stent onto the balloon may be used, especially when crimping larger profile stents on to small diameter balloons. During crimping, the guide wire should be left in the catheter-balloon shaft in order to straighten the system and avoid damage to the balloon and crushing of the shaft. Manual crimping of the covered CP stent onto the catheter balloon and loading it into the long sheath requires extra care. Wetting of the ePTFE layer should be avoided so that it keeps its original shape around the stent, preventing unfolding and damage. A cutoff short sheath (with the same profile of the long sheath) is used to protect the covered CP stent while advancing it through the hemostatic valve and to prevent it billowing.

The balloon-stent assembly is back-loaded into the sheath and advanced to its tip. The sheath is slowly retracted, exposing the stent in the vascular lumen. Repeat angiograms via the side arm of the long sheath during retraction or via a second angiographic catheter positioned in the arch are performed to ensure proper stent position prior to balloon inflation.

Although the use of the BIB balloon can facilitate precise stent deployment, additional maneuvers can also be used. Reduction of the pulse pressure in a controlled manner by rapid right ventricular pacing at 180 bpm 220 bpm during stent deployment is useful, particularly in transverse arch stenting.[30] The rate of pacing varies between 180 and 220 beats per minute and the exact rate is determined at the outset by monitoring the pressure in the ascending aorta while pacing the heart at different rates. The rate for pacing that reduces the pulse pressure in the aorta is used. The authors

often use the sheath to buttress the balloon, once inflated, to prevent it being pushed down to the descending aorta with the predilation of the lesion is controversial and has been associated with a higher incidence of aortic wall abnormalities at follow-up in the report from the Congenital Cardiovascular Interventional Study Consortium (CCISC) multicenter study.[5,6] In the presence of a critical lesion, however, the coarctation may be predilated using a 5-mm to 6 mm diameter balloon, just to make enough room for the passage of the long sheath. Predilation of the coarctation is a prerequisite in the Coarctation of the Aorta Stent Trial (COAST) protocol (http://clinicaltrials.gov/ct2/show/NCT00552812). From the authors' viewpoint, although postsurgical lesions may be noncompliant, almost all native coarctations, except those that are part of a middle aortic syndrome, are compliant and do not need to be routinely predilated. When using the BIB balloon, the inner balloon is inflated first and the stent repositioned, if needed, before inflation of the outer balloon.[18] Most patients require only 1 or 2 dilations for stent deployment and it is recommended that the second inflation of the outer balloon is performed while keeping the inner balloon deflated because the dilation force is better distributed in this way.

The authors have described[24] a method for covered CP stent implantation using the lowest profile system possible by anchoring the stent in the coarctation with an 8-mm to 10-mm high-pressure single balloon and then carefully removing this balloon and further dilating the stent through the same sheath with a Maxi LD balloon. The authors have managed to implant and dilate stents up to 16-mm in this way, on a regular basis, using a 9F Brite-Tip 55-cm sheath.

The low-profile Advanta V12 LD stent can be implanted on a 12-mm balloon through an 8F sheath (manufacturer's recommendation is 9F) and the 14-mm and 16-mm delivery systems need an 11F sheath.[26] The methods for implantation are similar to those described previously.

Assessment and Further Dilation

After implantation, the pressure gradient is measured and aortography performed to assess the stent position, adequacy of dilation, and presence of aortic wall complications. Further dilation of the stent can be performed during the current procedure or scheduled at a later date when there is a large mismatch of initial size of coarctation to the diameter required. When using a covered stent, the authors try to dilate the stent so that the covering is apposed to the dilated aortic wall immediately adjacent to the coarcted segment to maximize the protection of the ePTFE in preventing aneurysm formation. Although some investigators have advocated flaring the ends of stents to optimize endothelialization,[45] it is unlikely that complete stent apposition in the poststenotic region can be achieved without distorting the stent, and this may be detrimental to stent stability without any evidence that it is neccessary. The main goal of stenting coarctation is for gradient relief and this is attained regardless of complete apposition of the stent in the poststenotic area. With covered stent implantation, the flow in the poststenotic area is contained within the stent and directed toward the lumen and not the aortic wall, thereby protecting the wall. The formation of clots between the stent and aortic wall in the poststenotic area has not been reported[46,47] or found in the authors' experience.

After stent deployment, care should be taken to not dislodge the stent. Once the balloon is deflated, the sheath is gently advanced over it, followed by balloon withdrawal.

Excessive catheter and wire manipulation over the recently stented area should be avoided; however, if needed to match the aortic contour, the stent can be shaped by the same or additional balloons (as seen in **Fig. 6**).

Sheath Removal

When the ACT is prolonged (>200 s), the effect of can be partially neutralized using protamine. A Perclose or Prostar (Abbott Vascular) suture has been used to close the arteriotomy but needs to be inserted in the femoral artery prior to the introduction of the large sheath. This method helps achieve hemostasis quickly at the end of the procedure and prevent hemorrhagic complications at the puncture site.[30] Occasionally 2 sutures are needed to repair the artery, especially when a large (14F) sheath is used. Reliable hemostasis can usually be achieved, however, by judicious manual compression.

Patients are usually discharged home the following day on aspirin (5 mg/kg/d; maximum 300 mg) and instructed to avoid contact sports for 6 months. A chest radiograph, a 12-lead electrocardiogram, and a transthoracic echocardiogram are obtained before discharge and scheduled after 1 to 3 months, 6 months, 12 months, and yearly thereafter along with the clinical visits.

Due to the possibility of late aneurysm formation after stenting, follow-up imaging is mandatory in all patients.[46–50] Therefore, a repeat catheterization, MRI, or CT should be scheduled approximately 12 months after the procedure and probably at fixed periods during the patient's

lifetime, especially before and after pregnancy. Elective recatheterization is performed after 6 to 12 months to carry out stent redilation when there is residual stenosis as a result of the stent having been intentionally underinflated initially.[51,52]

OUTCOMES

Since the first cases of coarctation stenting were reported in the 1990s, the encouraging outcome of this procedure has been described in a considerable number of individual series reporting both short-term and intermediate-term results.[5,6,15–19] In 2007, one large multicenter retrospective series[5] was reported by the CCISC on 565 procedures of stent implantation performed in 555 patients with coarctation between 1989 and 2005, of which 553 (97.9%) were successful in reducing the gradient to less than 20 mm Hg. Among the successful cases, there was a mean reduction of the peak-to-peak gradient from 31.6 ± 16.0 to 2.7 ± 4.2 mm Hg, a mean increase in diameter from 7.4 ± 3.0 to 14.3 ± 3.2 mm, and a mean increase in the ratio of the coarctation of the aorta diameter to the descending aorta diameter measured at the level of the diaphragm (CoA:DAo) from 0.43 ± 0.17 to 0.85 ± 0.15. These results, showing a high degree of success, are similar to those reported in other smaller series.[15–19] These series and the CCISC in a follow-up study reported that the relief of the pressure gradient persisted in the majority of patients at medium-term follow-up.[6] Significant pressure gradients on follow-up were associated with suboptimal/restricted expansion of the stent at the time of implantation, stent recoil, and neointimal growth within the stent. In-stent restenosis was associated with a smaller poststent diameter and a higher poststent systolic gradient and in the main this occurred in those of a younger age and lower weight at the time of implantation[5,6,47] This is, as expected, due to the vascular lumen being larger in the adult aorta and a mild intrastent proliferation usually does not result in flow obstruction and local gradient generation. The stents could be dilated further in most instances to resolve these issues, although questions have been raised as to the feasibility, safety, and effectiveness of redilation.[30,51] It is the authors' experience and that of others that both bare and covered stents can be successfully redilated late at follow-up with no untoward effect.[52]

The efficacy of coarctation stenting is, therefore, high but the safety of the procedure has been a cause of concern with significant complications occurring in 14.3% of cases in the CCISC acute study.[5] The complications were broadly divided into the technical and aortic wall categories. Technical complications included stent migration, stent fracture, and balloon rupture and occurred in 10.9% of cases whereas acute aortic wall complications included intimal tears, dissection, and aneurysm formation and were present in 3.9%. These complications were treated by conservative, transcatheter methods, including the implantation of additional stents or surgery. Unfortunately, 2 of the patients died after having suffered severe neurologic damage. The investigators noted that there was a significant decrease in technical complications after January 2002 and related this to improvements in catheter and stent technology (eg, sharp-edged Palmaz 8 series stents causing balloon rupture), providing the interventionalists with greater options, and, in addition, "a learning curve phenomenon could not be excluded."[5]

In the intermediate follow-up CCISC study,[6] 144 of 578 (24.9%) patients had follow-up imaging (CT, MRI, or aortography) of whom 18 of 144 (12.5%) had an aneurysm or developed a dissection/intimal tear. Most aneurysms were small and were managed conservatively although 4 patients required further intervention, such as the implantation of a covered CP stent. The results reported in the CCISC studies are of particular interest with reference to the results reported by Chakrabarti and colleagues[49] on 88 patients with coarctation who underwent 102 stent procedures from 2002 to 2008. There were 4 acute complications (3.7%) of which 2 (1.9%) were aortic wall related. A follow-up CT was performed on 95.9% of the patients of whom only 1 developed an aneurysm associated with redilation of a stent that had fractured. This was successfully treated with a covered stent.

Chakrabarti and colleagues[49] and the CCISC[5,6] have similar percentages of native coarctations in their series and used the same definition for aneurysm formation. Therefore, the marked differences in the rates of aneurysm formation between the groups may be explained by the small percentage of the CCISC cohort who underwent follow-up imaging. This imaging was presumably performed due to clinical concerns and, therefore, the group is probably unrepresentative and biased. Another observation, however, is that in the CCISC group, 14 of 511 (2.7%) stents implanted were covered as opposed to 26 of 94 (27.7%) of the stents used in Chakrabarti and colleagues' series.

The use of covered stents for coarctation has gained popularity affter an initial case report[21] and small series[22,23] in treating native and recoarctations associated with, or at risk for, aneurysms. A larger experience was published by Ewert and colleagues,[53] in 2005, with the use of the CP stent in a broad spectrum of heart malformations, of which 37 had coarctation and 11 of these were successfully treated with covered stents. The indications included subatretic or severe lesions, aneurysm formation, and previously implanted stent fracture. All stents were placed in the lesion without complications. During follow-up, one covered stent fractured at 6 months and required the implantation of an additional covered stent. Similarly, in 2005, the authors' group (CACP) in Sao Paulo, Brazil,[23] reported on 9 patients with coarctation who received covered stents (10 CP stents and 2 self-expandable Braile stent grafts). The indications included severe or atretic coarctation, aneurysm formation, a coexistent patent arterial duct, and circumferential fracture of a previously implanted stent. Median age and weight were 31 years and 65 kg, respectively, and the procedure was successful in all subjects. However, 2 patients developed aneurysms, 1 requiring conservative management and the other successfully treated using a second covered custom-made self-expandable Braile stent. During follow-up, all patients had either reduced the dose or suspended the use of antihypertensive drugs.

After these early experiences several larger series were reported of 30 to 40 patients[25,27] who underwent implantation of covered stents for mainly complex coarctations with aneurysms, previous stent-related complications, recurrent coarctation after surgical treatment, aortobronchial fistula, previous stent fracture, an associated patent arterial duct, or coarctations at risk of because of complex coarctation anatomy or advanced age. All series reported a significant reduction in pressure gradients and improvement in the coarctation diameter with a low rate of acute complications. When available, short-term follow-up with imaging, including CT, MRI, and aortography, demonstrated maintained position and patency of the stent and exclusion of aneurysms present at the time of implantation.

In light of this success in complex coarctations, the authors (EB) decided to implant covered CP stents[24] in simple native coarctations in order to potentially benefit from the additional protection of the material covering to the acutely disrupted aortic wall in the short term and protection of the dilated segment and the downstream area of poststenotic dilation in the long-term. Initially, to create a small delivery system of 9F to 10F, the authors implanted the stents on balloons of diameter just sufficient to anchor the stent in the coarctation site and then performed subsequent serial dilations with larger diameter balloons until the pressure gradient was less than 20 mm Hg and the stent was apposed to the aortic wall; 22 patients with native coarctation were treated successfully with no complications and 9 patients underwent further dilation at an average of 5 months later. Complications included a small tear at further dilation, which was treated with a second stent and a femoral pseudoaneurysm treated conservatively. At short-term follow-up, all patients were alive and well with no evidence of recoarctation or aneurysm.

Recently, the authors and colleagues[26] reported the acute results on 25 patients with coarctation treated in a similar manner with the large diameter covered Advanta V12 premounted stent placed through 8F to 11F delivery systems. The technique again included an initial inflation on balloons of a diameter sufficient to anchor the stent in the coarctation site using the smallest available delivery system followed by a secondary dilation using larger diameter balloons until the pressure gradient was less than 20 mm Hg and the stent was apposed to the aortic wall. The procedure was successful in all patients with the stent reaching the planned diameter and there were no complications. Median follow-up was 4.9 months with no complications or evidence of recoarctation.

These series, and other recent reports,[54–56] have shown good procedural and midterm safety and effectiveness of stent implantation for coarctation. These reports are retrospective analyses, however, and are limited by nonrandomized study design, small sample size, absence of systematic prospective data collection, and planned follow-up imaging.[57]

Follow-up imaging is of paramount importance to the evaluation of the outcomes for coarctation interventions, including surgery. Apart from Chakrabarti and colleagues' series[49] and a smaller one by Tanous and colleagues,[54] however, there are no large studies with complete long-term imaging and, therefore, the true incidence of aneurysms is unknown. Imaging is complicated by the presence of the stent, which causes artifact in the MRI, making the evaluation of in-stent stenosis and stent fracture impossible.[50] MRI black blood imaging can be used to evaluate aneurysms, stent position, and dissections extending beyond the stent but there are a limited number of centers that can perform these procedures on a routine basis. CT scanning is quick and produces high-quality images but carries a significant radiation dose. If serial scans are performed during a patient's lifetime, the accumulated radiation dose is prohibitive. Aortography is usually confined to patients requiring reintervention and is both invasive and involves exposure to radiation.

A recent editorial[50] suggested 3 to 5 yearly follow-up by MRI imaging and if the scan is suggestive of a complication, then a CT scan or direct evaluation by catheterization is performed.

There are currently 2 ongoing prospective clinical trials to evaluate the safety and efficacy of covered stenting for coarctation of the aorta: the COAST II trial (NCT01278303) and the Large Diameter Advanta V12 Covered Stent Trial for Coarctation of the Aorta (NCT00978952). The results of these trials are eagerly awaited.

FUTURE PERSPECTIVES

Future directions in stent design should include a reduction of the stent profile while maintaining radial strength, flexibility, and maximal expandable diameter to prevent injury to the vascular access site and development of recapturable and repositionable devices as well as the capability of the stent to adapt to somatic growth (growth stent).[58] Biodegradable stents[59] may provide an alternative treatment of coarctation in infants.

SUMMARY

Stent implantation for native or recurrent coarctation of the aorta has progressed from an acceptable alternative to surgical therapy to be the primary intervention in older children, adolescents, and adults in many institutions. Stents have proved highly effective for intermediate-term relief of the obstruction and covered stents, and, in particular, may minimize the incidence of aortic wall complications. Although the implantation technique can be challenging and demanding, it is safe in experienced hands. Follow-up imaging is essential on a long-term basis to assess for aortic wall damage, in particular aneurysm formation. Reinterventions, including further dilations to match somatic growth, and additional stent placement are often required.

REFERENCES

1. Izukawa T, Mulholland HC, Rowe RD. Structural heart disease in the newborn. Arch Dis Child 1979; 54:281–5.
2. Benson L, McLaughlin PR. Coarctation of the aorta. In: Freedom R, Yoo SJ, Mikailian H, et al, editors. The natural and modified history of congenital heart disease. New York: Blackwell; 2004. p. 251–75.
3. Fyler DC. Coarctation of the aorta. In: Fyler DC, editor. Nadas' pediatric Cardiology. Philadelphia: Hanley & Belfus, Inc; 1992. p. 535–56.
4. Carr JA. The results of catheter-based therapy compared with surgical repair of adult aortic coarctation. J Am Coll Cardiol 2006;21(47):1101–7.

5. Forbes TJ, Garekar S, Amin Z, et al. Congenital Cardiovascular Interventional Study Consortium (CCISC). Procedural results and acute complications in stenting native and recurrent coarctation of the aorta in patients over 4 years of age: a multi-institutional study. Catheter Cardiovasc Interv 2007;70:276–85.

6. Forbes TJ, Moore P, Pedra CA, et al. Intermediate follow-up following intravascular stenting for treatment of coarctation of the aorta. Catheter Cardiovasc Interv 2007;70:569–77.

7. Egan M, Holzer RJ. Comparing balloon angioplasty, stenting and surgery in the treatment of aortic coarctation. Expert Rev Cardiovasc Ther 2009;7:1401–12.

8. Crafoord C, Nylin G. Congenital coarctation of the aorta and its surgical treatment. J Thorac Surg 1945;14:347–61.

9. Kouchoukos NT, Blackstone EH, Doty DR, et al. Kirklin/Barratt-Boyes cardiac surgery. 3rd edition. Philadelphia: Churchill Livingstone; 2003. Chapter 34, Coarctation of the aorta and interrupted aortic arch. p.

10. Singer MI, Rowen M, Dorsey TJ. Transluminal aortic balloon angioplasty for coarctation of the aorta in the newborn. Am Heart J 1982;103:131–2.

11. Tynan M, Finley JP, Fontes V, et al. Balloon angioplasty for the treatment of native coarctation: results of Valvuloplasty and Angioplasty of Congenital Anomalies Registry. Am J Cardiol 1990;65:790–2.

12. Fontes V, Esteves C, Braga S, et al. It is valid to dilate native aortic coarctation with a balloon catheter. Int J Cardiol 1990;27:311–6.

13. Maheshwari S, Bruckheimer E, Fahey JT, et al. Balloon angioplasty of postsurgical recoarctation in infants: the risk of restenosis and long-term follow-up. J Am Coll Cardiol 2000;35:209–13.

14. Isner JM, Donaldson RF, Fulton D, et al. Cystic medial necrosis in coarctation of the aorta: a potential factor contributing to adverse consequences observed after percutaneous balloon angioplasty of coarctation sites. Circulation 1987;75:689–95.

15. O'Laughlin MP, Perry SB, Lock JE, et al. Use of endovascular stents in congenital heart disease. Circulation 1991;83:1923–39.

16. Bulbul ZR, Bruckheimer E, Love JC, et al. Implantation of balloon-expandable stents for coarctation of the aorta: implantation data and short-term results. Cathet Cardiovasc Diagn 1996;39:36–42.

17. Pilla CB, Fontes VF, Pedra CA. Stenting for aortic coarctation. Expert Rev Cardiovasc Ther 2005;3:879–90.

18. Cheatham JP. Stenting of coarctation of the aorta. Catheter Cardiovasc Interv 2001;54:112–25.

19. Golden A, Hellenbrand W. Coarctation of the aorta: stenting in children and adults. Catheter Cardiovasc Interv 2007;69:289–99.

20. Ohkubo M, Takahashi K, Kishiro M, et al. Histological findings after angioplasty using conventional balloon, radiofrequency thermal balloon, and stent for experimental aortic coarctation. Pediatr Int 2004;46:39–47.

21. Gunn J, Cleveland T, Gaines P. Covered stent to treat coexistent coarctation and aneurysm of the aorta in a young man. Heart 1999;82:351.

22. De Giovanni JV. Covered stents in the treatment of aortic coarctation. J Interv Cardiol 2001;14:187–90.

23. Pedra C, Fontes V, Esteves C, et al. Use of covered stents in the management of coarctation of aorta. Pediatr Cardiol 2005;26:431–9.

24. Bruckheimer E, Dagan T, Amir G, et al. Covered Cheatham-Platinum stents for serial dilation of severe native aortic coarctation. Catheter Cardiovasc Interv 2009;74:117–23.

25. Qureshi SA, Zubrzycka M, Brzezinska-Rajszys G, et al. Use of covered Cheatham-platinum stents in aortic coarctation and recoarctation. Cardiol Young 2004;14:50–4.

26. Bruckheimer E, Birk E, Santiago R, et al. Coarctation of the aorta treated with the Advanta V12 large diameter stent: acute results. Catheter Cardiovasc Interv 2010;75:402–6.

27. Kenny D, Margey R, Turner MS, et al. Self-expanding and balloon expandable covered stents in the treatment of aortic coarctation with or without aneurysm formation. Catheter Cardiovasc Interv 2008;72:65–71.

28. Feltes TF, Bacha E, Beekman RH 3rd, et al. American Heart Association Congenital Cardiac Defects Committee of the Council on Cardiovascular Disease in the Young; Council on Clinical Cardiology; Council on Cardiovascular Radiology and Intervention. Indications for cardiac catheterization and intervention in pediatric cardiac disease: a scientific statement from the American Heart Association. Circulation 2011;123:2607–52.

29. Snider AR, Serwer GA, Ritter SB. Echocardiography in pediatric heart disease. 2nd edition. St Louis (MO): Mosby Year Book; 1997. Chapter 11, Coarctation of the aorta. p. 479–82.

30. Qureshi SA. Stenting in aortic coarctation and transverse arch/isthmus hypoplasia. In: Sievert H, Qureshi SA, Wilson N, et al, editors. Percutaneous interventions for congenital heart disease. London: Informa Healthcare; 2007. p. 475–86.

31. Zabal C, Attie F, Rosas M, et al. The adult patient with native coarctation of the aorta: balloon angioplasty or primary stenting? Heart 2003;89:77–83.

32. Marshall AC, Perry SB, Keane JF, et al. Early results and medium-term follow-up of stent implantation for mild residual or recurrent aortic coarctation. Am Heart J 2000;139:1054–60.

33. Qureshi AM, McElhinney DB, Lock JE, et al. Acute and intermediate outcomes, and evaluation of injury to the aortic wall, as based on 15 year experience of implanting stents to treat aortic coarctation. Cardiol Young 2007;17:307–18.

34. Pedra CA, Fontes VF, Esteves CA, et al. Stenting vs. balloon angioplasty for discrete unoperated coarctation of the aorta in adolescents and adults. Catheter Cardiovasc Interv 2005;64:495–506.

35. Forbes TJ, Kim DW, Du W, et al. Comparison of surgical, stent, and balloon angioplasty treatment of native coarctation of the aorta: an observational study by the CCISC (Congenital Cardiovascular Interventional Study Consortium). J Am Coll Cardiol 2011;58:2664–74.

36. Białkowski J, Szkutnik M, Fiszer R, et al. Percutaneous dilatation of coarctation of the aorta, stenotic pulmonary arteries or homografts, and stenotic superior vena cava using Andrastents XL and XXL. Kardiol Pol 2011;69:1213–9.

37. Oberhuber A, Muehling BM, Orend KH, et al. Endovascular repair of aortic isthmus coarctation with a self-expanding covered stent. Ann Vasc Surg 2012;26:573.

38. Ing F. Stents: what's available to the pediatric interventional cardiologist? Catheter Cardiovasc Interv 2002;57:374–86.

39. Peters B, Ewert P, Berger F. The role of stents in the treatment of congenital heart disease: current status and future perspectives. Ann Pediatr Cardiol 2009;2:3–23.

40. Kenny D, Cao QL, Kavinsky C, et al. Innovative resource utilization to fashion individualized covered stents in the setting of aortic coarctation. Catheter Cardiovasc Interv 2011;78:413–8.

41. Holzer R, Concilio K, Hijazi Z. Self-fabricated covered stent to exclude an aortic aneurysm after balloon angioplasty for post-surgical recoarctation. J Invasive Cardiol 2005;17:177–9.

42. Matsuda H, Fukuda T, Iritani O, et al. Spinal cord injury is not negligible after TEVAR for lower descending aorta. Eur J Vasc Endovasc Surg 2010; 39:179–86.

43. Tsai SF, Hill SL, Cheatham JP. Treatment of aortic arch aneurysm with a NuMED-covered stent and restoration of flow to excluded left subclavian artery: perforation and dilation of e-PTFE can be done! Catheter Cardiovasc Interv 2009;72:385–9.

44. Eicken A, Kaemmerer H, Ewert P. Treatment of aortic isthmus atresia with a covered stent. Catheter Cardiovasc Interv 2008;72(6):844–6.

45. Hamdan M, Maheshwari S, Fahey J, et al. Endovascular stents for coarctation of the aorta: initial results and intermediate-term follow-up. J Am Coll Cardiol 2001;38:1518–23.

46. Harrison DA, McLaughlin PR, Lazzam C, et al. Endovascular stents in the management of coarctation of the aorta in the adolescent and adult: one year follow up. Heart 2001;85:561–6.

47. Lezo S, Pan M, Romero M, et al. Immediate and follow-up findings after stent treatment for severe coarctation of aorta. Am J Cardiol 1999;83:400–6.

48. Collins N, Mahadevan V, Horlick E. Aortic rupture following a covered stent for coarctation: delayed recognition. Catheter Cardiovasc Interv 2006;68: 653–5.

49. Chakrabarti S, Kenny D, Morgan G, et al. Balloon expandable stent implantation for native and recurrent coarctation of the aorta: prospective computed tomography assessment of stent integrity, aneurysm formation and stenosis relief. Heart 2010;96:1212–6.

50. Rosenthal E, Bell A. Optimal imaging after coarctation stenting. Heart 2010;96:1169–71.

51. Duke C, Rosenthal E, Qureshi S. The efficacy and safety of stent redilatation in congenital heart disease. Heart 2003;89:905–12.

52. Butera G, Gaio G, Carminati M. Redilation of e-PTFE covered CP stents. Catheter Cardiovasc Interv 2008;72:273–7.

53. Ewert P, Schubert S, Peters B, et al. The CP stent—short, long, covered—for the treatment of aortic coarctation, stenosis of pulmonary arteries and caval veins, and Fontan anastomosis in children and adults: an evaluation of 60 stents in 53 patients. Heart 2005;81:948–53.

54. Tanous D, Collins N, Dehghani P, et al. Covered stents in the management of coarctation of the aorta in the adult: initial results and 1-year angiographic and hemodynamic follow-up. Int J Cardiol 2010; 140:287–95.

55. Butera G, Manica JL, Chessa M, et al. Covered-stent implantation to treat aortic coarctation. Expert Rev Med Devices 2012;9:123–30.

56. Krasemann T, Bano M, Rosenthal E, et al. Results of stent implantation for native and recurrent coarctation of the aorta-follow-up of up to 13 years. Catheter Cardiovasc Interv 2011;78:405–12.

57. Pádua LM, Garcia LC, Rubira CJ, et al. Stent placement versus surgery for coarctation of the thoracic aorta. Cochrane Database Syst Rev 2012;16:5.

58. Ewert P, Peters B, Nagdyman N, et al. Early and midterm results with the Growth Stent–a possible concept for transcatheter treatment of aortic coarctation from infancy to adulthood by stent implantation? Catheter Cardiovasc Interv 2008;7:120–6.

59. Waksman R, Maluenda G. Polymer drug-eluting stents: is the future biodegradable? Lancet 2011; 378:1900–2.

Catheter Interventions for Pulmonary Artery Stenosis
Matching the Intervention with the Pathology

Asra Khan, MD[a], Frank F. Ing, MD[b],*

KEYWORDS

- Pulmonary artery stenosis • Catheter intervention • Dilation balloons • Angioplasty

KEY POINTS

- Pulmonary artery (PA) stenosis represents a heterogeneous defect with a wide morphology and etiology.
- Types of interventions to treat PA stenosis should be based on the location, severity, and cause of stenosis as well as the size of patient at presentation.
- A variety of specialized dilation balloons including ultrahigh-pressure and cutting balloons are available to treat PA stenosis.
- There are many types of stents available, and many delivery techniques have been developed to treat a variety of PA stenoses in small infants through adulthood.
- Early and intermediate results of angioplasty and stenting are superior to surgical results, while long-term data on angioplasty and stenting now becoming available show these techniques to be safe and effective.

INTRODUCTION

Pulmonary artery (PA) stenosis is a common but heterogeneous defect associated with multiple forms of congenital heart disease and genetic syndromes. Surgical repair may itself cause or exacerbate PA stenosis. Treatment options include surgical repair, angioplasty using standard angioplasty balloons, cutting balloons, high-pressure or ultrahigh-pressure balloons, and stent implantation, each with its own set of advantages and disadvantages. Surgical repair had been the primary option offered until the 1980s when dilation balloons became available. Over time, PA angioplasty and stent implantation have become the preferred treatment option for patients of all ages. However, careful consideration should be given to the anatomy and cause of the stenosis as well as its relationship to adjacent anatomy when planning these interventions. The purpose of this article is to review the diversity of PA stenosis and discuss the treatment options based on the anatomy of the stenosis.

TREATMENT OPTIONS
Surgical Repair

Surgical techniques used to repair PA stenosis include excision of a focal stenosis and reanastomosis for discrete lesions, "V-Y" advancement flaps, patch augmentation using pericardium, Gortex, or even azygous venous grafts, and use of intraoperative dilators. Careful planning to address pulmonary stenosis while tackling associated

a Baylor College of Medicine, One Baylor Plaza, Houston, TX 77030, USA; b Cardiac Catheterization Laboratory, Pediatric Cardiology, Children's Hospital Los Angeles, University of Southern California, 4650 Sunset Boulevard, Mailstop #34, Los Angeles, CA 90027, USA
* Corresponding author.
E-mail address: frankfing@gmail.com

Intervent Cardiol Clin 2 (2013) 131–151
http://dx.doi.org/10.1016/j.iccl.2012.09.013
2211-7458/13/$ – see front matter © 2013 Elsevier Inc. All rights reserved.

lesions can avoid any additional procedure. Occasionally, aortopulmonary shunts are used to enhance growth in patients with severely hypoplastic pulmonary vasculature, before surgical repair.[1,2] Such a strategy is especially useful for patients with significant size discrepancy between the 2 branches or with stenosis secondary to ductal constriction. However, such shunts including the Blalock-Taussig shunt are also associated with significant stenosis and distortion, and subsequent decreased interval growth of the branch PA.[3] Extensive reconstruction of severe bilateral PA stenosis has also been achieved using a staged approach with pericardial rolls.[4] In addition to the risk of bypass and high rates of restenosis at the anastomotic site, the surgical approach is limited primarily to hilar vessels proximal to the lobar branches. Patients with more distal stenosis or diffusely hypoplastic systems are less suitable for surgical repair, especially if the procedure is a reoperation whereby significant scarring may increase morbidity (ie, bleeding and injury to the recurrent laryngeal nerves). There are few published data on the success rates of surgical repair, which perhaps is a testament of its rather poor outcome. In the 1960s to 1980s, restenosis rates ranged from 50% to 60%. In the 1990s, the few articles on this topic suggest that an overall success rate for surgical repair remains approximately 30% with a 35% to 40% recurrence rate, and long-term follow-up is lacking.[4,5]

Catheterization Laboratory Interventions

In general, all being equal, a lesser invasive intervention is preferred. That is, whenever angioplasty alone is effective, one should avoid implanting a stent. However, this decision is not always clear cut. Studies have shown that whereas angioplasty compared with stenting may have comparable immediate outcomes at best, intermediate and long-term effectiveness is less ideal because of vascular recoil. On the other hand, stenting in an infant or young child would commit the patient to repeated trips to the catheterization laboratory (cath lab) for further dilation as the patient grows to adult size. Furthermore, the smaller-sized patients may render the need for the larger delivery system for stenting difficult, if not impossible. A decision for angioplasty versus stenting may also depend on the skill level and experience of the interventionist.

Angioplasty

Angioplasty was first introduced as an alternative to surgery to address proximal stenosis in the late 1980s.[6,7] Early results were comparable with those of surgery. With the availability of a wider range of

sizes and lower-profile balloons, almost all types of lesions can be accessed by angioplasty. Using angioplasty alone in adults with isolated, multifocal PA stenosis has also shown symptomatic improvement, sustained over a medium-range follow-up.[8] However, data also show angioplasty alone to have a success rate of only 50% to 60%, with a recurrence rate of 15% to 35%.[5,9–12] Predictive factors for restenosis are yet to be identified in this population. Recent studies suggest a difference in response to angioplasty between the proximal and distal lesions.[13] Although balloons can successfully expand to the desired diameter, the proximal vessels are often compliant with higher recoil rate once the balloon is removed. Distal lesions may require dilation with larger-sized and higher-pressure balloons, but show an improved and more sustained response to angioplasty.

Ultrahigh-pressure angioplasty

High-pressure balloons made of noncompliant polyethylene terephthalate or nylon were initially introduced in the early 1970s, and have been used to treat resistant hemodialysis-related venous stenosis[14] and coronary lesions.[15,16] Currently available high-pressure balloons can achieve pressures as high as 17 to 27 atm or more, as opposed to the more compliant low-pressure balloons that normally generate 3 to 12 atm. Availability of smaller sizes and lower-profile balloons has allowed used in smaller patients. Initial experience with high-pressure angioplasty for resistant lesions showed an increase in success rates from 59% using low-pressure balloons to 72%.[17] Nevertheless, mid-term follow-up has shown a high (44%) restenosis rate.[18]

High-pressure angioplasty seems to be more successful in postsurgical sites.[17] Such angioplasties have been extremely useful in treating in-stent or peri-stent restenosis resistant to standard angioplasty.[19] The special arrangement of the woven fibers surrounding the balloons prevents eccentric expansion and therefore prevents asymmetric dilation of previously placed stents during redilation. Recent reports have shown that these balloons can be used to intentionally fracture previously implanted small stents in patients who have outgrown their stents, thus allowing for further expansion beyond their maximal diameters.[20,21]

Cutting balloon

Cutting balloons have added a new facet to angioplasty, especially when dealing with resistant lesions. Angioplasty relies on creating tears in the intima and media of the stenotic vessel, but high-pressure balloons can cause uncontrolled tears in the area of interest as well as in the adjacent vascular lumen. Cutting balloons are designed with 3 to 4 microblades mounted on a noncompliant balloon to provide precise scoring at the area of stenosis (**Fig. 1**).[22] These microtomes offer several controlled, longitudinal tears in the arterial lumen, decreasing the risk of dissection or intimal flaps. However, care must be taken to refrain from oversizing such balloons. Long sheaths positioned adjacent to the stenotic segment and slow inflation and deflation, 1 atm at a time, are required to unfold and fold the microtomes properly to avoid injury to the vasculature. Care must also be taken to withdraw the balloon into the protective long sheaths to avoid dislodging the microtomes.

Cutting balloons have been shown to be more effective than angioplasty using high-pressure balloons in a recent randomized trial,[23] similar to results seen when using cutting balloons for other noncardiac lesions.[24] Cutting balloons can be used to initially "score" the resistant lesion, followed by angioplasty with a larger balloon to further increase luminal size. This technique can also be applied before stenting of complex stenoses[25] or in patients with Williams and Alagille syndrome, who traditionally have poor responses to angioplasty and with a higher complication rate.[26,27] Unfortunately, owing to the limited sizes available (2–8 mm), use of cutting balloons is limited to smaller vessels at this time.

Stent implantation

Stent implantation is usually reserved for lesions unresponsive to angioplasty or as a bail-out to treat dissections and intimal flaps. Unfortunately, this is more often the rule than the exception. Lesions not responsive to angioplasty alone can be simply resistant to the inflation pressure used. Alternatively, they are complaint but have a tendency to recoil or are created by complex folds or external compression. In the first scenario, the resistant lesion can be treated with a high-pressure or cutting balloon followed by stent implantation. In the latter situation, stent implantation provides more structural support against recoil or external compression. Studies evaluating the effects of stent implantation report success rates as high as 90% to 100% with good medium-term and long-term follow-up.[28–31]

One major disadvantage to stent implantation is the need for serial further dilation to match somatic growth. Stented patients require follow-up with echocardiograms, magnetic resonance imaging (MRI), or lung perfusion scans to assess for restenosis and regional flow. Currently available stents come in all sizes ranging from coronary size (dilatable to 4 mm) to extra-large (dilatable to 25 mm in diameter). Proper selection is crucial. In general, the stent selected should have the capability of expanding to the native adult size of the vessel in which it is implanted. In the proximal branch PA, the "large" size stent (dilatable to 18 mm) should be selected whereas "medium" size stents (dilatable to 12–14 mm) can be used in lobar branches. However, in infants and small children, implanting large stents may be difficult if not impossible because of the relatively larger and stiffer delivery systems required. Various new techniques to overcome the size mismatch are beyond the scope of this article. There have been several recent reports advocating the use of premounted medium-size and even small coronary stents in infants, which is discussed later in this article. It should be kept in mind that there is considerable stent foreshortening (up to 60%) when stents are dilated to their maximal diameters.

HETEROGENEITY OF PULMONARY ARTERY STENOSIS

Branch PA stenosis presents in a variety of locations along the pulmonary arterial tree, starting from the main trunk to the right and left main branch to the lobar branches to segmental and subsegmental branches. In addition, the stenosis can be located at the ostia of the main branch, and ostia of the lobar and segmental branches. The stenoses can be quite complex, involving a variety of combinations of involved branches, unilaterally or bilaterally. The morphology of the stenosis can also be diverse, ranging from single discrete lesions to long segments to a hypoplastic pulmonary vascular bed (**Fig. 2**). The stenosis can

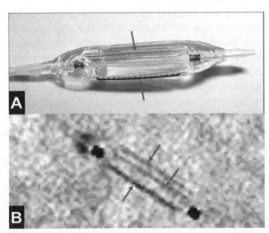

Fig. 1. (*A*) Cutting balloon with 4 longitudinally mounted microtomes (*red arrows*) with working height of 0.005 inch (0.0127 cm). (*B*) Magnified fluoroscopic image of inflated cutting balloon. Microtomes are identified by red arrows.

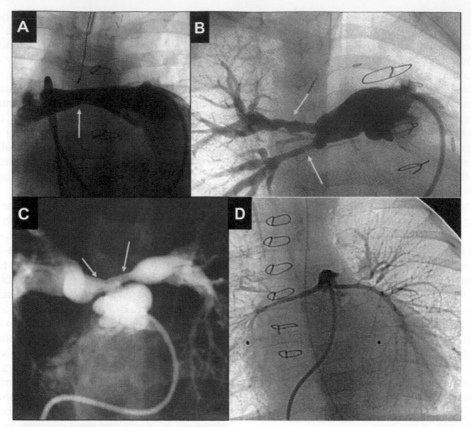

Fig. 2. (*A*) Simple mid-branch discrete stenosis. (*B*) Upper and lower lobar stenosis. (*C*) Bilateral ostial stenosis following arterial switch for d-transposition of the great arteries (d-TGA). (*D*) Williams syndrome with severe hypoplastic pulmonary arterial tree.

also be due to a fold or kink at a branch point, most commonly seen at the take-off of a main branch from the main PA (MPA). Long-segment stenosis starting at a branch orifice can also be due to "stretching" of the branch PA after a LeCompte maneuver. Other causes include external compression usually caused by a dilated pulsatile ascending aorta. Postsurgical stenosis may be due to scar formation over time or unintended twists of the segment at the time of the surgical anastomosis. Congenital stenosis is associated with a variety of syndromes such as Williams and Alagille syndromes or unidentified arteriopathies. These types of stenoses can represent the most complex and severe stenoses found, because they often involve multiple levels of branching (see **Fig. 2**D).

Proximal Main Branch Pulmonary Artery Stenosis

Proximal PA stenosis is commonly seen in tetralogy of Fallot, d-transposition of the great arteries (d-TGA), truncus arteriosus, and pulmonary atresia with or without ventricular septal defects, both before and after surgical repair. Isolated branch PA stenosis or isolation secondary to ductal constriction is a rare entity, requiring a high index of suspicion. When treating proximal PA stenosis, the 3-dimensional relationship of the stenotic segment to its side branches and adjacent anatomy need to be fully evaluated to successfully relieve the stenosis without compromising flow to other branches. Obtaining a second venous access to position an angiographic catheter proximally for repeat angiograms before and after interventions can be helpful in such situations. Recent introduction of rotational angiography has also helped to improve the understanding of the anatomy of the stenosis, especially in relation to adjacent side branches.[32,33]

When deciding on the appropriate intervention for proximal branch PA stenosis, several anatomic factors need consideration:

Discrete stenosis

Discrete branch PA stenosis is relatively uncommon but, when found in the mid segment, it is most commonly due to anastomotic scars from a Blalock-Taussig shunt or at the anastomotic site of a patch-plasty. These types of stenoses are most amenable but not always to angioplasty alone. Balloon size chosen should be based on the adjacent segment with a normal diameter. General sizing should range between 100% and 120% of the normal diameter but no more than 3 to 4 times the minimal diameter. Stenting can be considered if angioplasty fails to adequately relieve the obstruction. Discrete stenosis located at the ostium is more common and can be due to a fold/kink that develops as the main PA dilates and forms an angle between the main and branch PAs. Multiple angulations may be needed to fully assess the ostial stenosis because it may be superimposed by a dilated MPA (**Fig. 3**). These types of stenoses are not amenable to angioplasty and almost always require a stent to provide structural support. This aspect is discussed this later in this article.

Long-segment stenosis

This type of stenosis is more commonly found at the main left and right branches. The length may span from the ostium to the take-off of the upper lobes and even into the lower lobes in severe cases. Long-segment stenoses can be found in the congenital form or postoperatively after patch-plasty. Angioplasty alone is rarely effective beyond short-term results, and stenting is almost always the better option to relieve the obstruction. However, it is reasonable to attempt angioplasty first if only to assess the vessel resistance to dilation before stenting. If a long-segment stenosis is highly resistant to dilation, primary stenting may result in balloon-stent slippage as the balloon expands and in potential stent embolization. By "softening" the stenosis with angioplasty first, the stent may be more stable as it expands in the

intended position. In infants and small children who may not tolerate a large delivery system for stenting, one option is to palliate with angioplasty to allow time for somatic growth before stenting. However, this strategy is suboptimal because it may require repeated and frequent redilations, usually with only marginal benefits. The author advocates early and aggressive stenting in this situation to optimize flow to the distal pulmonary parenchyma for maximal growth and development of the distal small vessels (**Fig. 4**). Choosing the appropriate stent and balloon is beyond the scope of this article.

Ostial stenosis and bilateral branch stenosis with closely related ostia

Bilateral PA stenoses that involve the ostia or in the presence of closely related ostia can be found after truncus arteriosus repair or after LeCompte repair for d-TGA. The stenosis may appear as "Y" shaped, involving the distal main PA or conduit and both ostia and proximal branches. This type of stenosis presents a unique problem and can be technically challenging. Angioplasty is usually ineffective. However, stenting one branch will risk jailing the contralateral branch. In this situation, simultaneous stent implantation in both branches is the preferred option (**Fig. 5**).[34] By implanting both stents simultaneously, future access to both branches is ensured. It is equally important to inflate and deflate both balloons simultaneously to avoid compressing either stent. In smaller children who may not tolerate two large delivery systems, a hybrid approach may be necessary. One additional advantage of the hybrid approach is that the implanted stents can be adjusted or trimmed precisely to avoid jailing of either branches. Occasionally, trimming the medial

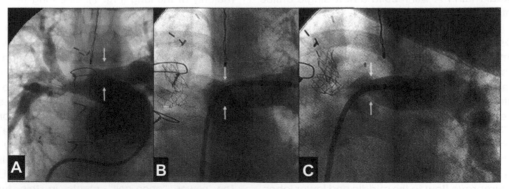

Fig. 3. Multiple angiograms may be needed to accurately assess pulmonary artery (PA) anatomy. (*A*) right PA (RPA) stenosis at distal branch and at lobar branches are easily seen, but left PA (LPA) orifice stenosis (*red arrows*) is obscured by anterior main PA in the standard anteroposterior (AP) projection. (*B*) At 20° right anterior oblique (RAO)/20° cranial angulation, LPA orifice stenosis does not appear to be severe. (*C*) At 30° RAO/30° cranial angulation, LPA orifice stenosis is finally noted to be significant.

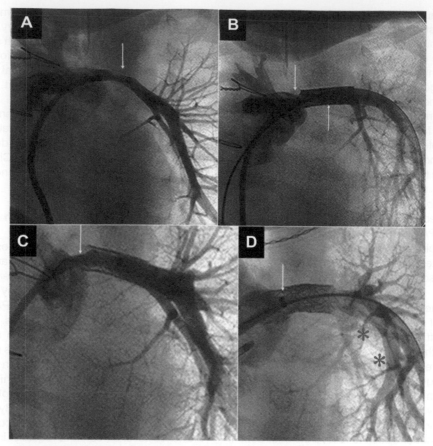

Fig. 4. (*A*) Severe hypoplasia of the left pulmonary arterial tree with 2.0-mm minimum diameter proximally (*red arrow*) in this infant. (*B*) Post stent implant with small residual stenosis proximally measuring 4.8 mm (*red arrow*). Stent diameter measures 6 mm (*yellow arrow*). (*C*) Follow-up catheterization 6 months later: intimal proliferation is noted proximally with minimum diameter now at 2.4 mm (*red arrow*). (*D*) After implantation of additional stent. Minimum diameter is now 6.8 mm (*red arrow*). Note distal vessels have grown significantly with improved flow (*red asterisks*).

edges and folding back the lateral edges against the distal main PA will rebuild a new single orifice for both branch PAs (**Fig. 6**).

Stenosis adjacent to a major side branch

Treatment of a main-branch stenosis that spans across a major side branch (usually the upper lobe) also presents a unique problem. Again, these are almost always long-segment stenoses and require a stent for long-term relief of the obstruction. The major problem in this type of stenosis is that any implanted stent will jail the adjacent side branch. One strategy used early in the stent experience was to intentionally stent across the upper lobe to improve flow to the middle and lower lobes. Because there are more segments in the middle and lower lobes, even if the upper lobe segments were completely jailed and obstructed the overall effect would still lower the pressure load on the

right ventricle and improve overall flow to the majority of the lung (**Fig. 7**). One long-term study reported 27 of 55 stents (49%) resulted in partial or complete jailing of a side branch with 16% showing no compromise in flow, 24% diminished flow, and only 9% complete obstruction.[28] Of interest, the right ventricular (RV) pressure of this cohort improved from 86 ± 14 mm Hg to 60 ± 18 mm Hg ($P = .005$) at 6.5 ± 3.9 years, similar to the group that did not have a jailed side branch. Although intentionally jailing the upper lobe is not an ideal approach, this long-term study does show it is an effective method to relieve this type of stenosis and lower the RV pressure. Use of the newer "open-cell" stents in this type of anatomy allows dilation of the jailed side branch through the side cells of the stent (**Figs. 8 and 9**). The open-cell configuration in the Mega LD stent can be dilated to 12 mm diameter. Another newly

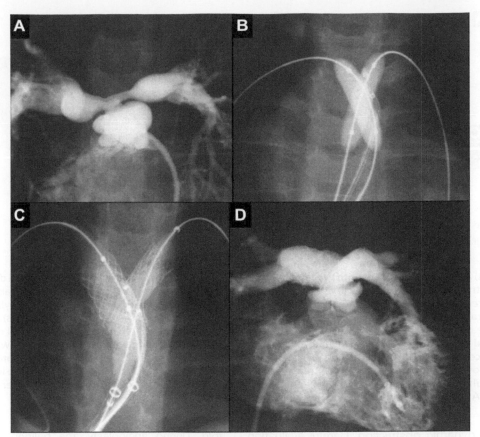

Fig. 5. (*A*) Bilateral proximal branch PA stenosis with closely related ostia following arterial switch with LeCompte maneuver in a 2-year-old with d-TGA. (*B*) Simultaneous angioplasty of both branch PAs to test balloon stability. (*C*) Simultaneous implantation of 2 Palmaz XD stents into proximal branches. (*D*) Poststent angiogram shows significant improvement in caliber of both branch PAs. Bilateral stents prevent jailing to either branch and permit future access for further dilations.

described technique is to trim the stent length to fit the anatomy of the patient. This technique is particularly useful for smaller patients in whom the stenotic length between the branch orifice and the take-off of the upper lobe is short (**Fig. 10**) (author's personal experience).

Stenosis caused by external compression

Another common cause of proximal branch PA stenosis in congenital heart disease is extrinsic compression from a dilated aorta, especially in patients with tetralogy of Fallot with a right aortic arch. The right PA is often compressed as it passes between the ascending and descending aorta (**Fig. 11**). The Norwood operation in hypoplastic left heart syndrome can also result in a dilated neo-aorta that can anteriorly compress the left PA. The LeCompte maneuver for repair of d-TGA results in the branch PAs anteriorly straddling the ascending aorta. Occasionally, this configuration can cause proximal compression of

both branch PAs by the pulsating ascending aorta. Cardiac imaging such as MRI or a computed tomographic angiogram can demonstrate all of these types of compression well. Angioplasty is of limited benefit in such anatomy, and stent implantation is often required to provide structural support. However, there are a few case reports of stent implantation in branch pulmonary stenosis due to extrinsic compression by a dilated aorta that later erodes into the aorta or causes an aorto-pulmonary communication.[35,36] Fortunately, these erosions can be treated with a covered stent.

Stenosis caused by folding/kinking/twisting

Occasionally, the main PA in patients with tetralogy of Fallot who have undergone a transannular patch repair become dilated and pulsatile. The geometric change caused by the dilation results in a posterior shift, which causes an angle to be formed between the main and branch PAs. A fold at the branch orifice develops, which can

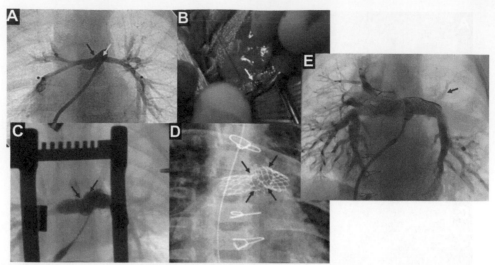

Fig. 6. (*A*) A 2-month-old infant with Williams syndrome with severe bilateral stenosis of branch PAs and depressed right ventricular (RV) function. Distal vessels are also hypoplastic. Note that ostia of both branch PAs are also closely related (*red arrows*). (*B*) Implantation of stents into both branches using a hybrid approach. (*C*) Post–hybrid stent intraoperative angiogram. Notice significant improvement in caliber of proximal branch PAs (*red arrows*). (*D*) Post-operative chest radiograph showing intraoperative modification of proximal stent struts with removal of medial edges and flaring of lateral struts to create a single opening at the distal main PA (MPA). This technique will permit future access to both PAs for further rehabilitation in the cath lab. (*E*) After 3 follow-up catheterizations and further dilations over a 26-month period, the PA tree is tediously rehabilitated. Note LPA stent that has jailed the left upper lobe, resulting in compromise of flow and less vessel growth in that lobe (*red arrow*). However, left lower lobe and entire RPA has grown significantly and overall RV pressure has normalized.

cause a dynamic obstruction. Careful evaluation with angiograms obtained in multiple views and careful assessment in systole and diastole are required to delineate such lesions. One clue of such an obstruction is straightening of the angle when a stiff wire or sheath is passed across the

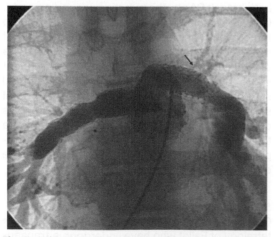

Fig. 7. Bilateral stents placed in this patient with bilateral branch pulmonary stenosis (PS). The LPA stent is intentionally implanted across the left upper lobe to improve the flow to the larger lower lobe. Although LPA flow is compromised (*red arrow*), the overall effect is still decreased pressure load on the right ventricle.

fold. During angioplasty, the balloon will fully inflate without any obvious waist under low pressures. This angle along with the obstruction will recur once the balloon is deflated and the wire is removed. Follow-up angiograms will show the same fold. In fact, it is also not uncommon for the surgeon to misinterpret patency in a stenotic ostial fold when he easily passes a dilator into an ostium of a branch PA that straightens out the bend temporarily, but once the dilator is removed, the fold returns and ostial stenosis recurs postoperatively. Such folds or kinks are not caused by a restrictive potential circumference of the ostium, and the best way to relieve such obstructions is to implant a stent to straighten out and provide structural support for the bend at the ostium (**Fig. 12**).

Infants and small children

Proximal PA stenosis in infants and toddlers is an especially challenging situation. Current technology limits the use of large stents in these cases because of a high risk of vascular injury from the large sheath sizes, the tight curve of the RV outflow tract, and the limited lengths of the stents available. Small coronary or medium-sized premounted stents have been used in certain cases as palliative measures until future surgeries. However, because these small stents cannot be

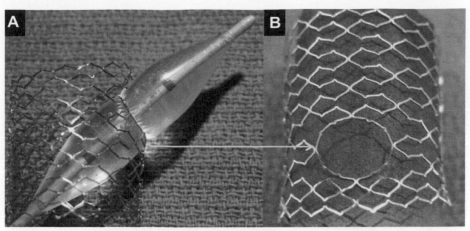

Fig. 8. (*A*) A 12-mm balloon inflated across a side cell of a Mega LD stent. (*B*) "Open-cell" design of this stent allows creation of a 12-mm diameter side orifice as a result of balloon dilation across the side cells.

dilated to the adult diameters, these stents will have to be surgically removed or cut to provide large diameters for the growing child. A few case reports show that high-pressure balloons can be used to intentionally fracture these stents to allow for further expansion beyond the intrinsic stent diameters. However, the area of further circumferential expansion in a fractured stent is limited to the site of the fracture, and dissection or aneurysm formation is a risk. There are no long-term studies showing the safety and efficacy of this technique at present, especially regarding further expansion from infant to adult size. "Tailoring" the stent by trimming and folding can be done using a hybrid approach, while shortening the stent length can allow better matching of the stent to the PA length in the cath lab (see **Figs. 6** and **10**). Various interventional options are discussed here.

Angioplasty A common approach is to palliate these small patients with serial angioplasties,

followed by surgical repair or stent implantation once they are older and larger. Repeated catheterizations and angioplasties may be required in such cases. This strategy includes the use of cutting balloons, which have shown promising results in short-term and medium-range follow-up when used in smaller vessels.[37] However, angioplasty in neonates less than 1 month old is associated with almost 2.5 times higher odds of complications.[38] A subset of infants benefiting from such interventions are those in the immediate postoperative period especially involving surgical sites. Such lesions can be effectively dilated using a balloon/stenosis ratio of 2.5:1 or less.[39,40]

Coronary and premounted stents Another strategy is to use the smaller coronary or medium-sized premounted stents for intermediate palliation in patients for whom larger stent delivery systems are limited by vascular access. In certain circumstances such as having to traverse an aortopulmonary shunt

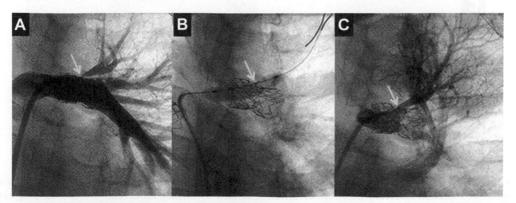

Fig. 9. (*A*) Example of a Mega LD stent implanted in the LPA jailing a left upper lobe. (*B*) Balloon dilation through a side cell into the left upper lobe. (*C*) Left upper lobe orifice diameter and distal flow improved significantly.

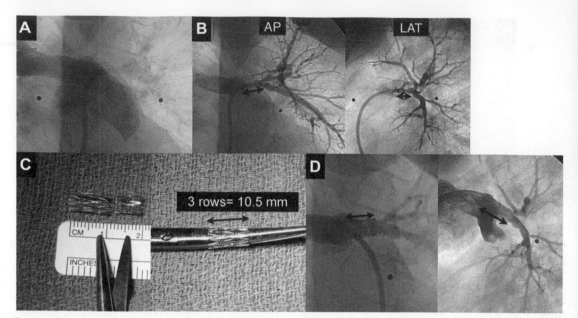

Fig. 10. (*A*) A 3-year-old (11.9 kg) boy status post repair for pulmonary atresia, ventricular septal defect (VSD), and AP collaterals with severe stenosis of LPA and significant decreased flow to the left lung. (*B*) Left anterior oblique and lateral projections show a very short landing zone (10 mm) between the LPA orifice and takeoff of left upper lobe (*red arrow*). (*C*) 1910 Genesis XD stent is cut to match the required length of stenosis. Three rows of this stent (*red arrow*) equals 10.5 mm, which will match the 10-mm landing zone in the LPA. (*D*) Poststent implant showing the stent does not protrude into the MPA and does not jail the left upper lobe (*red arrow*).

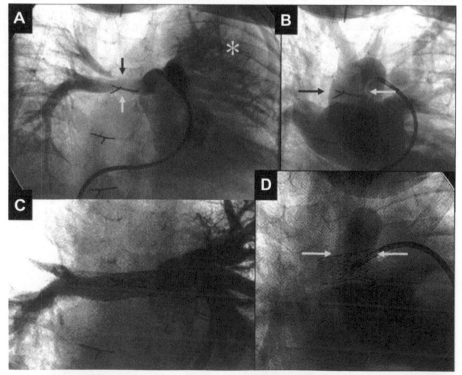

Fig. 11. (*A*) Severe RPA stenosis (*red arrows*) resulting in flow discrepancy favoring left lung (*red asterisk*). (*B*) Levophase of injection showing position of anterior dilated ascending aorta (*red arrows*) causing external compression of proximal RPA. (*C*) Poststent angiogram showing improvement in RPA diameter. (*D*) Levophase showing position of ascending aorta (*red arrow*) relative to stent position.

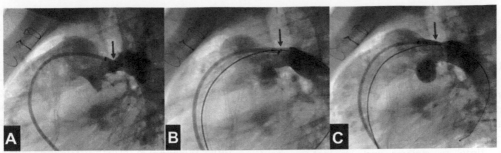

Fig. 12. (*A*) Lateral projection of an LPA ostial stenosis caused by a superior fold (*red arrow*). (*B*) Angiography demonstrating the fold to have to be straightened out by the stiff wire and an uninflated stent in position. (*C*) Poststent angiogram shows resolution of ostial fold.

to reach a stenotic PA, these premounted stents may be the only option to effectively relieve an obstruction. While stent dilation offers better acute and long-term outcomes when compared with angioplasty in these patients, the obvious limitation is that that these stents have limited maximal size and eventually would require surgical removal. Ideally, removing these stents should be coordinated with planned future surgery such as a conduit revision or Glenn and Fontan completion.[40,41] Coronary stent diameters can be dilated to around 4 to 5 mm and the medium-sized stents can go up to 10 to 12 mm. A more recent option is to use ultrahigh-pressure balloons to intentionally fracture an implanted stent beyond its intrinsic maximal diameter.[38] However, significant foreshortening of these stents often results in a napkin-ring configuration on further dilation to maximal sizes. It should be cautioned that intentional fracturing of a stent does not lead to a consistent result, and failure to "crack" such stents despite using ultrahigh-pressure balloons has been reported (**Fig. 13**). Nevertheless, limited intermediate-term studies indicate a low degree of in-stent restenosis and successful further dilation to match somatic growth.[42,43] Pass and colleagues[44] reported successful implantation of premounted stents without the use of a long sheath. This technique combined with the lower profile of the delivery system allows for more hemodynamic stability during stent implantation.[44,45] However, this is a controversial technique because there is no long sheath to retrieve or reposition stents if an adverse event (ie, balloon rupture, stent malposition) occurs. At present, the author does not advocate this potentially dangerous technique. The recent introduction of biodegradable stents may prove to be the best option for these younger patients in the future.[46]

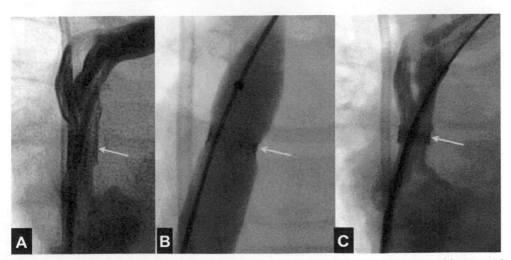

Fig. 13. (*A*) Premounted stent placed in a stenotic superior vena cava (*red arrow*). (*B*) Further dilation with larger balloon. Stent has expanded to its maximal diameter, which appears to take on a "napkin-ring" configuration (*red arrow*). (*C*) Balloon unable to fracture stent beyond its intrinsic diameter, which becomes the limiting size. (*Courtesy of* Dr Henri Justino.)

Stents If technically possible, implanting a large-size stent into a branch PA is the best option, and can be achieved in the cath lab in sizes down to 4 to 5 kg using currently available stents and balloons going through 7F-long sheaths (**Fig. 14**) Placement of stiff sheaths and wires can cause tricuspid and pulmonary valve regurgitation, resulting in hypotension. The hemodynamic derangement can often be treated at least transiently with administration of volume and systemic vasoconstrictors to "buy" enough time to deliver and implant a stent. However, this should be attempted only by experienced operators who know how to handle adverse events to avoid further complications. A tedious technique of cutting off a dilator tip and mounting it onto the tip of a balloon to act as a dilator, and front-loading a stent onto a long sheath for delivery, has allowed delivery of large-size stents through 7F sheaths into infants as small as 5 to 10 kg (**Fig. 15**).[47] This technique became obsolete when Genesis stents were introduced, which could be mounted on small (6 mm diameter) balloons and delivered through 7F sheaths. Nevertheless, it is a useful technique to use when implanting large stents in small infants with fragile hemodynamics.

Hybrid stenting Another alternative is a combined hybrid approach, which allows for not only easy access but also placement of large stents without compromising peripheral vessels.[48,49] Direct access into the main or proximal branch PA allows stent implantation without sheaths. Stents can also be customized to fit the anatomy and can be precisely implanted into proximal lesions under direct vision (see **Fig. 6**). However, careful planning with quality presurgical imaging and collaboration with surgeons is crucial.

Lobar Branch Pulmonary Artery Stenosis

Stenoses involving the distal branches, including lobar, segmental, and subsegmental branches, can be especially difficult to treat. Careful evaluation of their anatomy and their association with other branches is required. Whereas echocardiograms are essentially useless, MRI and 3-dimensional dynamic computed tomography can be extremely helpful when assessing these lesions. Multiple power injections and hand angiograms, performed at various nonstandard angles, may be required to understand the severity and nature of the lesion and its relationship to the unaffected segments. Careful assessment of proximal and distal vasculature to determine target dimension for the affected vessels is also important in planning the intervention.

Although stents can offer long-term efficacy, stenting lobar stenoses is associated with the risk of jailing off multiple segmental branches, and hence is not the first option. Cutting balloons and high-pressure balloons may be needed to dilate highly resistant lesions, although restenosis can occur. Unfortunately, most of these cases have stenoses at multiple levels and represent the most difficult lesions to treat. If angioplasty fails repeatedly, stents may be the only option even if it risks jailing off some of the segmental branches. In such cases, multiple small stents of

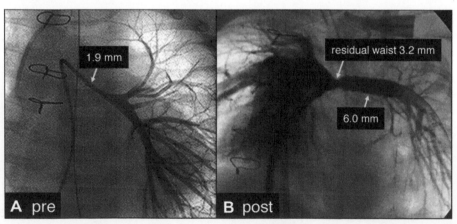

Fig. 14. (A) Angiogram of a 2-month-old (4.7 kg) with double-outlet right ventricle, aortic coarctation, and d-TGA with severe LPA stenosis after surgical repair. (B) Angiogram following implantation of a 16-mm long Doublestrut stent with a 6-mm balloon via 7F sheath. Note residual stenosis at the LPA orifice. During stent implantation, hypotension developed because of transient tricuspid and pulmonary insufficiency caused by a stiff sheath. This hypotension was treated with ephedrine, giving enough time for rapid stent delivery and implantation and very little time for precise positioning. Stiff wire and sheath were removed immediately following stent implant and angiography. Despite residual waist, the patient's hemodynamics improved significantly, allowing for successful extubation. Follow-up catheterization was performed for additional stent implants to treat residual stenosis.

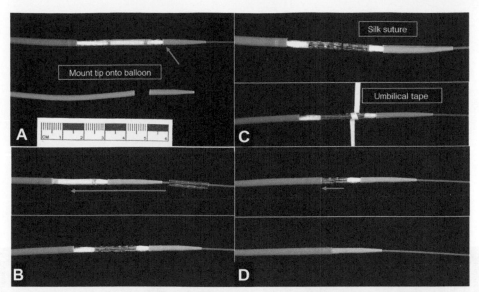

Fig. 15. Dilator-tipped balloon with front-loading technique. (*A*) Dilator tip of a long sheath cut and mounted onto the tip of a balloon that is front-loaded through the long sheath (*red arrow*). (*B*) Large stent is then mounted and crimped onto the balloon (*red arrow*). (*C*) The stent is secured onto the balloon using either a silk suture or an umbilical tape. (*D*) The entire "balloon-dilator tip-stent" unit is withdrawn into the sheath (*red arrow*) leaving only the dilator tip exposed at the end of the sheath to allow a smooth transition for passage into the femoral veins. Stent and balloon is front-loaded so that there is no need to advance the stent through the entire sheath once the sheath is in position, which minimizes stent slippage off the balloon during delivery.

varying lengths may be implanted simultaneously to treat the lobar stenosis and minimize the risk of jailing off some segmental branches (**Fig. 16**). Again, open-cell stents should also be considered in such situations, especially when redilation of side struts is required to improve flow in jailed-off branches while maintaining the overall integrity and radial strength of the stent (see **Fig. 9**).

Segmental and Subsegmental Pulmonary Artery Stenosis

Multilobar and subsegmental stenoses are frequently associated with Williams and Alagille syndromes as well as nonsyndromic ill-defined arteriopathies (**Fig. 17**). Often these branches are hypoplastic down to the pulmonary vasculature

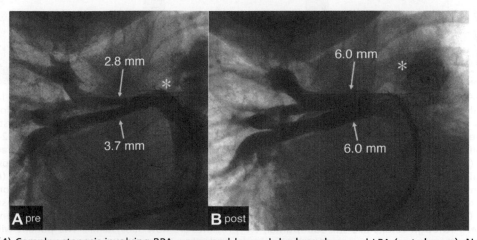

Fig. 16. (*A*) Complex stenosis involving RPA, upper and lower lobe branches, and LPA (not shown). Note stents already implanted into proximal RPA (*red asterisk*). (*B*) Simultaneous stents placed into right upper and lower lobes increase lobar diameters significantly and permit future access to both lobes for further dilation. An additional LPA stent is placed as well (*yellow asterisk*).

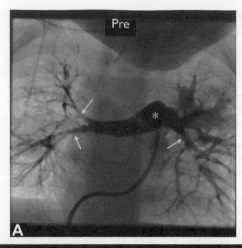

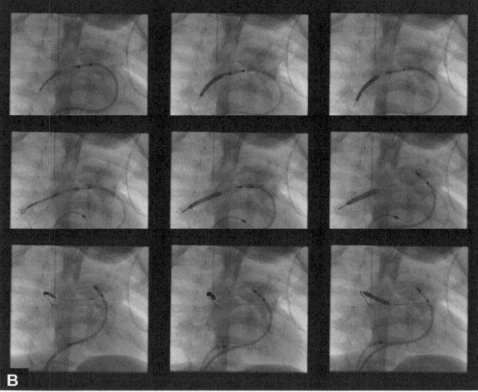

Fig. 17. (A) Alagille syndrome in a 2-month-old infant with severe bilateral branch PS involving lobar and segmental branches of RPA and branches of the left lower lobe (LLL) (red arrows). In the left upper lobe, there are areas of variable perfusion at the pulmonary vascular bed (red asterisk). RV pressure suprasystemic. (B) Tedious sequential angioplasty in the RPA lower and middle lobes and segmental branches using 2-, 3-, and 4-mm balloons. (C) Sequential angioplasty of right upper lobe segmental branches using 2-, 3-, and 4-mm balloons. (D) Angiogram after angioplasty of 10 segments in the RPA and LPA (red arrows). There is improvement in angioplastied lobar and segmental branches. Note the improvement in perfusion (red asterisks). (E) Lateral projection of RPA before and after angioplasty. For segmental branch dilations, lateral projection is more helpful to separate out anterior and posterior segments. Note the improvement in diameters of the dilated segmental branches (red arrows). (F) Pressure tracings of RV and fractional area before and after this 8-hour angioplasty procedure. Although results are still suboptimal, RV pressures are now subsystemic. The patient will require multiple interventions over years to rehabilitate this hypoplastic pulmonary arterial tree.

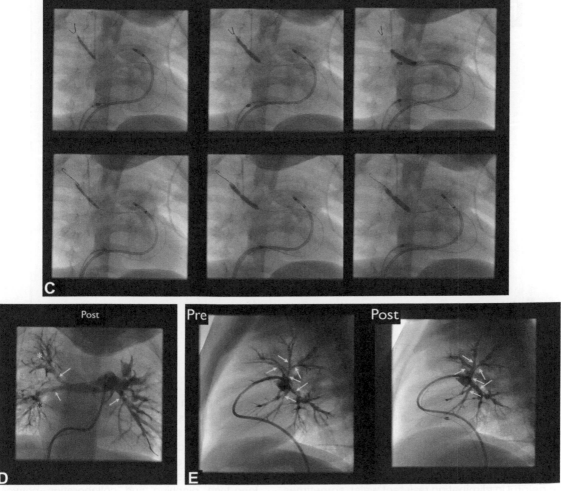

Fig. 17. (*continued*)

bed, but may be interspersed with normal vessels. These vessels are often resistant to dilation, with a higher rate of neointimal proliferation and restenosis. Cutting balloons and high-pressure balloons are often needed, but risks of dissection and aneurysm formation are reported. Hand injections performed in the small segmental and subsegmental branches in nonconventional projections can be extremely helpful in understanding the 3-dimensional nature of the stenosis as well as the relationship of the affected vessels with the surrounding vasculature. Biplane angiography is essential. Angioplasty is the preferred option at this level of stenosis because stents will certainly jail off multiple small but important side branches. Angioplasty of multiple vessels over many hours in the cath lab is the norm. Vascular access from bilateral femoral veins is highly recommended.

Unifocalized Aortopulmonary Collaterals

Subsets of patients requiring special consideration are those with pulmonary atresia with ventricular septal defect requiring unifocalization of aortopulmonary collaterals. Often these collaterals are attached to the native vessels in an end-to-side fashion that puts them at a risk of restenosis in the future. In addition, the sharp angles at the anastomosis make accessing these vessels very difficult. Another problem in such patients can be dual supply to segments, with stenosis of one or both of the limbs. Natural history of such vessels indicates progressive stenosis, secondary to intimal proliferation worsened by polycythemia seen in most patients. These vessels resemble bronchial arteries and are usually highly vasoreactive with variable wall thickness, resulting in a risk of complete obstruction or dissection on

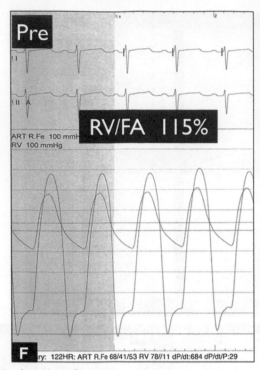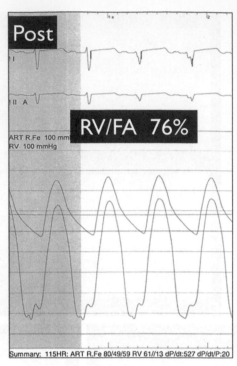

Fig. 17. (*continued*)

manipulation (**Fig. 18**). Such vessels generally require high-pressure angioplasty or cutting balloons to effectively score the fibrotic layers to allow further dilation.[50] However, care must be taken to avoid aggressive dilation and oversizing the balloon. Long inflation times can sometimes be helpful in eliminating resistant waist, sometimes requiring a few minutes. "Milking" of the balloon during inflation is a common problem encountered in such vessels, and this can be avoided by using long sheaths and refraining from oversizing the balloons. Predilation with a cutting balloon, if applicable, prevents suboptimal dilation of the stent. Management of this anatomy requires long-term planning and collaboration between the surgeon and interventionist. One strategy is

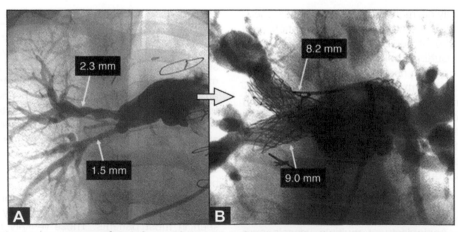

Fig. 18. (*A*) Initial angiogram of an infant with PA/VSD and major aortopulmonary collateral arteries status post unifocalization. Notice variable stenoses along 2 of the unifocalized collaterals to the RPA (*red arrow*). (*B*) Angiogram taken 3 years and 7 catheterizations later, after multiple angioplasties, stent implantations, and further dilations, shows that collaterals and distal perfusion are near normal.

early surgical repair with unifocalization and placement of an RV to PA conduit to provide a pathway to the stenotic pulmonary branches. The interventionist will use this pathway to perform rehabilitation of the pulmonary arterial tree over time. Pulmonary atresia with major aortopulmonary collateral arteries along with congenital branch pulmonary stenosis are the anatomic substrates that provide for some of the most tedious and painstakingly long interventional procedures encountered (see **Fig. 18**). A hybrid approach can be useful in younger patients or those with diffusely hypoplastic pulmonary vasculature. Occasionally, these collaterals are found to be nearly or completely atretic with no collateral supply, before or after unifocalization, resulting in loss of valuable lung segments. Recanalization of such vessels requires the use of hydrophilic wires (Glide wire) followed by serial dilation and possibly stent implantation (**Fig. 19**). Techniques using rotational ablation assisted balloon angioplasty have also been reported.[51] Because of the risk of rupture, covered stents are recommended as backup for such procedures.

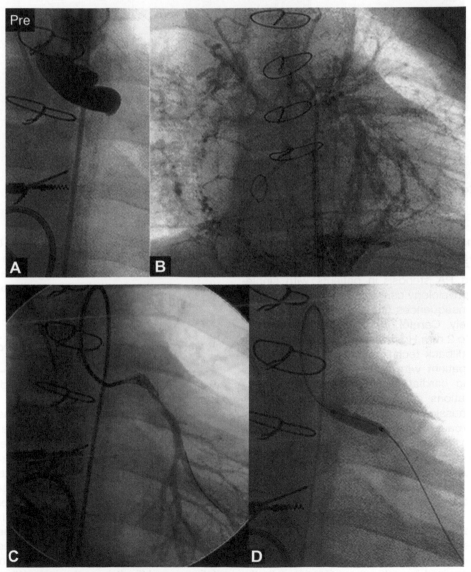

Fig. 19. (*A*) Complete occlusion of proximal LPA following unifocalization and aortopulmonary shunt. (*B*) Aortogram showing residual small vessel collateral flow to distal LPA. (*C*) Recannulated occluded vessel. (*D*) Angioplasty with 4-mm balloon. (*E*) Implantation of 2 Genesis premounted stents on 5-mm balloons. (*F*) Postintervention angiogram showing reestablishment of flow to LLL.

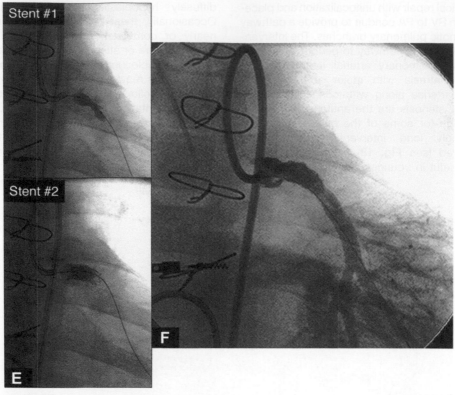

Fig. 19. (*continued*)

Pulmonary Artery Stenosis in Single-Ventricle Physiology

Even mild PA stenosis in patients with single-ventricle physiology can have significant hemodynamic consequences and should be addressed aggressively. Careful evaluation for gradients as low as 1 to 2 mm Hg measured simultaneously or using a pullback technique should be performed in every patient with single-ventricle physiology undergoing cardiac catheterization. Stenosis is such situations can be secondary to previous Blalock-Taussig or other aortopulmonary shunts, which can cause significant distortion of the branch PAs. It can also be a result of extrinsic compression by a dilated aorta or other surrounding structures.[52] For patients scheduled for surgical palliation, aggressive angioplasty can be helpful. However, occasionally these segments remain stenotic despite extensive reconstruction and patch augmentation at the time of surgery. Such patients should be closely followed up after surgical repair to assess for residual stenosis. Stent implantation is often required in such cases. Occasionally the upper lobe branches may become stenotic or completely occluded after cavopulmonary anastomosis. Flow to these segments should be carefully

assessed at the time of catheterization. Choice of angioplasty or stenting depends on the anatomy and nature of the stenosis, but aggressive intervention is essential to optimize flow into the pulmonary arterial tree in these patients who do not have a pulmonary pumping chamber (**Fig. 20**).

Pulmonary Artery Stenosis Associated with Genetic Syndromes

Genetic syndromes such as Alagille and Williams syndromes are often associated with complex stenoses, ranging from diffuse hypoplasia of the entire pulmonary circulation to multisegmental involvement (see **Fig. 17**). Owing to the inherent elastic nature of these pulmonary vessels, they are often extremely resistant to intervention. Surgical repair is limited to the proximal segments, with some benefit. Catheter-based interventions have therefore become the primary therapy in such cases.[26,27,53–55] Because of the diffuse involvement, intervention in such cases can be difficult and time consuming, making stent implantation very difficult in such cases. When dealing with diffusely hypoplastic vessels, a careful evaluation of the goal for dilation is important. These vessels are at a higher risk of injury or dissection,

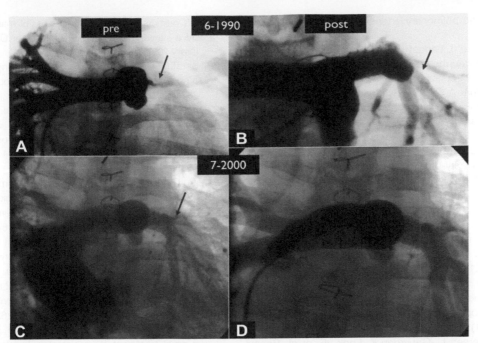

Fig. 20. (*A*) Severe stenosis and apparent hypoplastic LPA (*red arrow*) in a Fontan patient despite no gradient across stenosis because of lack of a pulmonary pumping chamber and essentially no flow to the LPA. (*B*) Angiogram following stent implant showing a small but well developed distal LPA (*red arrow*). (*C*) Ten-year follow-up showing excellent persistent flow to the LPA, especially LLL (*red arrow*). (*D*) Angiogram after further dilation of LPA stent (*red arrow*).

and aggressive overdilation should be avoided. Frequent serial dilation using high-pressure and cutting balloons may be required. These patients should be closely monitored and scheduled for redilation in 6 to 12 months as needed.

SUMMARY

Branch PA stenosis is a heterogeneous disease ranging from simple to complex, presenting at many levels along the pulmonary arterial tree. The causes are also varied, from congenital to postsurgical scars, inadequate surgery, folds, kinks, and external compression. These stenoses can present as mild discrete stenosis all the way to severe hypoplasia of the entire lung bed. The physiology can also vary depending on whether it is unilateral or bilateral, or in the presence of a 2-ventricle or single-ventricle circuit. Transcatheter interventions available to treat these stenoses include angioplasty, use of high-pressure or cutting balloons, and stenting. These interventions can be performed in the cath lab or in the operating room as a hybrid procedure. Careful consideration of the type of intervention and approach should be made based on the PA anatomy, the severity, and important adjacent structures. Finally, the interventionist should be fully familiar with all the tricks of the trade, the various pitfalls

of each procedure, and how to avoid and manage adverse events associated with these procedures.

REFERENCES

1. Brandt B 3rd, Camacho JA, Mahoney LT, et al. Growth of the pulmonary arteries following Blalock-Taussig shunt. Ann Thorac Surg 1986;42(Suppl 6):S1–4.
2. Potapov EV, Alexi-Meskishvili VV, Dähnert I, et al. Development of pulmonary arteries after central aortopulmonary shunt in newborns. Ann Thorac Surg 2001;71:899–905.
3. Gladman G, McCrindle BW, Williams WG, et al. The modified Blalock-Taussig shunt: clinical impact and morbidity in Fallot's tetralogy in the current era. J Thorac Cardiovasc Surg 1997;114:25–30.
4. Fraser CD Jr, Latson LA, Mee RB. Surgical repair of severe bilateral branch pulmonary artery stenosis. Ann Thorac Surg 1995;59(3):738–40.
5. Trant CA Jr, O'Laughlin MP, Ungerleider RM, et al. Cost-effectiveness analysis of stents, balloon angioplasty and surgery for the treatment of pulmonary artery stenosis. Pediatr Cardiol 1997;18:339–44.
6. Lock JE, Niemi T, Einzig S, et al. Transvenous angioplasty of experimental branch pulmonary artery stenosis in newborn lambs. Circulation 1981;64(5):886–93.
7. Lock JE, Castaneda-Zuniga WR, Fuhrman BP, et al. Balloon dilation angioplasty of hypoplastic and

stenotic pulmonary arteries. Circulation 1983;67(5): 962–7.

8. Kreutzer J, Landzberg MJ, Preminger TJ, et al. Isolated peripheral pulmonary artery stenoses in the adult. Circulation 1996;93:1417–23.

9. Rothman A, Perry SB, Keane JF, et al. Early results and follow-up of balloon angioplasty for branch pulmonary artery stenoses. J Am Coll Cardiol 1990;15(5): 1109–17.

10. Kan JS, Marvin WJ Jr, Bass JL, et al. Balloon angioplasty-branch pulmonary artery stenosis: results from the Valvuloplasty and Angioplasty of Congenital Anomalies Registry. Am J Cardiol 1990;65(11): 798–801.

11. Zeevi B, Berant M, Blieden LC. Midterm clinical impact versus procedural success of balloon angioplasty for pulmonary artery stenosis. Pediatr Cardiol 1997;18:101–6.

12. Bush DM, Hoffman TM, Del Rosario J, et al. Frequency of restenosis after balloon pulmonary arterioplasty and its causes. Am J Cardiol 2000; 86(11):1205–9.

13. Bergersen L, Gauvreau K, Lock JE, et al. Recent results of pulmonary arterial angioplasty: the differences between proximal and distal lesions. Cardiol Young 2005;15(6):597–604.

14. Glanz S, Gordon D, Butt K, et al. Stenotic lesions in dialysis-access fistulas: treatment by transluminal angioplasty using high-pressure balloons. Radiology 1985;156:236.

15. Nakamura S, Hall P, Gaglione A, et al. High pressure assisted coronary stent implantation accomplished without intravascular ultrasound guidance and subsequent anticoagulation. J Am Coll Cardiol 1997;29:21–7.

16. Holmes DR Jr, Hirshfeld J Jr, Faxon D, et al. ACC expert consensus document on coronary artery stents. Document of the American College of Cardiology. J Am Coll Cardiol 1998;32:1471–82.

17. Gentles TL, Lock JE, Perry SB. High pressure balloon angioplasty for branch pulmonary artery stenosis: early experience. J Am Coll Cardiol 1993; 22(3):867–72.

18. Ettinger LM, Hijazi ZM, Geggel GL, et al. Peripheral pulmonary artery stenosis: acute and mid-term results of high pressure balloon angioplasty. J Interv Cardiol 1998;11(4):337–44.

19. Maglione J, Bergersen L, Lock JE, et al. Ultra-high-pressure balloon angioplasty for treatment of resistant stenoses within or adjacent to previously implanted pulmonary arterial stents. Circ Cardiovasc Interv 2009;2(1):52–8.

20. Bergersen LT, Gauvreau K, Marshall A, et al. Procedure type risk groups for pediatric and congenital cardiac catheterization. Circ Cardiovasc Interv 2011;4:188–94.

21. Knirsch W, Haas NA, Lewin MA, et al. Longitudinal stent fracture 11 months after implantation in the left pulmonary artery and successful management by a stent-in-stent maneuver. Catheter Cardiovasc Interv 2003;58(1):116–8.

22. Barath P, Fishbein M, Vari S, et al. Cutting balloon: a novel approach to percutaneous angioplasty. Am J Cardiol 1991;68:1249–52.

23. Bergersen L, Gauvreau K, Justino H, et al. Randomized trial of cutting balloon compared with high-pressure angioplasty for the treatment of resistant pulmonary artery stenosis. Circulation 2011;124(22): 2388–96.

24. Wu CC, Lin MC, Pu SY, et al. Comparison of cutting balloon versus high-pressure balloon angioplasty for resistant venous stenoses of native hemodialysis fistulas. J Vasc Interv Radiol 2008;19(6):877–83.

25. Bergersen LJ, Perry SB, Lock JE. Effect of cutting balloon angioplasty on resistant pulmonary artery stenosis. Am J Cardiol 2003;91(2):185–9.

26. Sugiyama H, Veldtman GR, Norgard G, et al. Bladed balloon angioplasty for peripheral pulmonary artery stenosis. Catheter Cardiovasc Interv 2004;62(1):71–7.

27. Gogola L, Veldtman GR. Endoarterial scoring— a novel treatment for resistant pulmonary arterial lesions associated with Williams-Beuren syndrome. J Invasive Cardiol 2010;22(4):E56–8.

28. Law MA, Shamszad P, Nugent AW, et al. Pulmonary artery stents: long-term follow-up. Catheter Cardiovasc Interv 2010;75(5):757–64.

29. Spadoni I, Giusti S, Bertolaccini P, et al. Long-term follow-up of stents implanted to relieve peripheral pulmonary arterial stenosis: hemodynamic findings and results of lung perfusion scanning. Cardiol Young 1999;9(6):585–91.

30. Kenny D, Amin Z, Slyder S, et al. Medium-term outcomes for peripheral pulmonary artery stenting in adults with congenital heart disease. J Interv Cardiol 2011;24(4):373–7.

31. Shaffer KM, Mullins CE, Grifka RG, et al. Intravascular stents in congenital heart disease: short- and long-term results from a large single-center experience. J Am Coll Cardiol 1998;31(3):661–7.

32. Berman DP, Khan DM, Gutierrez Y, et al. The use of three-dimensional rotational angiography to assess the pulmonary circulation following cavo-pulmonary connection in patients with single ventricle. Catheter Cardiovasc Interv 2012. [Epub ahead of print].

33. Fagan T, Kay J, Carroll J, et al. 3-D guidance of complex pulmonary artery stent placement using reconstructed rotational angiography with live overlay. Catheter Cardiovasc Interv 2012;79(3):414–21.

34. Stapleton GE, Hamzeh R, Mullins CE, et al. Simultaneous stent implantation to treat bifurcation stenoses in the pulmonary arteries: initial results and long-term follow up. Catheter Cardiovasc Interv 2009;73(4): 557–63.

35. Carano N, Agnetti A, Tchana B, et al. Descending thoracic aorta to left pulmonary artery fistula after

stent implantation for acquired left pulmonary artery stenosis. J Interv Cardiol 2002;15(5):411–3.

36. Ailawadi G, Lim DS, Peeler BB, et al. Traumatic ascending aortopulmonary window following pulmonary artery stent dilatation: therapy with aortic endovascular stent graft. Pediatr Cardiol 2007;28(4):305–8.

37. Bergersen L, Jenkins KJ, Gauvreau K, et al. Follow-up results of cutting balloon angioplasty used to relieve stenoses in small pulmonary arteries. Cardiol Young 2005;15(6):605–10.

38. Holzer RJ, Gauvreau K, Kreutzer J, et al. Balloon angioplasty and stenting of branch pulmonary arteries: adverse events and procedural characteristics: results of a multi-institutional registry. Circ Cardiovasc Interv 2011;4(3):287–96.

39. Zahn EM, Dobrolet NC, Nykanen DG, et al. Interventional catheterization performed in the early postoperative period after congenital heart surgery in children. J Am Coll Cardiol 2004;43(7):1264–9.

40. Rosales AM, Lock JE, Perry SB, et al. Interventional catheterization management of perioperative peripheral pulmonary stenosis: balloon angioplasty or endovascular stenting. Catheter Cardiovasc Interv 2002;56(2):272–7.

41. Zeidenweber CM, Kim DW, Vincent RN. Right ventricular outflow tract and pulmonary artery stents in children under 18 months of age. Catheter Cardiovasc Interv 2007;69(1):23–7.

42. Stanfill R, Nykanen DG, Osorio S, et al. Stent implantation is effective treatment of vascular stenosis in young infants with congenital heart disease: acute implantation and long-term follow-up results. Catheter Cardiovasc Interv 2008;71(6):831–41.

43. Hatai Y, Nykanen DG, Williams WG, et al. Endovascular stents in children under 1 year of age: acute impact and late results. Br Heart J 1995;74(6):689–95.

44. Pass RH, Hsu DT, Garabedian CP, et al. Endovascular stent implantation in the pulmonary arteries of infants and children without the use of a long vascular sheath. Catheter Cardiovasc Interv 2002;55(4):505–9.

45. Moszura T, Michalak KW, Dryzek P, et al. One center experience in pulmonary artery stenting without long vascular sheath. Cardiol J 2010;17(2):149–56.

46. Zartner P, Cesnjevar R, Singer H, et al. First successful implantation of a biodegradable metal stent into the left pulmonary artery of a preterm baby. Catheter Cardiovasc Interv 2005;66(4):590–4.

47. Ing FF, Mathewson JC, Cocalis M, et al. A new technique for implantation of large stents through small sheaths in infants and children with branch pulmonary artery stenoses. J Am Coll Cardiol 2000;35(2 Suppl A):500A.

48. Holzer RJ, Chisolm JL, Hill SL, et al. "Hybrid" stent delivery in the pulmonary circulation. J Invasive Cardiol 2008;20:592–8.

49. Ing FF. Delivery of stents to target lesions: techniques of intraoperative stent implantation and intraoperative angiograms [review]. Pediatr Cardiol 2005;26(3):260–6.

50. Brown S, Eyskens B, Mertens L, et al. Percutaneous treatment of stenosed major aortopulmonary collaterals with balloon dilatation and stenting: what can be achieved? Heart 1998;79(1):24–8.

51. Wilson N, White C. Rotational ablation assisted angioplasty of an obstructed aortopulmonary collateral artery. Heart 1998;79(2):203–4.

52. Kretschmar O, Sglimbea A, Prêtre R, et al. Pulmonary artery stent implantation in children with single ventricle malformation before and after completion of partial and total cavopulmonary connections. J Interv Cardiol 2009;22(3):285–90.

53. Reesink HJ, Henneman OD, van Delden OM, et al. Pulmonary arterial stent implantation in an adult with Williams Syndrome. Cardiovasc Intervent Radiol 2007;30(4):782–5.

54. Saidi AS, Kovalchin JP, Fisher DJ, et al. Balloon pulmonary valvuloplasty and stent implantation. For peripheral pulmonary artery stenosis in Alagille syndrome. Tex Heart Inst J 1998;25(1):79–82.

55. Geggel RL, Gauvreau K, Lock JE. Balloon dilation angioplasty of peripheral pulmonary stenosis associated with Williams syndrome. Circulation 2001;103:2165–70.

Complex Interventions in the Adult with Congenital Heart Disease

Percutaneous Solutions for Venous Baffles, Coronary Artery Fistulas, and Ruptured Sinus of Valsalva Aneurysms

Harsimran S. Singh, MD, MSc[a,b], Christian Nagy, MD[b],
Andrea W. Wan, MD[c], Mark D. Osten, MD[b],
Lee N. Benson, MD[c], Eric M. Horlick, MD, CM, FRCPC[b,*]

KEYWORDS

- Adult congenital heart disease • Venous baffles • Coronary artery fistula,
- Sinus of valsalva aneurysm

KEY POINTS

- Adult congenital heart disease (ACHD) cases challenge the operator's knowledge of native and surgical anatomy and pathophysiology.
- The ACHD interventionalist must review the primary imaging personally and confirm the details before proceeding to intervention.
- As a general rule of thumb, intervention in the patient with ACHD should not be performed on an ad hoc basis, but rather carefully planned and discussed in a collaborative multi-disciplinary fashion.
- patients with ACHD and their families have high expectations of their providers with regard to procedural expertise, appropriate and complete consent, and explanation of a holistic long-term plan. An honest and direct approach to managing patient expectations and concerns pays substantial dividends in the long-term relationships that must be fostered by the health care team.
- Three distinct ACHD lesions that are amenable to percutaneous repair are (1) venous baffle obstruction in transposition of the great arteries (d-TGA), (2) coronary artery fistulas, and (3) ruptured sinus of Valsalva aneurysms.

Interventions in complex adult congenital heart disease (ACHD) can be the most challenging procedures performed in the catheterization laboratory. In addition to technical concerns, ACHD cases challenge the operator's knowledge of anatomy and pathophysiology, further compounded by multiple surgeries that span over decades. Comorbidities, challenging vascular access, and additional acquired defects further complicate the milieu.

a Division of Cardiology, Department of Medicine, New York Presbyterian Hospital, Weill Cornell Medical College, New York, NY, USA; b Division of Cardiology, Department of Medicine, Toronto General Hospital, University Health Network, University of Toronto School of Medicine, Toronto, Ontario, Canada; c Division of Cardiology, Department of Pediatrics, The Labatt Family Heart Center, The Hospital for Sick Children, University of Toronto School of Medicine, Toronto, Ontario, Canada
* Corresponding author. Toronto General Hospital, University of Toronto, 200 Elizabeth Street, 6E-249, Toronto, Ontario M5G 2G4, Canada.
E-mail address: eric.horlick@uhn.ca

Intervent Cardiol Clin 2 (2013) 153–172
http://dx.doi.org/10.1016/j.iccl.2012.09.010

The medical records of patients with ACHD are long, complicated, and oftentimes sprinkled with multiple levels of misinformation. Conflicting reports of prior surgeries and interventions can result from a lack of source documents and notes. The original operative reports can be a treasure trove of the most reliable information. It is a necessity for the ACHD interventionalist to review the primary imaging personally and confirm the details before proceeding to intervention. Even with experienced radiologists, the technical details and measurements required for a particular intervention or device are not always present in the radiology report. In addition, questions of when and how to intervene are not easily answered when outcomes data are lacking.

As a general rule of thumb, intervention in the patient with ACHD should not be performed on an ad hoc basis, but rather carefully planned and discussed in a collaborative multidisciplinary fashion. These procedures represent unfamiliar territory for adult cardiologists with little or no congenital heart disease (CHD) experience and, in our opinion, should remain that way. The skill sets of both pediatric and adult cardiologists who specialize in ACHD are invaluable, in addition to consultation with congenital heart surgeons, radiologists, and anesthesiologists. Whether discussed in a weekly meeting or multidisciplinary conference, a consensual team approach should be sought when performing procedures that are far removed from routine. No single interventionalist has the skill set to perform every possible type of intervention that a patient with ACHD may require, and collaboration in the laboratory (the pediatric and adult interventionalist) is central to accomplishing a safe and effective procedure.

The average complex patient with ACHD is an experienced and often savvy consumer of health care who has been in the medical system since birth. Although patients may or may not fully understand their own physiology and diagnosis, such patients and their families have high expectations of their providers with regard to procedural expertise, appropriate and complete consent, and explanation of a holistic long-term plan. An honest and direct approach to managing patient expectations and concerns pays substantial dividends in the long-term relationships that must be fostered by the health care team.

In the course of this review, we describe 3 distinct ACHD lesions amenable to percutaneous repair: (1) venous baffle obstruction in transposition of the great arteries (d-TGA), (2) coronary artery fistulas, and (3) ruptured sinus of Valsalva aneurysms. For each entity, we chronicle the typical clinical scenario and indications for intervention to supplement the technical approach and potential pitfalls with treatment.

VENOUS BAFFLES IN TRANSPOSITION OF THE GREAT ARTERIES
Introduction: Nature of the Problem

Complete transposition of the great arteries, also known as d-TGA is one of the most common forms of cyanotic congenital heart disease.[1] In 1957, Dr Ake Senning first described an atrial switch procedure for surgical palliation by creating an intra-atrial baffle from autologous tissue.[2] This baffle redirected blood from the superior (SVC) and inferior vena cava (IVC) to the left ventricle and hence to the pulmonary arteries, while pulmonary venous blood is directed toward the right ventricle and aorta. In 1963, Dr William T. Mustard performed a modification of the atrial switch procedure using an interatrial baffle to redirect blood flow to the concordant great artery.[3] These surgeries led to dramatic improvements in intermediate to long-term survival of transposition patients, but also created a unique set of clinical problems specific to the altered surgical anatomy.[4–9]

For the past several decades, the atrial switch procedure has been superseded by the Jatene arterial switch operation; however, there remain a large population of patients living with prior atrial switch procedures. Throughout their lives, these patients encounter a number of cardiac complications, including (1) arrhythmias, such as sinus node dysfunction, atrial arrhythmias, and sudden cardiac death; (2) systemic atrioventricular-valve (ie, tricuspid valve) regurgitation; (3) subpulmonary obstruction; (4) heart failure sequelae secondary to long-term cardiac dysfunction of the subaortic right ventricle; and (5) problems related to the surgical baffle including baffle leaks, baffle stenosis, and pulmonary vein stenosis.[1,8,10,11] Interventional cardiologists with the appropriate ACHD training are often called on to provide catheter-based solutions for baffle-related problems.

Baffle leaks are reported to occur in approximately 3% to 35% of patients with prior atrial switch procedures.[12,13] They are typically located along baffle suture lines with a higher prevalence in the superior limb over the inferior limb.[14] Although most leaks are small and not hemodynamically significant, approximately 2% of such left-to-right shunts may be large enough to warrant intervention. In addition to considerations of chamber volume loading, the specter of paradoxic embolism and cerebrovascular events looms large in a population, with approximately 30% prevalence of atrial arrhythmias and 10% to 20% requirement for pacemaker implantation.[15] Symptomatic desaturation (ie, reversal of the shunt) with exercise can occur and supports efforts to close the baffle leak. As expected, the presence of a baffle stenosis distal to a baffle leak often leads to profound cyanosis.

Estimates of baffle stenosis range from 5% to as high as 55%; with a higher prevalence of stenosis reported after the Mustard compared with the Senning operation.[5,6,16,17] The associated clinical syndrome can be slow and insidious, as a patent's azygous vein from the SVC will allow adequate venous decompression modifying symptoms (if any). That said, baffle stenosis can also present with classical symptoms of SVC syndrome with venous congestion of upper extremity and head or IVC syndrome with ascites and hepatic congestion. Focal stenosis in the venous system also increases the predisposition for thrombus formation. Indications for percutaneous or surgical intervention of baffle stenosis include symptoms, evidence of SVC or IVC syndrome, or SVC baffle stenosis in the setting of a planned permanent transvenous pacemaker. In this setting, a stenotic superior baffle will complicate transvenous wire implantation and can be simplified with baffle enlargement. As the absence of symptoms does not exclude baffle stenosis, venous assessment using angiography, MRI, or echocardiography is important before placement of a transvenous pacemaker.[16]

Preprocedure Planning

Clear delineation of anatomy, physiology, and clinical indications for therapy is a basic requirement before embarking on interventions on an atrial baffle. Case or conference discussion with a multidisciplinary team cannot be overemphasized, as noted previously.

At a minimum, preprocedural noninvasive imaging should include transthoracic echocardiography with a bubble study to assess for shunting in addition to visualizing both SVC and IVC baffles with color and continuous-wave Doppler. Often echocardiographic windows are inadequate to visualize both superior and inferior baffles in addition to pulmonary vein inflow. The addition of cardiac magnetic resonance imaging (MRI) (or computed tomography [CT] when MRI is contraindicated) greatly enhances the diagnosis of baffle obstruction or leak.[18,19]

Procedure Techniques

Although the approach to any case is variable and dependent on operator experience, there are certain axioms that should be considered. For an outline of the basic procedure for baffle stenting and device closure of baffle leaks, refer to **Boxes 1** and **2**. The procedural team may include

anesthesiology support. Although baffle stenting or leak closure can be safely performed using moderate sedation alone, patients with atrial switch typically have comorbidities, such as reduced sub-aortic right ventricular function or significant systemic deconditioning, increasing the risk of peri-procedural complications. A transesophageal echocardiogram may help to guide device or stent placement and identify impingement on cardiac structures (eg, pulmonary vein obstruction after device closure of a large baffle leak).

Venous access will depend on the location of the baffle obstruction. Leak or stenosis in the SVC baffle is best approached from the internal jugular vein, whereas procedures on the IVC baffle are best approached from the femoral vein. In many cases, formation of a veno-venous loop facilitates positioning and control of the stenting procedure; this is our preferred approach for SVC baffle stenting. Patient draping and table arrangements should be made accordingly. Heparin and antibiotics should be administered.

Irrespective of noninvasive imaging, all patients should undergo a complete hemodynamic, oxi-metric, and angiographic evaluation, either staged before or immediately before any planned intervention. This not only provides confirmation of the baffle stenosis or leak, but also ensures that no additional pathology contributing to patient symptoms is missed. A balloon-tipped catheter is typically used to enter the pulmonary arteries (PA) and can be facilitated by curving the stiff end of a standard 0.035-inch wire to point the catheter toward the PA as it is maneuvered into the morphologic left ventricle. Accurate measurement of pulmonary capillary wedge pressure is especially pertinent because of a propensity toward significant systemic AV-valve regurgitation. A modified JR4 (with side holes) can be used to cannulate the superior baffle and exchanged for a Gensini catheter for imaging.

For baffle stenosis, optimal angiographic visualization of the superior baffle is usually in the 30° left anterior oblique and 15° cranial projections; for the inferior baffle often the best projection is a straight anteroposterior view. Baffle leaks require more individual angle adjustment for maximal visualization.[20]

Crossing a chronically stenosed baffle limb can require patience, adequate guide support, and the use of several different wires (with varying degrees of stiffness and lubricity). There remain instances when no wire will cross a calcified stenotic segment; in such instances, the use of a transseptal needle or radiofrequency ablation wire have been shown to be effective means to cross the lesion.[21]

Box 1
Basic procedure for SVC or IVC baffle stenting

1. Access: Typically 11 to 12 Fr adequate for 18-mm to 20-mm balloon with stent.

   a. Femoral vein for inferior vena cava (IVC) baffle stenosis; internal jugular (or both internal jugular and femoral vein) for superior vena cava (SVC) baffle stenosis.

   b. Long sheath (80 cm).

   c. Heparin/antibiotics/regular continuous flushing.

2. Balloon/Stent selection:

   a. Balloon choice appropriate for stent deployment, usually ZMED-2/BIB.

   b. Aspirate balloon and fill with 30:70 contrast: flush and flush wire port.

   c. Stent sized to baffle dimensions—compensate for stent shortening on large balloon.

3. Stent preparation:

   a. Use a sheath dilator to expand the end of the stent for placement on balloon.

   b. Crimp firmly. Rotate and squeeze along length.

   c. Make an introducer (to pass stent through long sheath valve) so valve on long sheath does not displace stent. Score to allow introducer removal.

4. Stent delivery:

   a. Delivery over stiff wire; distal wire may be curved and placed in the left ventricle.

   b. Key to appropriate stent delivery is SLOW and STEADY inflation (typically to 3–8 mm Hg depending on the stent).

5. Final angiogram and hemodynamic assessment:

   a. Assess final gradient across stent (should be approximately 0 mm Hg).

   b. Final angiogram to ensure correct stent placement and relief of obstruction.

Baffle stenting has been described in the literature using both self-expanding and balloon-expandable stents.[22,23] Predilation before using a self-expanding stent is advised, whereas it may not be necessary for balloon-expandable stents. **Figs. 1** and **2** illustrate an example of stenting SVC baffle stenosis and IVC baffle stenosis respectively. Baffle leaks alone can be closed by either covered stents or by plugging the leak using a device such as and atrial septal defect (ASD) occluder or plug (**Fig. 3**). When using a covered stent only to close a leak, it is imperative that the stent be well apposed to the baffle wall. Failure to do so will result in a persistent leak that will then be challenging for percutaneous closure. Our preference in the presence of both baffle leak and stenosis is to balloon size and close the leak first with an Amplatzer Septal Occluder (St Jude Medical, St Paul, MN), leaving the device attached until the long sheath for the stent is positioned across the stenosis. In instances with multiple levels of obstruction and/or leak, several stents or devices may be used to recreate the baffle anatomy.

Stent type and size should take into account stent shortening, adequate diameter, and overall durability. There are no published studies comparing different stent platforms for baffle reconstruction. It is our institutional preference to use a balloon expandable system with Palmaz XL series, Palmaz Genesis (J&J Interventional Systems Co., Warren, NJ), or Cheatham Platinum (NuMED, Hopkinton, NY). It is important to note that the Genesis XD series stents will expand to only 18 mm and thus these might be a better choice for the superior as opposed to inferior baffle. For baffle leaks, we prefer using closure devices such as the Amplatzer Septal Occluder appropriately sized for the baffle defect. Such devices can be delivered with the wire position in a left pulmonary vein using the standard techniques for device closure of ASDs.

Hemodynamics after stenting or device closure should document no significant gradient across the venous baffle. It is important to use echocardiography when delivering a closure device for baffle leaks to ensure secure placement and no additional leaks that require treatment. We routinely

---

Box 2
Basic procedure for device closure of SVC or IVC baffle leak

1. Access: Typically 8–12 Fr adequate for closure device placement.
   a. Femoral vein for IVC baffle leak; internal jugular for SVC baffle leak.
   b. Long sheath (80 cm).
   c. Heparin/antibiotics/regular flushing.

2. Measuring the defect:
   a. Typically cross defect using a straight-tip 0.035-inch or Terumo glide wire (Somerset, NJ) in a JR4 or using a Goodale-Lubin (Medtronic Vascular, Santa Rosa, CA).
   b. Exchange for stiff wire positioned in left pulmonary vein.
   c. Use sizing balloon to estimate defect diameter and anatomy.

3. Device delivery:
   a. Deliver appropriately sized device to close defect; our preference is Amplatzer septal occlude (St Jude Medical, St Paul, MN).
   b. Prior to device release, check stability with Minnesota wiggle and by using both fluoroscopy and echocardiography. Occasionally more than one leak is present.

4. Final angiogram and hemodynamic assessment:
   a. Assess final gradient across baffle (should be ~0 mm Hg) with angiogram to ensure that device does not obstruct the baffle.
   b. Final angiogram: likely see contrast leak through device, but important to check for additional leaks or baffle obstruction from the device.

---

perform completion angiography after the conclusion of the procedure to assess for development of or residual baffle leak and patency of the systemic and pulmonary veins.

Postprocedural Care and Recovery

After the procedure, patients may be discharged home the same day after stenting. We generally monitor patients who receive an ASD device overnight and routinely perform a transthoracic echocardiogram to document SVC/IVC baffle velocities and elimination of any prior leak. Patients are typically placed on single antiplatelet therapy (either aspirin or clopidogrel) after stenting or closure device for 6 months. Occasionally, long-term anticoagulation may be indicated depending on associated comorbidities (ie, atrial arrhythmias or history of thrombus).

The patient is counseled for empiric low-level activity limitations for 72 hours after the procedure and endocarditis prophylaxis before dental procedures is recommended. Routine ACHD follow-up at 2 to 6 months after the procedure is arranged with transthoracic echocardiography and additional imaging as needed.

If patients were symptomatic with SVC or IVC syndrome or desaturation with exercise, one expects an improvement in symptoms relatively quickly. When baffle stenting is performed in preparation for a transvenous pacemaker, we typically recommend a 2-week waiting period, if clinically possible, allowing for the access sites to heal before pacemaker implantation.

Clinical Results and Complications

Most literature related to percutaneous treatment of baffle leaks and/or stenosis is in the form of case reports or case series.[13,21,24–31] Surgical treatment of baffle stenosis has been reported to be associated with high rates of perioperative morbidity and mortality.[32] Balloon angioplasty alone has a limited long-term impact on baffle patency, with rates of baffle restenosis ranging from 30% to 100%.[24] However, stenting for venous baffle stenosis does maintain high rates of patency, with 6-month to 12-month imaging-based or angiographic follow-up.[7,24] In most published case series, baffle stenting or leak closure carry a very low incidence of periprocedural complications.[24] Short-term to long-term complications include stent fracture, restenosis, and need for reintervention.

CORONARY ARTERY FISTULAS
Introduction

Coronary artery fistulas (CAFs) in adults represent an uncommon clinical problem with an unknown

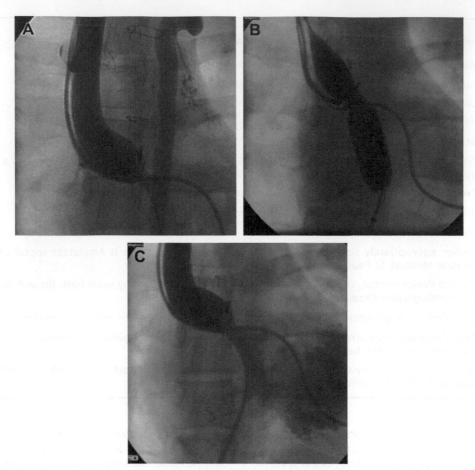

Fig. 1. SVC baffle stenosis stenting. (*A*) SVC angiography shows distal baffle stenosis. (*B*) Stent with 59-mm Palmaz Genesis (5910) stent (Cordis, Miami, FL) on 18-mm balloon. (*C*) Follow-up angiography with resolution of stenosis.

true incidence,[33] with reports ranging between 0.3% and 0.8% during diagnostic cardiac catheterization.[34,35] These fistulas are characterized by an abnormal connection from the coronary arteries, draining to a cardiac chamber or vessel without traversing the usual capillary network.[36] They can form almost anywhere in the coronary artery system, terminating in any cardiac chamber, great vein, or pulmonary artery. Roughly half originate from the right coronary and half from the left coronary artery often with multiple origins.[35] Small, asymptomatic fistulas arise much more commonly from the left coronary system (87%).[37]

The vast majority of CAFs (more than 90%) drain to the right side of the circulation. Drainage to the left ventricle is the least common. CAFs that drain to the right side of the circulation create a left-to-right shunt of oxygenated blood to the pulmonary circulation. Those that drain to the systemic veins or right atrium have a circulatory physiology similar to an ASD. Those that drain to the pulmonary arteries display similar hemodynamics to a patent arterial duct. A CAF that drains to the left atrium represents a left-to-left shunt that can cause volume loading similar to mitral regurgitation. A fistula that drains to the left ventricle produces hemodynamic changes comparable to aortic insufficiency.[33]

Frequently asymptomatic, CAF can cause chest pain (especially if there is concomitant coronary artery disease), myocardial infarction, dyspnea, congestive heart failure, palpitations, arrhythmias, infective endocarditis, hemopericardium, and sudden death. CAF can result in a coronary artery "steal" phenomenon, with coronary blood preferentially passing through the fistula instead of the more distal myocardial capillaries. Angina has been reported in many patients with large fistulas and may be aggravated by distal coronary artery disease. Anginal symptoms have disappeared with closure of the fistula in most patients with no distal disease.[38] There are typical differences

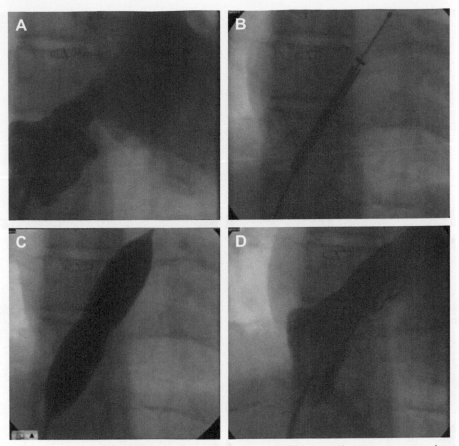

Fig. 2. IVC baffle stenosis stenting. (*A*) IVC angiography shows baffle stenosis; 11-mm narrowing with 8-mm gradient. (*B, C*) Stent with a J & J (P5014) XL series stent on a 20-mm balloon. (*D*) Follow-up angiography with resolution of stenosis. No gradient on postprocedural measurement.

in symptom presentations of CAF between adults and children (see **Table 1** for comparison).[39]

Symptoms are more likely to develop with advancing age, although the treatment of asymptomatic patients with a CAF still poses management difficulties for the adult cardiologist and interventionalist in terms of indications and timing of the intervention (if at all). An optimal strategy for management of a CAF would provide the greatest probability of event-free survival over a lifetime.[33] One must weigh the risks of intervention versus observation. Factors to consider include fistula size and anatomy, presence of symptoms or related complications, patient's age, and whether there are other indications present for an invasive procedure. Complicating matters, there is a small percentage of fistulas that occlude spontaneously with time in children. There is also a small (several percent per year) risk of spontaneous fistula rupture seen mostly in adult patients.[40]

CAFs are often tortuous and irregularly shaped. The smallest diameter of a fistula is frequently located near the exit point or at a sharp bend of a tortuous vessel. The increased flow through a CAF tends to cause dilation of the proximal portion of its associated coronary artery. Very distal coronary artery fistulas are associated with dilation and significant tortuosity throughout the coronary length. CAFs that arise near the origin of the coronary do not lead to distal coronary dilation,[33] and small fistulas will typically not dilate the proximal coronary segment with the maximal diameter of the proximal coronary less than twice normal. These small CAFs are usually clinically silent and are generally detected incidentally.[41] Fistulas that measure between 2 and 3 times the expected proximal normal coronary artery diameter are considered to be medium sized. Fistula with larger dimensions are considered large.[33]

The most common symptoms in adults include angina, palpitations, and dyspnea. Heart failure related to myocardial ischemia is more common in patients with concomitant coronary artery disease. Intervention is indicated in any patient with evidence of myocardial ischemia. At least 2 separate modalities for ischemia detection should

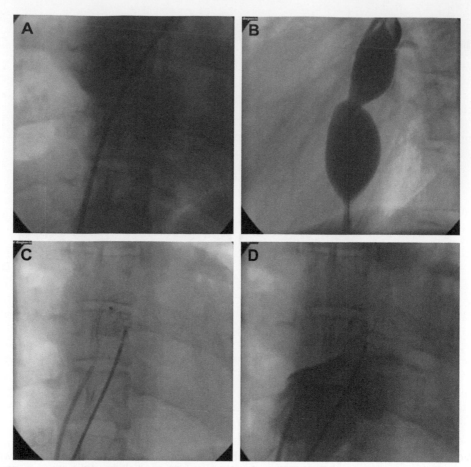

Fig. 3. Baffle leak from IVC baffle. (*A*) Catheter has crossed IVC baffle leak from femoral vein approach directed toward the left upper pulmonary vein. (*B*) A 34-mm sizing balloon used to measure defect size as 5 mm. (*C*) A 7-mm Amplatzer septal occluder partially delivered. (*D*) Angiography in IVC documenting of baffle leak closure before device release.

Table 1
Comparison of coronary artery fistula presentation between adults and children

	Adults (n = 107)	Children (n = 129)
Age, y	56	0.5
Years of data collection	1973–2001	1968–98
Murmur	none 48%, CM 32%	none 27%, CM 54%
Unilateral CAF	85%	88%
Associated defects	13%	21%
Spontaneous rupture	4%	0%
Spontaneous closure	3%	9%
Aneurysm	14%	9%
Coronary artery disease	19%	0%

Abbreviations: CAF, coronary artery fistula; CM, continuous murmur.
  Adapted from Said SA, Lam J, van der Werf T. Solitary coronary artery fistulas: a congenital anomaly in children and adults. A contemporary review. Congenit Heart Dis 2006;1:63–76.

be used to determine the clinical significance of any particular coronary fistula. We prefer a combination of perfusion imaging and a functional assessment with stress echocardiography.

Endocarditis is a potential complication with arteriovenous fistulas and has also been reported in approximately 3% of patients with a medium or large CAF.[38] The risk of endocarditis in patients with clinically silent CAF detected incidentally by echocardiography or angiography appears to be much less. Intervention should be offered to any patient with a CAF and a history of endocarditis or if the patient has a large-sized or medium-sized fistula that is clinically detectable. An invasive procedure is not warranted in patients with small and silent CAFs for the lone indication of endocarditis prevention, especially if the anatomy is difficult for catheter closure.

Up to 57% of patients with a CAF also have another congenital cardiovascular anomaly,[35] with the most common associated cardiac lesion being an ASD (21%) and moderate left ventricular dysfunction (14%). Intervention for even a small CAF may be justified in an adult who is undergoing a concomitant surgical or catheter procedure for an acquired cardiovascular problem, such as coronary artery or valvular disease. Treatment of small fistulas should always be carefully considered, as one is unlikely to modify a benign natural history.

Once the decision has been made that a CAF warrants treatment, options include surgical or percutaneous interventional approaches. Although surgical series have demonstrated excellent long-term results,[42] a surgical strategy is not without risk of morbidity and mortality. Various percutaneous methods of closure have been used with catheter embolization.

Since the first transcatheter occlusion of a CAF reported in 1983,[37] there have been numerous successful procedures reported in the literature.[33] Transcatheter results have generally been comparable to surgical, with an expected mortality rate of less than 1%. Potential complications include periprocedural ST changes, myocardial infarctions, and arrhythmias. Occluder device and coil embolization has been reported in some cases; however, the devices can typically be retrieved using percutaneous means.

Improved devices and delivery systems have made catheter closure applicable to more than 90% of patients.[33] Catheter techniques may have limitations in a small percentage of adult patients owing to extreme vessel tortuosity and inability to deliver a catheter far enough distally, presence of multiple drainage sites, or the presence of normal coronary branches too close to the drainage site to allow selective occlusion. Multiple feeding vessels may similarly pose a challenge. Because of a much shorter recovery time and avoidance of surgical morbidity, transcatheter closure is currently considered the procedure of choice in applicable patients.

Preprocedure Planning

Before percutaneous closure of a CAF it is imperative to have a clear rationale. Indications for intervention include symptoms attributable to the fistula, a hemodynamically significant left-to-right shunt, ventricular volume loading, evidence of myocardial ischemia, arrhythmias, or a history of endocarditis. It is our routine practice to perform 2 independent imaging modalities (eg, stress echo and nuclear myocardial perfusion) in assessing for ischemia from a CAF.

Depending on number and extent of collaterals, patient consent should include a discussion of the time such procedures often require. Although many patients note clinical improvement after closure, they must understand that symptomatic improvement is difficult to predict.

We perform diagnostic coronary angiography days to weeks before the planned fistula closure date. This allows time for strategy formulation and to understand the individual anatomy, crucial to procedural success. Most patients are referred based on the finding of a fistula during an angiogram performed because of symptoms or abnormal functional testing. In our experience, angiography remains the gold standard, as CT and MRI do not provide much in the way of additional information required for closure.

Any interventionalist considering coronary fistula closure should have expertise in percutaneous coronary interventions (PCI) so as to manage potential complications, such as device embolization, coronary dissection, thrombosis, vessel rupture, or microcatheter or wire entrapment. It is uncommon for adult interventionalists to possess the advanced structural heart disease skills required to perform this procedure and thus a pediatric and adult cardiologist working together may be beneficial depending on the experience of each individual. Any bleeding diathesis must be reviewed, as full anticoagulation (with activated clotting time levels >200) should be maintained throughout the procedure. We recommend heparin sulfate anticoagulation to allow for protamine reversal in the event of a bleeding-related complication.

Procedural Technique

The technical approach for CAF closure depends on the individual anatomy, degree of coronary dilation, and associated atherosclerosis. No one technique can be applied, and procedural flexibility is a necessity (see **Box 3** for basic procedure). **Figs. 4–6** illustrate case examples of percutaneous CAF closure.

Procedures should begin with a clear delineation of the anatomy. Sometimes this may require large-volume injection through a guiding catheter or balloon occlusion angiography using a wedge catheter advanced distally into the coronary. This technique halts flow distal to the balloon and clarifies the presence of branches that may serve working myocardium and the anatomy of the outlet. Advancing a balloon catheter retrograde through a larger guiding catheter or anterograde (over a retrograde wire that has been snared and exteriorized) also allows for a prolonged inflation at the intended site of occlusion. Monitoring for wall motion abnormalities and electrocardiogram (ECG) changes is important during test occlusion to predict the risk for postprocedural ischemia/infarction.

A wide array of coils, plugs and covered stents of multiple sizes should be readily available. Commonly used coils for coronary fistula closure can be mechanically detachable or pushable; coils can be made from stainless steel, platinum, or alloys, such as nitinol or inconel. Vascular occluders that have been described for CAF closure include the Amplatzer Vascular Plug, Vascular Plug II, Vascular Plug 4 and Duct Occluder (St Jude's Medical, St. Paul, MN). One consideration in device selection may be MRI-compatibility (eg, MReye Coils, Cook, Bloomington, IN, or any Amplatzer Vascular Plug).

A retrograde arterial approach is the preferred method to use, as it is straightforward and uses skills relevant to PCI procedures. Venous approaches have also been described in which a coronary wire directed from the venous outlet can be snared to create an arteriovenous rail for device delivery.[43] It is preferable to place the occlusion device as close to the venous outlet as possible, this may minimize the risk of backward propagation of thrombus. From an arterial approach, either a small-caliber catheter (eg, 4 or 5 Fr) can be deep seated into the fistula or a microcatheter (eg, 3-Fr Tracker, Boston Scientific, Natick, MA, or 4-Fr Renegade, Boston Scientific) can be used within a larger-diameter guide catheter (7 or 8 Fr) using a "telescoping catheter" technique. These microcatheters come in different shapes and can be delivered over a 0.014-inch wire to make it easier to pass through tortuous anatomy to the location of coil delivery.[35]

One key goal is to aim for complete fistula occlusion in the laboratory, which may require multiple coils or devices. Clear delineation of the anatomy is important, as many fistulas have

---

Box 3
Basic procedure for coronary artery fistula closure from retrograde arterial approach using coils

1. Access: Typically 6–8-Fr femoral arterial.

   a. Pretreatment with aspirin and clopidogrel/heparin/regular flushing.

   b. Heparin/antibiotics/regular flushing.

2. Catheter placement

   a. 7-Fr or 8-Fr coronary guide specific for vessel (right vs left main).

   b. Microcatheter brought into coronary to position over 0.014-inch coronary wire if coils are anticipated.

   c. Carefully choose position for coil delivery: narrowest distal diameter before multiple points of egress.

3. Coil selection and delivery:

   a. Coils should be selected to be ~1.3–1.5 × larger than the target vessel diameter.

   b. Coil selection: our institutional preference is MRI-compatibility coils (eg, MReye Coils; Cook, Bloomington, IN) with mechanical detachment.

   c. Deliver coils into place through microcatheter; often multiple coils will be required.

4. Final angiogram and hemodynamic assessment:

   a. Ensure adequate coil stability on fluoroscopy.

   b. Final angiogram should achieve complete occlusion in the catheter laboratory. Check multiple views to assess for additional fistulas or points of egress.

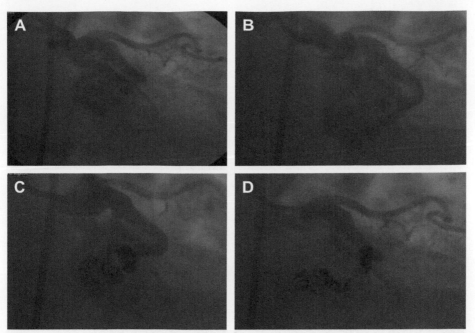

Fig. 4. Percutaneous coiling of CAF from circumflex artery. (*A*) Selective coronary angiogram of the left main coronary artery shows a large tortuous CAF arising from proximal circumflex artery and feeding distally into the pulmonary artery. This patient presented with atypical chest pain syndrome, a continuous murmur on examination, and a stress test with antero-lateral ischemia at peak stress. (*B*) An 8-Fr coronary guide is used to cannulate the left main. Using a telescoping catheter technique, a 4-Fr microcatheter is fed into the CAF over a 0.014-inch coronary wire into the body of the fistula to the chosen location for coil delivery. (*C*) Multiple fibered pushable coils are delivered into the fistula. (*D*) Final angiogram documenting near-complete occlusion of the CAF after coil placement without damage to remaining coronary system.

multiple points of egress. Thus, multiple coils in several branches are at times required. The optimal site for closure is at the narrowest distal diameter before multiple points of egress. There is some concern for an increased risk of long-term vessel thrombosis when a proximal cul-de-sac remains after closure.[44] Coils should be selected to be approximately 1.3 to 1.5 times larger than the target vessel diameter. When using a device such as an Amplatzer vascular plug, a tapered device waist after delivery is indicative of secure placement. Occasionally the use of a covered stent can simplify the procedure, covering the ostium of a vascular branch with potentially multiple fistulas. This technique must be tempered by the high rates of in-stent restenosis seen with covered stents in the coronary arteries and should generally be avoided.

Postprocedural Care and Recovery

Patients are typically monitored overnight with telemetry, serial ECGs, and clinical symptoms of coronary thrombosis. It is our routine to treat such patients with dual antiplatelet therapy (aspirin and clopidogrel) for an empiric 6 months (followed by aspirin alone). When distal fistulas are closed,

usually a long segment of severely dilated artery is left behind. The flow in these segments, where there is a mismatch between ingress and egress, results in swirling nonlaminar flow and may be prone to thrombosis. We suggest long-term anticoagulation for these patients. There are reports of other institutions recommending empiric anticoagulation with warfarin in addition to antiplatelet agents for a minimum of 1 year, with continuation of anticoagulation in "high-risk" anatomy with significant coronary dilation.[33,44]

There are no standards for follow-up after closure and it is our institutional preference to routinely perform diagnostic angiography in all adults 1 year after closure. The utility of follow-up functional imaging to assess for ischemia has not been clearly documented in the absence of recurrent symptoms. Gated CT scanning may be an acceptable modality for follow-up; however, especially for large distal fistulas, late image acquisition is critical to avoid misinterpreting a slow-filling vessel with one that is occluded.

Clinical Results and Complications

Transcatheter closure of CAFs has emerged as a less invasive alternative to surgery with high

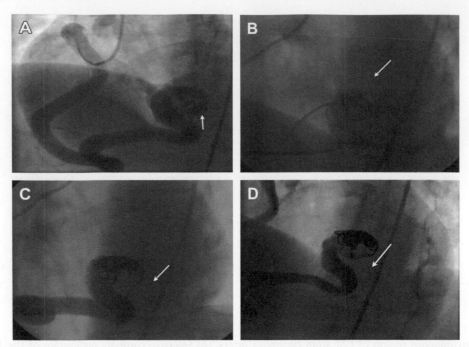

Fig. 5. Percutaneous coiling of CAF from right coronary artery. (*A*) Selective coronary angiogram of the right coronary artery shows a distal CAF (from the right posterior lateral branch) with severe proximal dilation of the proximal artery. This patient presented with symptoms of exertional dyspnea and right heart catheter measurements with PA pressure 24/12 (18) and a calculated Qp:Qs of 1.4:1. (*B, C*) Document coil delivery to right-posterior lateral and distal right coronary artery. Final angiogram (*C*) shows near occlusion of the CAF. After this procedure, the patient had a creatine kinase rise to 1400 with mild inferobasal hypokinesis on echo with preserved LV ejection fraction 60%. (*D*) A 3-month follow-up angiogram confirms complete closure of CAF with decrease in the proximal artery dilation. The patient noted significant improvement in symptoms.

treatment efficacy and overall low morbidity. When the fistula is an isolated cardiac lesion, a percutaneous approach should be the preferred option for therapy. Case series from experienced centers with follow-up angiography suggest complete closure to be possible in approximately 75% of patients.[45–47] In patients for whom complete closure is not achieved, repeat intervention can be offered. After closure, studies describe a reduction in left ventricular volumes and cardiothoracic ratios in addition to improvement in associated symptoms.[45]

Manipulation of catheters, wires, and devices in the often dilated and tortuous vasculature of CAF portends a tangible risk of complications, including dissection, vascular trauma, spasm, and thrombosis. Nearly all large case series of percutaneous closure report 0% procedural mortality. Device embolization remains the most commonly described complication in approximately 2% to 7% of case series.[35,45,47] Coil or device embolization remains a very real possibility, especially when either the precise anatomy or vessel size is not appreciated or the chosen device or coil is too small. In our clinical experience, most embolized devices can be successfully snared and removed via percutaneous means.

There are limited long-term data after percutaneous CAF closure. In one large mixed surgical and percutaneous closure study, fistulas that drained into the coronary sinus, in addition to comorbidities such as diabetes, smoking, hypertension, hyperlipidemia, and older age at diagnosis, were linked with higher rates of major complications including myocardial infarction, coronary thrombosis, ventricular tachycardia, or symptomatic heart failure.[48] There are reports of both early and late coronary thrombosis after CAF closure, which may be associated with distal fistulae with significant coronary dilation.[44]

SINUS OF VALSALVA RUPTURE
Introduction

Sinus of Valsalva aneurysms (SVAs) have been described in the literature since the 1800s and can be either congenital or acquired. They are hypothesized to arise from a loss of structural integrity in the focal tunica media or the junction between the media and annulosa fibrosa.[49,50]

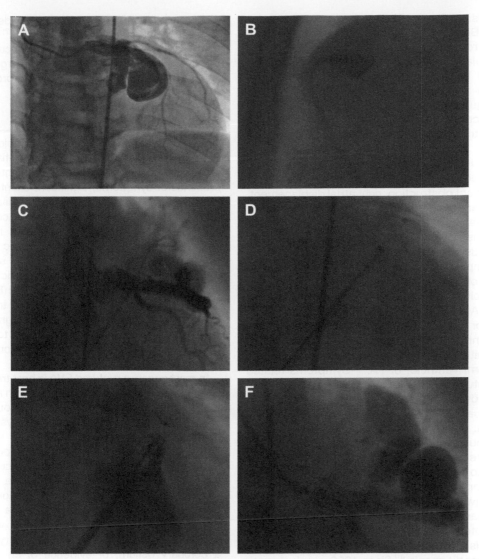

Fig. 6. Device closure of CAF using venous approach. (*A*) Selective coronary angiogram of the left main coronary artery shows a large tortuous CAF arising from proximal circumflex artery and feeding distally into the RV outflow tract. This patient presented with recurrent emergency department visits with chest pain in addition to a continuous murmur on examination. (*B*) A diagnostic catheter is used to cannulate the CAF from its exit point into the RV. (*C*) Balloon occlusion is attempted from the venous side with simultaneous injection of the coronary artery to confirm that there are no other points of fistula egress. (*C, D*) An Amplatzer duct occluder is delivered from a venous approach. (*E*) An RV angiogram documents that the device is not impinging on the pulmonary valve. (*F*) Final angiogram shows the device in place. Despite demonstrating that occluding the venous outflow was successful in reducing fistula flow, the PDA device was minimally helpful in reducing flow. This patient later required several additional coiling procedures from the retrograde approach and placement of an Amplatzer vascular plug from the retrograde approach into the left anterior descending fistula.

They represent an uncommon type of congenital heart disease with an estimated prevalence of 0.09% in the general population from autopsy studies.[51] Congenital SVAs typically involve the right coronary sinus and are associated with outlet, doubly committed, subaortic, or rarely perimembranous ventricular septal defects (VSDs) (30%–60%) and less commonly with bicuspid aortic valve (~10%), ASD, pulmonary stenosis, aortic coarctation, or subaortic stenosis.[49,50] Valve tissue may participate in VSD closure, and the lesion may begin as an outpoaching of the sinus tissue in the VSD, which over time may increase in size and perforate. Acquired SVAs are linked to vascular infections (ie, endocarditis, syphilis, tuberculosis), deceleration trauma, connective tissue disorders (ie, Marfan syndrome), or vasculitis (ie, Behcet syndrome or Takayasu arteritis), or are iatrogenic (ie, associated with surgical aortic valve replacement).[52–56] Although SVAs have been reported in all 3 sinuses, they more commonly occur in the right coronary cusp ($\sim$70%) with less frequent reports in the noncoronary ($\sim$25%) and left coronary ($\sim$5%) cusps.[49]

Unruptured SVA may be asymptomatic and can be found as an incidental finding during cardiac imaging. However, there are case reports of large unruptured SVAs leading to symptoms from RV outflow tract obstruction, right atrial displacement, ventricular tachycardia, heart block, coronary compression, mitral valve obstruction, or thromboembolism.[52,57–59] Most patients with a ruptured SVA are usually symptomatic, although physiology and symptom severity depend on orifice size, rapidity of rupture development, and the chambers involved. Rupture occurs more commonly in right SVAs (60%) than either noncoronary SVAs (42%) or left SVAs (10%).[49] Most aneuryms rupture into the right ventricle (60%) or right atrium (29%) with significantly fewer examples into the left atrium, ventricle, or PA.[60] Symptoms related to a ruptured SVA include chest pain, dyspnea, fatigue, dysrhythmias, and edema. Occasionally, sudden cardiac death can be the first clinical manifestation. Physical examination reveals a harsh continuous murmur with a palpable thrill, similar to a patent arterial duct. Clinical signs may be related to heart failure from left to right shunting and secondary volume loading, aortic valve insufficiency (which occurs in 20%–45%), arrhythmias, or coronary compromise.[61]

Untreated ruptured SVAs typically have a poor prognosis with average survival estimates of 3.9 years after diagnosis.[49] Since 1956, surgical repair has been the gold standard for treating a ruptured aneurysm by removing the aneurysmal sac, patch closure, and repairing any associated defects (ie, a VSD) with cardiopulmonary bypass.[62] Occasionally aortic root replacement and coronary reimplantation are also required. Overall, surgical repair can usually be performed with low operative mortality (0%–4%) with 5-year survival between 80% and 95% in addition to improvement in symptoms.[49,63,64] However, there are cases in which patient comorbidities or the inherent surgical risk profile of sternotomy (ie, repeat sternotomy) and cardiopulmonary bypass make surgical repair prohibitive. In such instances of isolated rupture, a percutaneous approach can be considered. The first described percutaneous closure of ruptured congenital SVA was performed using the Rashkind occluder device in 1994.[65] Over the past several decades, there have been numerous case reports and case series describing successful percutaneous closure.[66,67] In the appropriately selected patient, percutaneous closure can offer an alternative to surgery with high rates of technical success and low procedural morbidity.[66]

Preprocedure Planning

A clear delineation of anatomy, physiology, and clinical indications for therapy are essential before embarking on a percutaneous intervention. The presence of symptoms, significant shunt fraction (Qp:Qs >1.5:1), cyanosis, cardiac dilation or dysfunction, or prior endocarditis are all acceptable indications for closure. The diagnosis must be clearly delineated by echocardiographic imaging with color-Doppler documenting a saccular-shaped aneurysm with continuous systolic and diastolic turbulent flow at the perforation site (**Fig. 7**). In addition to adequate transthoracic and transesophageal echocardiography, CT-angiography of the aorta (and possibly cardiac MRI) to further delineate the anatomy before intervention can be very helpful.[68]

In most cases, a ruptured SVA is best treated by surgery, especially when associated with a VSD or aortic valve disease (**Fig. 8**). Percutaneous repair is primarily suitable for those aneurysms that have ruptured into the right atrium or ventricle, although there have also been case reports with rupture into the PA.[69] Although a percutaneous procedure may occlude the shunt, the inherent weakness and abnormality of the aortic wall persists. Other instances that favor a surgical approach include rupture into the left ventricle, significant proximity of ruptured aneurysm into a coronary ostium, or evidence of an elevated pulmonary vascular resistance or reversal of shunt direction.[70]

Procedure Technique

The basic procedural steps for percutaneous closure are listed in **Box 4**. These procedures should be performed under general anesthesia. Real-time intraprocedural echocardiography with 3-dimensional reconstructions can be an excellent tool to help guide device placement and end-results (see **Fig. 7**).[71]

Both femoral arterial and venous access should be obtained. Aortic angiography in orthogonal views (or even rotation angiography) can help delineate the size and shape of the aneurysm, precise location of rupture, and distance from the coronary ostium (**Fig. 9**). The defect is most easily crossed retrograde from the aorta using a diagnostic coronary catheter (eg, multipurpose, JR4,

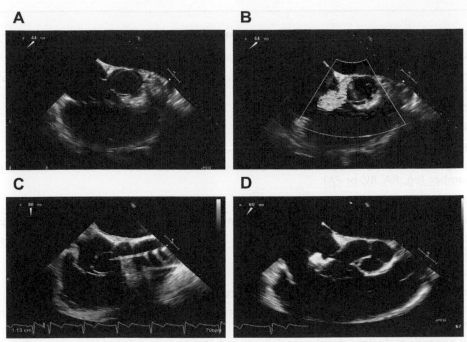

Fig. 7. Images from transesophageal echocardiogram of an SVA and percutaneous repair. (*A, B*) Short-axis view of the aortic valve documenting the SVA from the right coronary cusp into the right atrium. Color Doppler shows turbulent flow in the aneurysm. (*C*) With catheter across the SVA rupture, the echo measures the rupture site at 1.1 cm. (*D*) A 12-mm Amplatzer septal occluder is partially delivered into the SVA.

or IMA catheter) and a 0.035-inch Terumo Glide-wire (Somerset, NJ). The diagnostic catheter can follow over the glide wire across the defect.

Using a snare catheter introduced from the femoral vein, the exchange wire can be captured and gradually externalized from the femoral vein, creating a continuous rail between the arterial and venous systems. We recommend snaring the wire in the PAs to avoid damaging intracardiac structures (if the wire is snared in the right atrium (RA) it may traverse tricuspid valve chordae). The wire should remain housed in the catheter (ie, either diagnostic or snare retrieval catheter) to

prevent the wire from causing damage to the vasculature during wire externalization.

It is our institutional preference to estimate device size based solely on echocardiography and calibrated angiographic measurements and then select a device approximately 2 to 4 mm larger than the estimated diameter at the aortic end of aneurysm. Several investigators describe using a soft wedge catheter balloon to cautiously measure a "stop-flow" diameter.[70,72] Attempting to balloon size the defect can lead to its expansion and potentially worsen the clinical syndrome; however, balloon sizing can be helpful to confirm

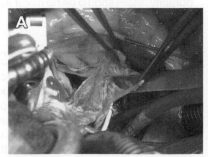
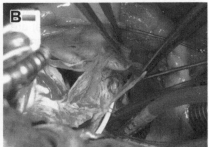

Fig. 8. Surgical visualization of SVA. (*A, B*) Surgical visualization of an SVA rupture before surgical repair. This patient was recommended surgery (as opposed to percutaneous repair) because of concomitant valvular disease requiring surgical repair.

Box 4
Basic procedure for device closure of ruptured sinus of Valsalva aneurysm

1. Access and angiography: Typically 8-Fr femoral arterial.

   a. Aortic angiography with and without selective coronary angiography to delineate anatomy of aneurysm.

   b. Heparin/antibiotics/regular flushing.

2. Crossing the defect

   a. 5-Fr or 6-Fr diagnostic coronary catheter (often JR4 or MP-1) positioned toward the aneurysm.

   b. Using a 0.035-inch, 260-cm Terumo Glidewire to thread through rupture site into draining chamber (eg, RA, RV, or PA).

3. Create arterio-venous rail

   a. Snare 260 cm wire (in main or branch pulmonary artery to avoid damage to tricuspid apparatus).

   b. Using kissing catheter technique, externalize 300 cm of wire through the femoral venous sheath, creating arterio-venous rail.

4. Device delivery

   a. Consider balloon sizing to confirm size and confirm that there is only a single defect.

   b. Choose device size (typically Amplatzer duct or septal occluder) based on imaging measurements (ie, echo or calibrated angiography).

   c. Use appropriately sized Amplatzer delivery catheter to deliver device from venous entry.

5. Final evaluation

   a. Before device delivery:

      i. Ensure that device is secure in placement before release.

      ii. Echo check to ensure no obstruction.

      iii. Selective angiograms should confirm patent coronary flow.

   b. Final angiogram after device delivery; should document no additional leaks or leaks around device (although may see left-to-right shunting through device).

---

that there is only a single and not multiple defects. The most commonly used devices for percutaneous closure of ruptured SVA are an Amplatzer duct occluder or Amplatzer septal occluder, although the use of coils has also been described with particularly tortuous and serpentine connections.[72] Typical device sizes for the Duct occluder range from 6/4 to 11/9.

The device and associated delivery catheter (eg, 6-Fr to 8-Fr Amplatzer delivery catheters) are introduced in to the femoral vein and taken anterograde across the aneurysm into the aorta. The aortic disk is exposed and positioned into the body of the aneurysm. After confirmation of position, the venous disk is then exposed across the length of the defect into the rupture opening.

Before release, the device should appear secure on fluoroscopy (a duct occluder device should have a central waist at the orifice of the aneurysm). Echo imaging should look for device impingement on cardiac structures, potential obstruction to blood flow, or worsening of aortic insufficiency. Aortic angiography, selective coronary angiography, and echocardiography all play important roles during and after device delivery. Final selective angiograms should confirm patent coronary flow. Although there may be initial evidence of left-to-right blood flow through the device on angiography, there should be no major leak noted from around the device.

Postprocedural Care and Recovery

Patients receive a dose of periprocedural antibiotics and are typically placed on antiplatelet therapy (either aspirin or clopidogrel) after the closure device for 6 months. These patients are managed in the cardiac care unit until hemodynamic improvement, depending on their initial clinical status. When percutaneous closure is performed for acute cardiogenic shock, recovery can be gradual.

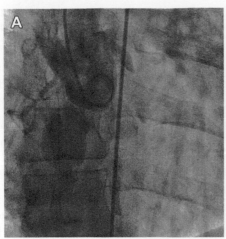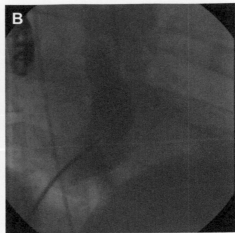

Fig. 9. Angiography from SVA percutaneous repair. (*A*) Aortic angiogram documenting the SVA from the right coronary cusp into the right atrium. The right coronary artery ostium is visualized in reference to the rupture site. (*B*) A 12-mm Amplatzer septal occluder is partially delivered into the SVA with aortic angiography; there remains aortic leak into the RA (although it now primarily is through the device).

The patient is counseled for empiric low-level activity limitations for 1 week after the procedure and endocarditis prophylaxis before dental procedures. Routine ACHD follow-up at 2 months after the procedure is arranged with additional transthoracic echocardiography and CT angiography of the aorta.

Clinical Results and Complications

Most of the literature related to percutaneous treatment of a ruptured SVA is in the form of case reports or case series.[66,72,73] A 20-patient case series reports approximately 90% procedural success, although 5 patients (20%) had residual shunts on discharge (4 small shunts; 1 moderate shunt).[74] Hemolysis and hemoglobinuria was described in the patient with moderate shunting; however, this improved on its own by the third postprocedural day. All 20 patients were followed for a median of 2 years, from which 15 (75%) remained New York Heart Association (NYHA) Class I, and 3 (15%) remained NYHA Class II. There was no progression of aortic insufficiency and no reported episodes of device embolization or endocarditis.

Potential procedural complications include aortic valve insufficiency either through directly damaging the aortic valve leaflets with the device or through tension/traction across the aortic annulus. Aortic insufficiency can worsen by the relative increase in afterload that happens after closing the left-to-right shunt.[74] Device encroachment on the ostium of the right coronary artery remains a potential complication that must be assessed for during the procedure. Despite these theoretical concerns, there have been very few

reports of aortic insufficiency or coronary compromise after closure of SVA rupture.

REFERENCES

1. Warnes CA. Transposition of the great arteries. Circulation 2006;114:2699–709.
2. Senning A. Surgical correction of transposition of the great vessels. Surgery 1959;45:966–80.
3. Mustard WT. Successful two-stage correction of transposition of the great vessels. Surgery 1964; 55:469–72.
4. Oechslin E, Jenni R. 40 years after the first atrial switch procedure in patients with transposition of the great arteries: long-term results in Toronto and Zurich. Thorac Cardiovasc Surg 2000;48:233–7.
5. Khairy P, Landzberg MJ, Lambert J, et al. Long-term outcomes after the atrial switch for surgical correction of transposition: a meta-analysis comparing the Mustard and Senning procedures. Cardiol Young 2004;14:284–92.
6. Moons P, Gewillig M, Sluysmans T, et al. Long-term outcome up to 30 years after the Mustard or Senning operation: a nationwide multicentre study in Belgium. Heart 2004;90:307–13.
7. Warnes CA, Somerville J. Transposition of the great arteries: late results in adolescents and adults after the Mustard procedure. Br Heart J 1987;58:148–55.
8. Dos L, Teruel L, Ferreira IJ, et al. Late outcome of Senning and Mustard procedures for correction of transposition of the great arteries. Heart 2005;91: 652–6.
9. Wilson NJ, Clarkson PM, Barratt-Boyes BG, et al. Long-term outcome after the Mustard repair for

simple transposition of the great arteries; 28-year follow-up. J Am Coll Cardiol 1998;32:758–65.

10. Kammeraad JA, van Deurzen CH, Sreeram N, et al. Predictors of sudden cardiac death after Mustard or Senning repair for transposition of the great arteries. J Am Coll Cardiol 2004;44:1095–102.

11. Gelatt M, Hamilton RM, McCrindle BW, et al. Arrhythmia and mortality after the Mustard procedure: a 30-year single-center experience. J Am Coll Cardiol 1997;29:194–201.

12. Helbing WA, Hansen B, Ottenkamp J, et al. Long-term results of atrial correction for transposition of the great arteries. Comparison of Mustard and Senning operations. J Thorac Cardiovasc Surg 1994; 108:363–72.

13. Bentham J, English K, Hares D, et al. Effect of transcatheter closure of baffle leaks following Senning or Mustard atrial redirection surgery on oxygen saturations and polycythaemia. Am J Cardiol 2012;110(7): 1046–50.

14. Hornung TS, Benson LN, McLaughlin PR. Catheter interventions in adult patients with congenital heart disease. Curr Cardiol Rep 2002;4:54–62.

15. Hayes CJ, Gersony WM. Arrhythmias after the Mustard operation for transposition of the great arteries: a long-term study. J Am Coll Cardiol 1986; 7:133–7.

16. Patel S, Shah D, Chintala K, et al. Atrial baffle problems following the Mustard operation in children and young adults with dextro-transposition of the great arteries: the need for improved clinical detection in the current era. Congenit Heart Dis 2011;6:466–74.

17. Bottega NA, Silversides CK, Oechslin EN, et al. Stenosis of the superior limb of the systemic venous baffle following a Mustard procedure: an under-recognized problem. Int J Cardiol 2012;154:32–7.

18. Fogel MA, Hubbard A, Weinberg PM. A simplified approach for assessment of intracardiac baffles and extracardiac conduits in congenital heart surgery with two- and three-dimensional magnetic resonance imaging. Am Heart J 2001;142:1028–36.

19. Ho JG, Cohen MD, Ebenroth ES, et al. Comparison between transthoracic echocardiography and cardiac magnetic resonance imaging in patients status post atrial switch procedure. Congenit Heart Dis 2012;7:122–30.

20. Benson L, Mikailian H. Angiography. In: Sievert H, Qureshi SA, Wilson N, et al, editors. Percutaneous interventions for congenital heart disease. New York: Informa Healthcare; 2010. p. 15–32.

21. Asgar AW, Miro J, Ibrahim R. Recanalization of systemic venous baffles by radiofrequency perforation and stent implantation. Catheter Cardiovasc Interv 2007;70.591–4.

22. Brown SC, Eyskens B, Mertens L, et al. Self-expandable stents for relief of venous baffle obstruction after the Mustard operation. Heart 1998;79:230–3.

23. Bu'Lock FA, Tometzki AJ, Kitchiner DJ, et al. Balloon expandable stents for systemic venous pathway stenosis late after Mustard's operation. Heart 1998; 79:225–9.

24. Ward CJ, Mullins CE, Nihill MR, et al. Use of intravascular stents in systemic venous and systemic venous baffle obstructions. Short-term follow-up results. Circulation 1995;91:2948–54.

25. Balzer DT, Johnson M, Sharkey AM, et al. Transcatheter occlusion of baffle leaks following atrial switch procedures for transposition of the great vessels (d-TGV). Catheter Cardiovasc Interv 2004;61:259–63.

26. Dragulescu A, Sidibe N, Aubert F, et al. Successful use of covered stent to treat superior systemic baffle obstruction and leak after atrial switch procedure. Pediatr Cardiol 2008;29:954–6.

27. Daehnert I, Hennig B, Wiener M, et al. Interventions in leaks and obstructions of the interatrial baffle late after Mustard and Senning correction for transposition of the great arteries. Catheter Cardiovasc Interv 2005;66:400–7.

28. Sharaf E, Waight DJ, Hijazi ZM. Simultaneous transcatheter occlusion of two atrial baffle leaks and stent implantation for SVC obstruction in a patient after Mustard repair. Catheter Cardiovasc Interv 2001; 54:72–6.

29. Apostolopoulou SC, Papagiannis J, Hausdorf G, et al. Transcatheter occlusion of atrial baffle leak after mustard repair. Catheter Cardiovasc Interv 2000;51:305–7.

30. Schneider DJ, Moore JW. Transcatheter treatment of IVC channel obstruction and baffle leak after Mustard procedure for d-transposition of the great arteries using Amplatzer ASD device and multiple stents. J Invasive Cardiol 2001;13:306–9.

31. Ebeid MR, Gaymes CH, McMullan MR, et al. Catheter management of occluded superior baffle after atrial switch procedures for transposition of great vessels. Am J Cardiol 2005;95:782–6.

32. Stark J, Silove ED, Taylor JF, et al. Obstruction to systemic venous return following the Mustard operation for transposition of the great arteries. J Thorac Cardiovasc Surg 1974;68:742–9.

33. Latson LA. Coronary artery fistulas: how to manage them. Catheter Cardiovasc Interv 2007; 70:110–6.

34. Gowda RM, Vasavada BC, Khan IA. Coronary artery fistulas: clinical and therapeutic considerations. Int J Cardiol 2006;107:7–10.

35. Collins N, Mehta R, Benson L, et al. Percutaneous coronary artery fistula closure in adults: technical and procedural aspects. Catheter Cardiovasc Interv 2007;69:872–80.

36. Sapin P, Frantz E, Jain A, et al. Coronary artery fistula: an abnormality affecting all age groups. Medicine (Baltimore) 1990;69:101–13.

37. Reidy JF, Sowton E, Ross DN. Transcatheter occlusion of coronary to bronchial anastomosis by detachable balloon combined with coronary angioplasty at same procedure. Br Heart J 1983;49:284–7.

38. Liberthson RR, Sagar K, Berkoben JP, et al. Congenital coronary arteriovenous fistula. Report of 13 patients, review of the literature and delineation of management. Circulation 1979;59:849–54.

39. Said SA, Lam J, van der Werf T. Solitary coronary artery fistulas: a congenital anomaly in children and adults. A contemporary review. Congenit Heart Dis 2006;1:63–76.

40. Misumi T, Nishikawa K, Yasudo M, et al. Rupture of an aneurysm of a coronary arteriovenous fistula. Ann Thorac Surg 2001;71:2026–7.

41. Sherwood MC, Rockenmacher S, Colan SD, et al. Prognostic significance of clinically silent coronary artery fistulas. Am J Cardiol 1999;83:407–11.

42. Cheung DL, Au WK, Cheung HH, et al. Coronary artery fistulas: long-term results of surgical correction. Ann Thorac Surg 2001;71:190–5.

43. Wax DF, MaGee AG, Nykanen D, et al. Coil embolization of a coronary artery to pulmonary artery fistula from an antegrade approach. Cathet Cardiovasc Diagn 1997;42:68–9.

44. Gowda ST, Latson LA, Kutty S, et al. Intermediate to long-term outcome following congenital coronary artery fistulae closure with focus on thrombus formation. Am J Cardiol 2011;107:302–8.

45. Zhu XY, Zhang DZ, Han XM, et al. Transcatheter closure of congenital coronary artery fistulae: immediate and long-term follow-up results. Clin Cardiol 2009;32:506–12.

46. Armsby LR, Keane JF, Sherwood MC, et al. Management of coronary artery fistulae. Patient selection and results of transcatheter closure. J Am Coll Cardiol 2002;39:1026–32.

47. Jama A, Barsoum M, Bjarnason H, et al. Percutaneous closure of congenital coronary artery fistulae: results and angiographic follow-up. JACC Cardiovasc Interv 2011;4:814–21.

48. Valente AM, Lock JE, Gauvreau K, et al. Predictors of long-term adverse outcomes in patients with congenital coronary artery fistulae. Circ Cardiovasc Interv 2010;3:134–9.

49. Ott DA. Aneurysm of the sinus of valsalva. Semin Thorac Cardiovasc Surg Pediatr Card Surg Annu 2006;165–76.

50. Feldman DN, Gade CL, Roman MJ. Ruptured aneurysm of the right sinus of valsalva associated with a ventricular septal defect and an anomalous coronary artery. Tex Heart Inst J 2005;32:555–9.

51. Smith WA. Aneurysm of the sinus of Valsalva, with report of 2 cases. JAMA 1914;62:1878.

52. Matsumoto Y, Kubo T, Tagawa H, et al. An autopsy case of the sinus of Valsalva aneurysm involved with tuberculous inflammation, leading to complete heart block. Kokyu To Junkan 1993;41:911–5 [in Japanese].

53. Nakano T, Okano H, Konishi T, et al. Aneurysm of the left aortic sinus caused by Takayasu's arteritis: compression of the left coronary artery producing coronary insufficiency. J Am Coll Cardiol 1986;7:696–700.

54. Nakagiri K, Kadowaki T, Morimoto N, et al. Aortic root reimplantation for isolated sinus of valsalva aneurysm in the patient with Marfan's syndrome. Ann Thorac Surg 2012;93:e49–51.

55. Incarvito J, Yang SS, Papa L, et al. Fungal endocarditis complicated by mycotic aneurysm of sinus of Valsalva, interventricular septal abscess, and infectious pericarditis: unique M-mode and two-dimensional echocardiographic findings. Clin Cardiol 1981;4:34–8.

56. Dong L, Pan C, Zhao W, et al. A traumatic rupture of valsalva sinus with dissection into the interventricular septum. J Am Coll Cardiol 2011;57:e373.

57. Abe T, Kada K, Murakami H, et al. Unruptured left coronary sinus of Valsalva aneurysm causing mitral valve obstruction. Circulation 2012;125:e389–91.

58. Saritas A, Unal EU, Caliskan A, et al. Unruptured sinus of Valsalva aneurysm displacing the right atrium. Eur J Cardiothorac Surg 2012. [Epub ahead of print].

59. Chadha S, Lodha A, Shetty V, et al. Sinus of Valsalva aneurysm: a rare presentation with ventricular tachycardia. J Am Coll Cardiol 2012;59:1729.

60. Mohite PN, Rohit MK, Thingnam SK. Ruptured right sinus of Valsalva into main pulmonary artery. J Cardiovasc Dis Res 2012;3:132–4.

61. Cuculi F, Rossi M, Bradley KM, et al. Rupture of a left sinus of valsalva aneurysm with coronary compression: a rare cause of ischemic chest pain. Ann Thorac Surg 2011;92:e97–9.

62. Taguchi K, Sasaki N, Matsuura Y, et al. Surgical correction of aneurysm of the sinus of Valsalva. A report of forty-five consecutive patients including eight with total replacement of the aortic valve. Am J Cardiol 1969;23:180–91.

63. Takach TJ, Reul GJ, Duncan JM, et al. Sinus of Valsalva aneurysm or fistula: management and outcome. Ann Thorac Surg 1999;68:1573–7.

64. Dong C, Wu QY, Tang Y. Ruptured sinus of valsalva aneurysm: a Beijing experience. Ann Thorac Surg 2002;74:1621–4.

65. Cullen S, Somerville J, Redington A. Transcatheter closure of a ruptured aneurysm of the sinus of Valsalva. Br Heart J 1994;71:479–80.

66. Kerkar P, Suvarna T, Burkule N, et al. Transcatheter closure of ruptured sinus of Valsalva aneurysm using the Amplatzer duct occluder in a critically ill post-CABG patient. J Invasive Cardiol 2007;19:E169–71.

67. Srivastava A, Radha AS. Transcatheter closure of ruptured sinus of valsalva aneurysm into the left ventricle: a retrograde approach. Pediatr Cardiol 2012;33:347–50.

68. Karaaslan T, Gudinchet F, Payot M, et al. Congenital aneurysm of sinus of valsalva ruptured into right ventricle diagnosed by magnetic resonance imaging. Pediatr Cardiol 1999;20:212–4.

69. Szkutnik M, Kusa J, Glowacki J, et al. Transcatheter closure of ruptured sinus of valsalva aneurysms with an Amplatzer occluder. Rev Esp Cardiol 2009;62: 1317–21.

70. Arora R. Catheter closure of perforated sinus of valsalva. In: Sievert H, Qureshi SA, Wilson N, et al, editors. Percutaneous interventions for congenital heart disease. New York: Informa Healthcare; 2010. p. 257–62.

71. Chandra S, Vijay SK, Dwivedi SK, et al. Delineation of anatomy of the ruptured sinus of valsalva with three-dimensional echocardiography: the advantage of the added dimension. Echocardiography 2012;29:E148–51.

72. Arora R, Trehan V, Rangasetty UM, et al. Transcatheter closure of ruptured sinus of valsalva aneurysm. J Interv Cardiol 2004;17:53–8.

73. Zhao SH, Yan CW, Zhu XY, et al. Transcatheter occlusion of the ruptured sinus of Valsalva aneurysm with an Amplatzer duct occluder. Int J Cardiol 2008; 129:81–5.

74. Kerkar PG, Lanjewar CP, Mishra N, et al. Transcatheter closure of ruptured sinus of Valsalva aneurysm using the Amplatzer duct occluder: immediate results and mid-term follow-up. Eur Heart J 2010; 31:2881–7.

Percutaneous Closure of Post-Myocardial Infarction Ventricular Septal Defect
Patient Selection and Management

Mark S. Turner, PhD, FRCP[a],*, Mark Hamilton, MRCP, FRCR[b],
Gareth J. Morgan, MPhil, MRCPCH[a],
Robin P. Martin, MB, ChB, FRCP, FRCPCH[a]

KEYWORDS

- Post-myocardial infarction ventricular septal defect • Percutaneous VSD closure
- Ventricular septal defect • Surgical repair of ventricular septal defect

KEY POINTS

- Post-myocardial infarction ventricular septal defects are uncommon but associated with significant mortality.
- Therapeutic options include surgical exclusion and transcatheter device closure.
- These defects occur secondary to rupture of the myocardium and are thus ragged and irregular in morphology.
- Preprocedural imaging with either cardiac computed tomography or magnetic resonance imaging provides highly detailed images of the defect and the surrounding tissues and adds significantly to patient selection and preprocedural planning.

INTRODUCTION

Development of a post-myocardial infarction ventricular septal defect (PIVSD) is an uncommon but potentially devastating event, historically occurring in 1% to 2% of patients after acute myocardial infarction.[1–3] Recent series suggest an incidence of 0.2% in thrombolysed patients.[4–6] The mean time from infarction to post-myocardial infarction ventricular septal defect (PIVSD) is 1 day in the thrombolysed patient, and 3 to 5 days in patients for whom no revascularization was performed, but rupture may occur up to 2 weeks after infarction.[6] Our own observation is that early reopening of the infarct-related artery (IRA) leads to early development of PIVSD that can occur within 24 hours.

Current literature suggests that the most patients have multiple vessel disease with anterior infarction being more prevalent with 60% to 75% of PIVSDs occurring in left anterior descending territory (anterior septum). However, we did not experience this rate, with inferior infarction present in 56% of our first 18 patients and only 21.4% had significant triple vessel disease (unpublished audit data 2012). Inferior defects are of a very different morphology, being more ragged and sometimes with an oblique tract through the septum.[7] Surgeons describe them as the septum being pulled off the floor of the heart.

At coronary angiography, patients who develop septal rupture are likely to have a total occlusion of the IRA, with minimal collateral flow,[5] because a full thickness infarction is needed for the rupture to occur.

Despite improvements in medical therapy and intensive care, mortality rate with PIVSD remains

[a] Brisstol Heart Institute, Bristol Royal Infirmary, Marlborough Street, Bristol BS2 8HW, United Kingdom;
[b] Department of Radiology, Bristol Heart Institute, Bristol Royal Infirmary, Marlborough Street, Bristol BS2 8HW, United Kingdom
* Corresponding author.
E-mail address: mark.turner@UHBristol.nhs.uk

Intervent Cardiol Clin 2 (2013) 173–180
http://dx.doi.org/10.1016/j.iccl.2012.09.012
2211-7458/13/$ – see front matter © 2013 Published by Elsevier Inc.

extremely high, exceeding 90% with medical management.[8] Factors associated with a poor prognosis include cardiogenic shock, and right ventricular (RV) dysfunction.[9] The reported 30-day mortality after surgery is 20% to 47%.[10–12] Experience with transcatheter device closure is limited, but so far, results compare favorably with surgery. The largest series using the Amplatzer PIVSD occluder (St Jude Medical, St Paul, Minnesota) (albeit with very few acutely presenting patients) achieved successful device deployment in 16 of 18 patients, with a 30-day mortality of 28%.[13]

Autopsy and surgical evidence suggests that the defects can be ragged, complex, ovoid, or serpiginous tracts rather than round, punched-out lesions making echocardiographic assessment difficult (especially when coupled with being critically ill with a balloon pump limiting the echo windows).[14]

PHYSIOLOGY

In the congenital ventricular septal defect (VSD), the left ventricle (LV) becomes volume loaded and may dilate. In the PIVSD, the problem is the acute pressure loading of the RV. For patients with inferior VSD caused by the occlusion of the right coronary artery, there may also be RV infarction compromising RV function.

RV infarction is less pronounced in anterior VSDs, caused by the occlusion of the left anterior descending artery (LAD), which may partly explain the observation that inferior VSDs have a higher mortality rate after surgical closure than anterior VSDs.

The LV is in a high-output state but with much of the ventricular output going through the VSD into the lower resistance pulmonary circulation. This low resistance flow also gives a false impression of the function of the LV. The venting of the LV blood into the RV, gives a measured ejection fraction that can be misleading, suggesting that the ventricular function is satisfactory, when it is actually poor.

CORONARY ANATOMY

Most patients presenting to our service have single vessel disease, and do not need revascularization. Because of the presence of a full thickness infarction revascularization of the IRA is rarely recommended. However, those with disease in the other vessels causing ischemia may benefit from revascularization. The surgical literature suggests that patients having surgical closure do better if concomitant coronary artery bypass graft is performed.[15]

SURGICAL TREATMENT

A variety of surgical techniques are described, but most involve a ventriculotomy through the infarcted area and suturing an exclusion patch to the LV edge of the defect around the septal margins of the defect and then the ventriculotomy is closed encompassing the patch sandwiched between the 2 sides of the ventriculotomy, thus completing the closure.[16] For patients with surgical coronary artery disease, rupture of the free wall of the RV or concomitant severe valve disease, surgery remains the treatment of choice.

TIMING OF INTERVENTION

In surgical practice, waiting for several weeks before undertaking PIVSD surgery is advocated to allow complete necrosis of the septum, and the edges of the VSD to fibrose, thereby allowing them to hold sutures better. The negative impact of this strategy is that some patients will die of pneumonia, right heart failure, or complications of long-term use of the intra-aortic balloon pump (IABP). The authors' practice has been to stabilize the patients, perform imaging, and then undertake percutaneous closure of the PIVSD, if possible within 48 hours. Although this practice has worked for some patients, the authors have undoubtedly seen patients who have had further necrosis and development of a leak around the device.

No data are available to determine whether percutaneous intervention should be performed acutely or after a period of weeks. The authors' approach is to perform the percutaneous PIVSD closure acutely, and if the need arises, they consider surgery after a few weeks if on-going necrosis causes a late leak, or device embolization.

ANATOMIC SUITABILITY AND IMAGING

Because of the complex shape and nature of the defects, two-dimensional echocardiography does not seem to fully describe the anatomy and three-dimensional (3D) echocardiography might be limited by the imaging window in such critically ill patients. In all other areas of structural heart disease practice the authors use the most appropriate imaging modality to inform decisions about intervention. The authors therefore use computed tomography (CT) or magnetic resonance imaging (MRI) to better delineate the anatomy of the defects.

CROSS-SECTIONAL IMAGE ACQUISITION

In our center, contrast enhanced cardiac CT is performed on a Siemens Sensation 16-slice CT

Somatom or Siemens 128-slice AS plus scanner, (Siemens Medical Systems, Erlangen, Germany), using a single breath hold at end inspiration. Multiphase reconstructions using retrospective echocardiography gating are obtained.

Cardiac MRI is performed on a Siemens Symphony 1.5 T MRI scanner. Balanced steady-state free precession is used to obtain short and long axis views of the ventricles and additional focused views of the VSD.

Examples of CT and MRI images are shown in **Fig. 1**.

DEVICE

The Amplatzer postinfarction muscular VSD occluder (AGA Medical; Golden Valley, Minnesota) is made of nitinol wire mesh shaped into 2 discs with a waist to fill the VSD. The waist is 10-mm long and the diameter of the waist provides the nominal size of the occluder. The LV and RV discs have a diameter 10 mm larger than the waist.

Polyester fabric inserts help to close the defect by promoting endothelization of the occluder. The devices were implanted using a 10F Amplatzer delivery sheath. Amplatzer PIVSD occluders are available from 16 to 24 mm in 2 mm increments. An example is shown in **Fig. 2**.

The authors decide on whether to offer a percutaneous procedure based on the clinical status and the imaging, with the emphasis being on the cross-sectional imaging reconstructed in the plane of the septum. If the defect is no more than 25 mm in its maximum diameter, the authors usually attempt percutaneous closure (based on the largest device available, having a 24-mm waist).

PROCEDURE DESCRIPTION
Patient Preparation and Team

The procedure is usually performed under general anesthesia to facilitate transesophageal echocardiography (TEE). An experienced TEE operator is important, and nonstandard views may be needed.

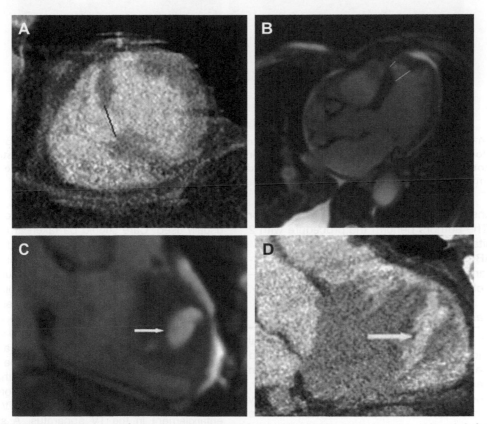

Fig. 1. (A) shows a short axis cut from a computed tomographic (CT) scan demonstrating a large defect which measured 41 mm in some planes excluding it from device closure. (B) demonstrates a funnel shaped defect on magnetic resonance imaging (MRI). The difference between the size of the opening to the funnel on the left ventricular side and the exit point on the right ventricular (RV) side is clearly demonstrated. The RV exit point measurement was used to confirm suitability for a successful device closure. (C) and (D) show enface views of 2 different defects on MRI and CT, respectively. They demonstrate a difference in morphology, which influenced the decision to perform percutaneous closure (C) or not to attempt this procedure (D).

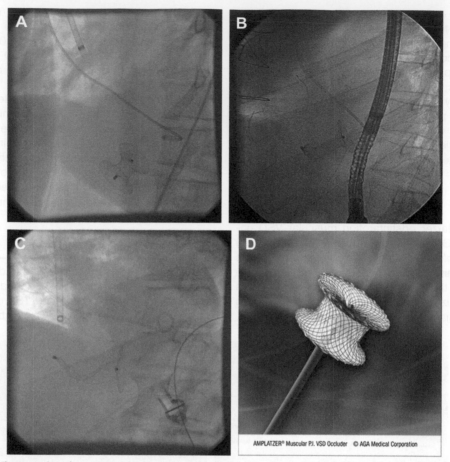

AMPLATZER® Muscular P.I. VSD Occluder   © AGA Medical Corporation

Fig. 2. (*A–C*) examples of variations in device conformity in 2 patients. (*B*) and (*C*) demonstrate the compressed morphology of the occluder which occurred in patients with long, funnel shaped defects. (*A*) demonstrates the typical conformation of the device, which is pictured before insertion in (*D*). ([*D*] *Courtesy of* St Jude Medical; with permission.)

The transgastric view can be useful for inferior VSDs. The authors perform the procedure with 2 congenital/structural interventionalists.

An IABP should be implanted before the induction of anesthesia to reduce the risk of hemodynamic collapse in case of hemodynamic instability.

Access and Angiography

Femoral artery, femoral vein, and right internal jugular access (RIJ) is obtained (using ultrasound guidance in our cath lab). LV angiography is then performed in a left anterior oblique view usually, but the best angle for profiling of the septum may be estimated from the cardiac CT. The patient is fully heparinized to an activated clotting time of 250 to 300 seconds.

Crossing and Formation of Guide Wire Circuit

A long (125 cm) right coronary catheter (JR4) is then placed in the LV and is manipulated to cross

the VSD. An exchange length Terumo wire is usually used. Care should be taken at this point as the wire can cause ventricular fibrillation because of the irritable peri-infarction border zone. Once across the VSD, the Terumo wire should be advanced to one of the pulmonary arteries (PA), or occasionally to the superior vena cava (SVC). Attempts should be made to avoid the tricuspid valve (TV) apparatus at this stage.

Once the Terumo wire is in the PA, a second catheter should be introduced from the internal jugular vein across the TV and into the same branch PA as the Terumo wire. A balloon-tipped catheter may be helpful in crossing the TV without entanglement in the TV apparatus. A standard stiffness, 0.035 in 260 cm length wire should be used to exchange the catheter from the RIJ for a snare catheter, and a 20-mm snare should be introduced. The Terumo wire then needs to be snared. Once captured the snare should be gently withdrawn, carefully watching for any appearance to suggest that the wire loop is trapped around a papillary muscle of the TV. The TEE operator should carefully observe the TV at this time for evidence of distortion or tricuspid regurgitation (TR). The operator at the groin and the operator at the neck need to work together to carefully control the wire loop. If there is evidence of compromise of the TV, the wire should be released from the snare and the catheters and wires should be passed again. This part of the procedure must be approached with caution. Entanglement of the wire in the tricuspid apparatus can cause temporary tricuspid regurgitation, and excessive force can cause serious damage to the valve, which could prove fatal in a patient with right heart failure.

Once a satisfactory wire loop is established through the VSD, the 125-cm JR4 should be advanced to the SVC, where the snare should be advanced over the wire to capture the JR4 catheter about 1 to 2 cm from its tip. The Terumo should then be removed from the leg and a 300-cm noodle wire from St Jude/AGA should be advanced from the femoral JR4 to protrude from the JR4 in the SVC. The snare can then be released from the catheter and slowly withdrawn to capture the noodle wire just below the J. The noodle wire can then be exteriorized in the neck by pulling it through the RIJ sheath. An 8F sheath makes this process easier.

CROSSING THE DEFECT WITH THE DELIVERY SHEATH FROM THE VENOUS SIDE

The noodle wire is then pulled through to give approximately 100 cm protruding from the neck. The 8F short sheath in the neck should be removed and hemostasis can be maintained by digital pressure. A St Jude/AGA 10F 80-cm delivery sheath should then be introduced into the internal jugular. The sheath and its dilator are then advanced to meet the JR4 catheter on the noodle wire. The 2 operators then need to work together to maintain the tension in the noodle wire and by advancing the 10F sheath, withdrawing the JR4 and pulling the whole assembly, the 10F sheath needs to be positioned with its tip well into the LV in the region of the lateral ventricular wall under the mitral valve, for inferior VSD. For anterior VSD the femoral vein approach can be used, but the authors still use the RIJ.

DEVICE IMPLANTATION

At this stage or before, the chosen device should be loaded. We use the 24 mm PIVSD device unless the defect is smaller than 18 mm. There

seems little downside to oversizing to allow for future necrosis in the infarcted area.

The sheath dilator can now be removed by the RIJ operator and the leg operator can pull back the noodle wire to allow the loader to be attached to the 10F sheath. Because the sheath is in the LV at this point, blood loss occurs from the sheath, so the loader needs to be attached quickly. The device is then advanced down the sheath while the leg operator gradually pulls the noodle wire back. When the device reaches the tip of the sheath, the noodle wire will be released and the circuit is broken, with the sheath in the LV and the device at the tip ready for deployment. As the device stiffens the sheath, care is needed to ensure that the stiffened sheath does not traumatize the lateral wall of the LV or the papillary muscle. If in doubt, the sheath may need to be withdrawn a little to the LV body. TEE can be useful to guide this process.

The device can now be delivered, which is usually guided by TEE. The device should be held in place, and the sheath gradually withdrawn to allow opening of the left-sided disc and some of the waist. The disc and waist should be pulled back together, toward the septum, but a large amount of force should not be applied to the recently infarcted septum. Once the left disc is in the plane of the left side of the septum, the right disc can be released from the sheath and can be allowed to conform to the right heart structures. If too much force is applied to the left-sided disc and waist, the device may rotate to allow it to be posted through the VSD, which is one of the reason for oversizing.

ASSESSMENT OF THE RESULT

Once the device is in place it can be evaluated by TEE and by LV angiography (with a pigtail catheter being re-introduced from the femoral artery). Residual shunt is to be expected at this stage, and assessment is to see if the shunt has been reduced significantly, but mainly to determine if the device is implanted with the left disc in the plane of the left side of the septum. If not the device may be recaptured and manipulated, but readvancing across the septum without the left disc being well into the LV is not always possible. If the device is positioned well, it can be released and consideration can be given to a second device, but the authors prefer to use 1 device. Implanting a second device can cause dislodgement of the first or other complications.

The authors aim to implant the left disc of the device flush with the LV aspect of the septum. The right side of the device can be constrained by the trabeculations in the RV. Examples of the variable conformations of the Amplatzer device are shown in **Fig. 2**, including an image of the device courtesy of St Jude Medical. **Fig. 3** shows a postprocedural CT scan of the device.

COMPLICATIONS

Complications include bleeding, stroke, ventricular rupture, hemodynamic deterioration, VF, damage to valves, device embolization, failure to close the shunt and hemolysis. Hemolysis on 2 occasions have been observed by the authors, one acutely after device closure, which led to acute renal failure due to the hemoglobinuria (and contributed to his death) and the other chronic, that started some months after the procedure and was managed medically with occasional transfusion.

Device embolization may occur because the defect size is underestimated or because further necrosis occurs to enlarge the defect and allows the device to move. Embolization is likely to result in a large residual shunt and may be an indication for surgery if the patient is operable.

Pacemaker therapy may be required for heart block.

Post-Procedure Care

Some patients show immediate improvement when the device is implanted, but in others it takes a little longer for the RV to recover. The IABP is left in situ and other inotropes are usually weaned first.

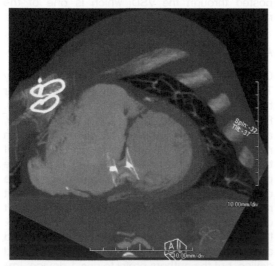

Fig. 3. A computed tomographic scan showing the Amplatzer device in place in an inferior post-myocardial infarction ventricular septal defect. Note the patient had undergone previous aortic valve replacement some years before; the sternal wires are related to the previous surgery.

Patients are usually managed on the surgical intensive care unit by specially trained cardiac anesthetists.

Usual post-MI medical therapy is then introduced. angiotensin-converting-enzyme (ACE) inhibitor therapy is often initiated before IABP withdrawal. Beta blockade is added if the blood pressure is sufficient to tolerate it, after ACE-inhibitor therapy is in place.

Anticoagulation/Anti-Platelet

If the patient is in sinus rhythm the authors give Aspirin and clopidogrel to prevent clot formation on the VSD occluder. If in atrial fibrillation the authors prescribe warfarin, with low dose aspirin. If the patient has had a coronary stent then the antiplatelet therapy is determined by the coronary interventionist.

Follow-up and Recurrent Leaks

As previously discussed, vigilance is needed to treat complications and identify residual or recurrent leaks. Small leaks are common and are to be expected.

Cross Over to Surgery for Late Residual Leak

For patients with recurrent or incomplete closure of the left to right shunt, surgical treatment may be performed later. The authors have treated 2 patients (one inferior and one anterior) who had an initially good result from transcatheter closure and later developed a further leak. Both underwent a second transcatheter procedure, but still with unacceptable residual shunt. Both patients were then treated surgically, one 4 weeks and other 3 weeks after percutaneous treatment. Both patients survived, and the surgeons commented that the margins of the defect were less friable than they usually see. In the anterior defect, the defect was clearly larger than at initial presentation, suggesting that there had been some necrosis of the surrounding myocardium. The device closure in these 2 patients allowed us to defer surgery to a time when the surgical risk would be expected to be lower.

TRANSCATHETER CLOSURE OF RESIDUAL DEFECTS AFTER SURGICAL CLOSURE

Residual defects after surgical closure of PIVSD are relatively common because the surgeon is often faced with a difficult repair with a limited view of the defect and the margins of the defect where sutures need to be placed are often friable. Sometimes there may be progression of the infarction area as the zone around the area of rupture extends during the postoperative period. Small residual defects are common and may be managed conservatively. However, if there is hemodynamic compromise or there is a large shunt during later follow-up, then transcatheter closure of the patch leak may be considered.

CLINICAL ASSESSMENT AND ECHOCARDIOGRAPHY FOR POSTSURGICAL PATCH LEAK

The clinical findings will typically be a persistent pansystolic murmur, cardiac failure, or a low cardiac output state postoperatively. Echocardiography will identify the presence of the residual defect and to assess its size based on the left to right color flow jet. Functional assessment will include either assessment of the Doppler velocity of the left to right shunt or the velocity of the TV regurgitation, to assess RV pressure and the presence of pulmonary hypertension. There may be multiple defects and sometimes identification of the anatomy of the defects can be difficult on echocardiography. Three-dimensional echocardiography and TEE gives a good assessment of the size of the defects but the anatomy is often very complex and cross-sectional MRI or CT imaging is usually needed if transcatheter closure is being considered. If the patient is not on a balloon pump, MRI flow imaging may identify areas of left to right shunt around the surgical patch. Many surgeons use large exclusion patches with Teflon patches to buttress sutures. MRI can also assess the left to right shunting by measuring pulmonary to systemic flow ratio. When MRI imaging is contraindicated gated CT imaging will give a good assessment of the anatomy.

Technique for Transcatheter Closure of Postsurgical Patch Leaks

The technique for closure will be similar to that for native defects described previously. A jugular approach is usually best for apical defects, but anterior defects may be easier to cross from a femoral venous approach, and sometimes in certain patients, the authors have found an arterial approach from the brachial artery to be the best (because the delivery sheaths are not long enough for femoral delivery). In the authors' limited experience with acute postoperative patients, multiple occluders may be required because of the multiple residual sites of shunting and to help reattach the patch at an area of dehiscence. Recurrent leaks may occur late after surgery, and in one case the patient was treated for heart failure 10 years after surgery.

Bristol VSD Strategy

In Bristol the authors have developed the following approach to PIVSD.

The patient's hemodynamics are assessed. If there is evidence of hypotension, hypoperfusion, renal dysfunction, or a need for inotropes, the authors immediately implant an IABP, usually in the left leg. If there is any evidence of ongoing ischemia the coronaries are imaged and percutaneous coronary intervention is performed if there are significant lesions in the noninfarct arteries (by definition there is a full thickness infarct in the IRA).

Echocardiography, including 3D echocardiography, if the imaging windows are satisfactory for this task, is performed to assess valve function, left and RV function, right heart pressures, presence of pericardial effusion and the anatomy of the ventricular septal defect.

Patients who do not need a balloon pump may be assessed by cardiac MRI to look for shunt, morphology of the VSD, and ventricular function. However, most patients have a balloon pump or find it difficult to lie flat for a cardiac MRI. Most patients therefore have gated cardiac CT to assess the VSD morphology, with image reconstructions being made in the plane of the septum.

Taking the 3D imaging together, percutaneous closure to patients with reasonable LV function and a VSD with the maximum diameter being less than 25 mm can be attempted. Because most defects are oval, this means that a 24 mm Amplatzer VSD device (with a 24 mm waist and 34 mm discs) should be just adequate to occlude the ruptured septum.

Exclusions are

> VSD >25 mm diameter
> Poor LV function
> Major sepsis
> Other surgical indication, significant valve disease, multi-vessel coronary disease, or coronary disease unsuitable for PCI.

After device implantation the patient is managed in intensive care and mechanical support and inotropes are weaned slowly. Regular echocardiography is performed and renal function is carefully managed. Deterioration prompts a detailed search for residual leaks.

Bristol Outcomes

The authors have treated 24 patients with acute PIVSDs, including those with shock, using percutaneous transcatheter devices with 15 patients surviving to 30 days (62.5%), and all were treated acutely. Twelve of 22 patients with more than one-year follow up, were alive at one year. The longest survivors had their procedure more than 7 years ago, so acute percutaneous PIVSD closure can provide a long-term result.

SUMMARY

Percutaneous closure of PIVSD is a technically challenging but feasible technique. The authors approach relies heavily on cross-sectional imaging to understand the morphology of the defect. Percutaneous treatment can be performed acutely with reasonable results.

REFERENCES

1. Di Summa M, Actis Dato GM, Centofanti P, et al. Ventricular septal rupture after a myocardial infarction: clinical features and long term survival. J Cardiovasc Surg (Torino) 1997;38(6):589–93.
2. Reeder GS. Identification and treatment of complications of myocardial infarction. Mayo Clin Proc 1995;70(9):880–4.
3. Held AC, Cole PL, Lipton B, et al. Rupture of the interventricular septum complicating acute myocardial infarction: a multicenter analysis of clinical findings and outcome. Am Heart J 1988;116(5 Pt 1):1330–6.
4. Crenshaw BS, Granger CB, Birnbaum Y, et al. Risk factors, angiographic patterns, and outcomes in patients with ventricular septal defect complicating acute myocardial infarction. GUSTO-I (Global Utilization of Streptokinase and TPA for Occluded Coronary Arteries) Trial Investigators. Circulation 2000; 101(1):27–32.
5. Yip HK, Fang CY, Tsai KT, et al. The potential impact of primary percutaneous coronary intervention on ventricular septal rupture complicating acute myocardial infarction. Chest 2004;125(5):1622–8.
6. Skehan JD, Carey C, Norrell MS, et al. Patterns of coronary artery disease in post-infarction ventricular septal rupture. Br Heart J 1989;62:268–72.
7. Feneley MP, Chang VP, O'Rourke MF. Myocardial rupture after acute myocardial infarction: ten year review. Br Heart J 1983;49:550–6.
8. Moore CA, Nygaard TW, Kaiser DL, et al. Postinfarction ventricular septal rupture: the importance of location of infarction and right ventricular function in determining survival. Circulation 1986;74: 45–55.
9. Montoya A, McKeever L, Scanlon P, et al. Early repair of ventricular septal rupture after infarction. Am J Cardiol 1980;45(2):345–8.
10. Skillington PD, Davies RH, Luff AJ, et al. Surgical treatment for infarct-related ventricular septal defects. Improved early results combined with analysis of late functional status. J Thorac Cardiovasc Surg 1990;99(5):798–808.
11. Jeppsson A, Liden H, Johnsson P, et al. Surgical repair of post infarction ventricular septal defects: a national experience. Eur J Cardiothorac Surg 2005;28(1):185–6.
12. Holzer R, Balzer D, Amin Z, et al. Transcatheter closure of postinfarction ventricular septal defects using the new Amplatzer muscular VSD occluder: results of a U.S. Registry. Catheter Cardiovasc Interv 2004;61(2):196–201.
13. Edwards BS, Edwards WD, Edwards JE. Ventricular septal rupture complicating acute myocardial infarction: identification of simple and complex types in 53 autopsied hearts. Am J Cardiol 1984; 54:1201–4.
14. Swithingbank JM. Perforation of the interventricular septum in myocardial infarction. Br Heart J 1959; 21:562–7.
15. Perrotta S, Lentini S. In patients undergoing surgical repair of post-infarction ventricular septal defect, does concomitant revascularization improve prognosis? Interact Cardiovasc Thorac Surg 2009;9(5): 879–87.
16. David TE, Dale L, Sun Z. Postinfarction ventricular septal rupture: repair by endocardial patch with infarct exclusion. J Thorac Cardiovasc Surg 1995; 110:1315–22.

Transcatheter Pulmonary Valve Replacement
Current Status and Future Potentials

Damien Kenny, MB, MD, MRCPCH,
Ziyad M. Hijazi, MD, MPH, FSCAI*

KEYWORDS

- Transcatheter • Valve • Stent • Pulmonary • Regurgitation

KEY POINTS

- Transcatheter pulmonary valve replacement has evolved into an attractive alternative to surgery in older children and adults with dysfunctional ventricular-to-pulmonary artery conduits.
- The learning curve with initial valve design has led to significant improvements to both valve design and procedural approach.
- Indications for implantation are evolving; however, a more aggressive approach may now be possible to prevent the longer-term effects of chronic right ventricular pressure and volume loading.
- Simplification of follow-up protocols may reduce both financial and time burden to patients.
- Future endeavors will focus on a percutaneous valve for the dilated native right ventricular outflow tract and tissue engineering that may promote valve growth and longevity.

INTRODUCTION

Endeavors in congenital heart disease are mirroring (often preceding) efforts in adult cardiology in providing less-invasive, but equally effective alternatives to surgery. In the context of transcatheter pulmonary valve replacement (tPVR), battle lines were drawn when Bonhoeffer and colleagues[1] reported successful transcatheter delivery of a valved stent into a 12-year-old boy with stenosis and insufficiency of a prosthetic conduit from the right ventricle to the pulmonary artery more than 10 years ago. This delivery set the platform for nonsurgical replacement or repair of other heart valves, which is proving to be the most exciting advancement in the treatment of valve disease in many years. In less than a decade, tPVR has evolved rapidly through the inevitable technical learning curve and design modifications to establish itself as an acceptable therapy for right ventricular (RV)-to-pulmonary artery conduit and bioprosthetic valve dysfunction. Limitations remain related to valve size in patients with native outflow tracts, and although tPVR has been described with both established and novel approaches in this setting,[2–5] surgery remains the preferred approach in most cases. Extensive data collection through early clinical experience and clinical trials was necessary to prove safety and efficacy of the approach. Evolving data from these studies have shown beneficial effects of tPVR in right ventricular (RV) volume reduction,[6] left ventricular filling properties,[7] exercise capacity,[8] and electrical remodeling.[9] This review discusses the evolution of tPVR,

Disclosure: Dr Hijazi is a non-paid consultant for Edwards Lifesciences, the company that manufactures the Edwards Sapien THV. He is also a consultant for Colibri and has stock options. Dr Kenny has no conflict of interest related to this study. This is an original manuscript and has not been previously published or submitted to another journal.
Rush Center for Congenital and Structural Heart Disease, Rush University Medical Center, 1653 West Congress Parkway, Chicago, IL 60612, USA
* Corresponding author.
E-mail address: ZHijazi@rush.edu

Intervent Cardiol Clin 2 (2013) 181–193
http://dx.doi.org/10.1016/j.iccl.2012.09.008
2211-7458/13/$ – see front matter Published by Elsevier Inc.

interventional.theclinics.com

the attempts and challenges to establishing itself as an acceptable and cost-effective alternative to surgery, and possible future endeavors in this field.

PROCEDURAL EVOLUTION

Initial work in animals was reported in 2000 by Bonhoeffer and colleagues,[10] in an ovine model with successful valve delivery in 7 of 11 attempts. Valve design consisted of a section of fresh bovine jugular vein attached to a platinum iridium stent. Initially, the stent was expanded to a radial diameter of 18 mm, and the length of jugular vein was sutured to span the entire axial length of the stent. The valved stent was then hand crimped onto the inflatable portion of an 18- to 22-mm balloon catheter. Five valves were delivered in the desired location, and macroscopic review after explantation at 2 months showed transparent, mobile, and competent valves in 4 of these. One stent was slightly stenotic and showed macroscopically visible calcifications. Reported experience in humans followed,[11] with the first detailed clinical study reporting on 59 consecutive patients with right ventricular outflow tract (RVOT) dysfunction associated with stenosis or significant pulmonary insufficiency, leading to RV dilatation or RV failure.[6] Successful valve implantation was achieved in 58 patients. Three patients required acute surgical intervention because of stent dislodgment or conduit rupture. During a mean follow-up of just less than 10 months, there was no mortality; however, device-related complications were seen in 14 of the 56 patients (25%). These included in-stent stenosis, referred to as the *hammock effect* in 7 because of lack of apposition of the valve to the stent. This observation led to a change in device design with suturing of the whole length of the bioprosthetic valve tissue to the stent. Stent fracture, which has continued to

be clinically relevant for this valve (Medtronic Melody Valve [Medtronic Inc, Minneapolis, MN]) (**Fig. 1**) was noted in 7 patients, with one patient undergoing a second valve-in-valve implantation. Overall freedom from surgical explantation for valve failure was 83% at 12 months.

More recent studies with the Melody Valve have found improved outcomes with reduction in adverse events.[12,13] Further follow-up data from Bonhoeffer's group after the initial report showed reduction in procedural complications from 6% to 2.9%.[12] Recently, a multicenter US clinical trial evaluating the Melody Valve found impressive medium-term outcomes in 124 patients with dysfunctional right ventricular-to-pulmonary artery conduits. Freedom from Melody Valve dysfunction or reintervention was almost 94% at 1 year.[13] An alternative transcatheter pulmonary valve has also become available, achieving CE marking in the European Union and undergoing trials in the United States. The Edwards SAPIEN transcatheter heart valve (Edwards Lifesciences LLC, Irvine, CA) (**Fig. 2**) was initially introduced as a transcatheter alternative to surgical valve replacement in elderly patients with severe aortic stenosis.[14] Reports describing implantation in the pulmonary position for RVOT conduit dysfunction, mirroring valve efficacy and durability in the aortic position, have followed.[15] Recently, a multicenter international clinical trial found effective reduction of RVOT gradient (27 mm Hg–12 mm Hg [P<.001]) with improvement in clinical symptoms and maintenance of pulmonary valvar competence at 6-month follow-up.[16]

INDICATIONS

Defining objective parameters of when to replace the pulmonary valve in the setting of chronic pulmonary regurgitation has been difficult. With

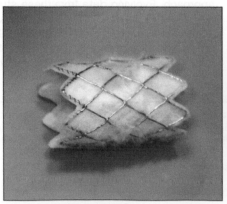 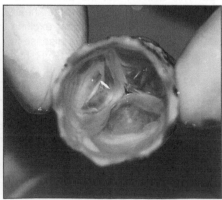

Fig. 1. The Medtronic Melody valve seen in 2 different views. (*Courtesy of* Medtronic, Mounds View, MN; with permission.)

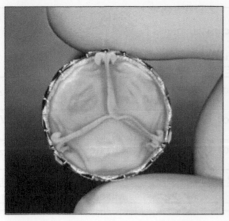 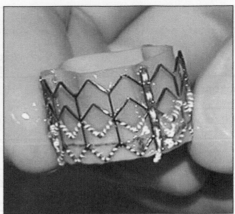

Fig. 2. The Edwards SAPIEN valve seen in 2 different views.

the advent of magnetic resonance imaging (MRI), right ventricular volumes greater than which normalization cannot be re-established after insertion of a competent pulmonary valve have been used as a general guide for surgical intervention.[17,18] This guide has been necessary to optimize timing of surgical valve replacement, especially considering the limited lifespan of these valves. Currently, surgical intervention is generally indicated with indexed right ventricular end-diastolic volumes (RVEDV) >150 mL/m^2 based on recently published data[18]; however, American Heart Association/American College of Cardiology guidelines for repeat surgery in this setting are not so prescriptive.[19] Other indications for surgical valve replacement have centered on presence of symptoms or right ventricular dysfunction. Guidelines for tPVR are even less clear cut with recently published guidelines for intervention in pediatric cardiac disease advocating tPVR in a patient with an RV-to-pulmonary artery conduit with associated moderate-to-severe pulmonary regurgitation

or stenosis provided the patient meets inclusion/exclusion criteria for the available valve.[20]

Thus, with 2 currently available valves, indications for tPVR are reflected in the inclusion/exclusion criteria of published clinical trials with these respective valves (**Table 1**).[13,16]

Some studies have also included patients with peak oxygen consumption less than 65% predicted as an indication.[21,22] Irrespective of variations in inclusion protocols, it is clear that tPVR is being performed at indexed RVEDVs significantly less than those being followed for surgical valve replacement. This may in part be because of conduit stenosis, which often is not encountered in patients with a dilated RVOT after a transannular patch. The contribution of outflow tract narrowing to symptoms should not be underestimated in this setting. In a study by Lurz and colleagues,[23] patients with predominantly stenotic conduits showed significant increases in RV ejection fraction after tPVR, changes not seen in those with predominant regurgitation. Exercise capacity also

Table 1
Published inclusion criteria for clinical trials with both the Melody and SAPIEN valves

Inclusion Criteria (Melody)[13]	Inclusion Criteria (Edwards)[16]
Age ≥5 y/Weight ≥30 kg Original conduit diameter ≥16 mm Echocardiographic RVOT conduit dysfunction: • Patients classified as NYHA class II, III or IV: Doppler mean gradient ≥35 mm Hg or ≥ moderate PR • Patients classified as NYHA class I: Doppler mean gradient ≥40 mm Hg or severe PR associated with TV annulus z-score ≥2 or RVEF <40%.	Weight >35 kg In situ conduit ≥16 mm and ≤24 mm ≥3 + PR (TTE) or PRF ≥40% (MRI) with or without stenosis.

Abbreviations: PRF, pulmonary regurgitant fraction; PR, Pulmonary regurgitation; RVEF, right ventricle ejection fraction; TTE, transthoracic echocardiogram; TV, tricuspid annulus.

Table 2
Cardiopulmonary exercise testing outcomes from clinical studies

Study	Journal	Patients Undergoing CPET (n)	Method	Results
Khambadkone et al,[6]	Circulation 2005	16 of 59	Bicycle	Improved V_{O2max}
McElhinney et al,[13]	Circulation 2010	93 of 124	Bicycle	Improved VE/VCO_2[a]
Vezmar et al,[22]	JACC Cardiovasc Interv 2010	19 of 28	Bicycle	Improved V_{O2max} and VE/VCO_2[b]
Eicken et al,[21]	Eu Heart J 2011	102	N/A	No change in V_{O2max}
Kenny et al,[16]	J Am Cull Cardiol 2011	34	Mixed	No change in V_{O2max}[a]

[a] Greater than 40% did not reach AT.
[b] Nonpaired data.

increased in the stenotic cohort but not in those with regurgitation. This is thought to be related to limiting effects of fixed obstruction on cardiac output during exercise, which is not seen in those with predominant pulmonary regurgitation.

Two other important indications for intervention should not be overlooked, namely, risk for longer-term arrhythmia and progressive left ventricular dysfunction. QRS duration ≥180 ms has been associated with 42-fold increased risk of sustained ventricular tachycardia developing and a 2.2-fold increased risk of sudden cardiac death during a 10-year follow-up study.[24] Further work by Oosterhof and colleagues,[25] suggested that

delayed postoperative increases in QRS duration may occur in patients with preoperative QRS greater than150 ms, again suggesting that earlier intervention may be beneficial on propensity for arrhythmia. Although mortality with ventricular tachycardia in this study was low, implantable cardiac defibrillators are problematic in the setting of tetralogy of Fallot with high rates of inappropriate shocks and lead to complications.[26] Transcatheter pulmonary valve replacement has been found to significantly reduce QRS duration in those with predominant regurgitation and therefore may affect arrhythmia burden in this patient group.[9]

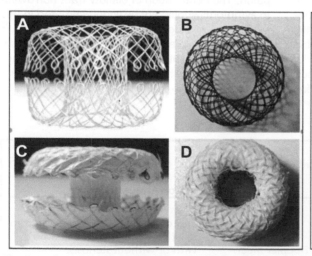 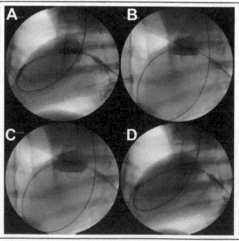

Fig. 3. *Left Panel,* The novel self-expanding nitinol stent with a central constriction. The device is shortened as both extremities curve backward, which also provides more stability. (*A, B*) The device shown in 2 different views. (*A–D*) The device with Polytetrafluroethylene covering to assure sealing of the device and prevent paravalvular leak. *Right Panel,* Series of fluoroscopic images outlining deployment of the Melody valve within a native RVOT with the novel self-expanding stent in place. (*[Left panel] From* Mollet A, Basquin A, Stos B, et al. Off-pump replacement of the pulmonary valve in large right ventricular outflow tracts: a transcatheter approach using an intravascular infundibulum reducer. Pediatr Res 2007;62:428–33; with permission.)

Table 3
Procedural outcomes from clinical studies

Study	No. of Patients	Success	Complications	Fracture	FFR (Follow-Up)
Lurz et al,[12]	163	155 (95%)	7 (4.5%)	21%	70% (70 mo)
McElhinney et al,[13]	136	124 (91%)	8 (6%)	22%	93.5% (12 mo)
Eicken et al,[21]	102	100%	2 (2%)	5%	89% (12 mo)
Kenny et al,[16]	36	33 (92%)	7[a] (20.5%)	0	97% (6 mo)
Butera et al,[43]	63	61 (97%)	9[a] (14%)	16%	81.4% (30 mo)

Abbreviation: FFR, freedom from reintervention.
[a] Includes major and minor complications.

Left ventricular (LV) dysfunction has been seen in approximately 20% of adult patients with repaired tetralogy of Fallot, particularly in those patients with significant RV dysfunction.[27] The exact mechanisms underlying the LV dysfunction are not clear, but ventricular diastolic interaction, along with prolonged abnormal electrical remodeling may be involved.[28] The impact of tPVR on LV dynamics has shown small but significant increases in left ventricular ejection fraction.[21,22] It is unclear if this represents a beneficial effect of earlier intervention, which may otherwise lead to lack of complete RV remodeling and continue to affect left ventricular filling properties. The other possibility is the impact of tPVR on concomitant stenosis. Relief of stenosis in this setting with tPVR has been shown to increase LV end-diastolic volumes.[29] Further work found improved left ventricular filling dynamics were secondary to reduction in interventricular mechanical delay (caused by leftward bowing of the interventricular septum), which may impede left ventricular filling.[7]

PROCEDURAL WORKUP AND TECHNICAL CONSIDERATIONS

Preprocedural workup assists in ensuring appropriate patient choice and in the evaluation of potential technical challenges during the procedure. Cardiopulmonary exercise testing (CPET) and cardiac MRI became established preprocedural diagnostic tools as part of the clinical trials that evaluated the safety and efficacy of the procedure.[13,16] However, as the procedure becomes more established and widespread, it is vital that these investigations are performed to similar standards as in the clinical trials. Cardiopulmonary exercise testing has been useful in stratifying patients with tetralogy of Fallot at risk for both hospitalization and death. Patients with peak oxygen uptake $\leq$36% of predicted value and those with VE/VCO^2 slopes greater than 39 have been shown to be at greater risk for cardiac-related death.[30] However, the cohorts of patients evaluated for tPVR usually have mixed stenosis/regurgitation, providing a different substrate, and concern to date has centered on intervening too early rather than too late. CPET may be useful in patients with predominant regurgitation being evaluated for tPVR when there is a question

Box 1
Complications associated with tPVR

Procedural

Pulmonary hemorrhage (2° to guide wire)

Ventricular arrhythmia

Stent embolization (prestenting)

Coronary artery compression

Conduit rupture

Valve embolization

Follow-up

Stent fracture

Infective endocarditis

Box 2
Classification of stent fractures

Type I: fracture of 1 strut without loss of stent integrity

Type II: fracture with loss of stent integrity

Type III: fracture associated with separation of fragments or embolization

Data from Nordmeyer J, Khambadkone S, Coats L, et al. Risk stratification, systematic classification, and anticipatory management strategies for stent fracture after percutaneous pulmonary valve implantation. Circulation 2007;115:1392–7.

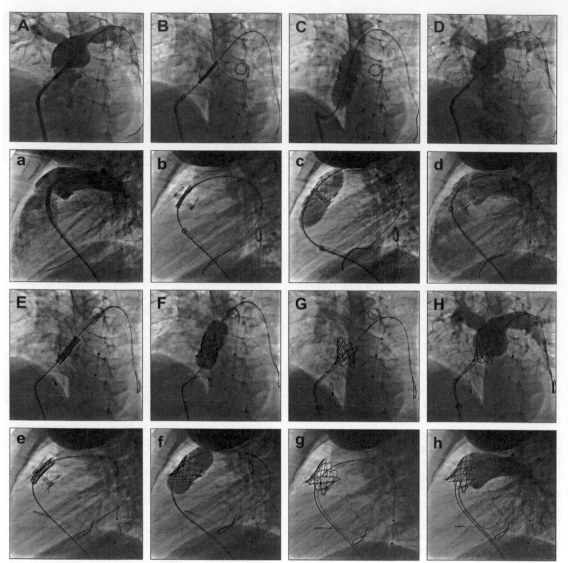

Fig. 4. Series of fluoroscopic (*A–H*) and intracardiac echocardiographic (*I–V*) images show tPVR in a patient with a preexisting bioprosthetic pulmonary valve with the Melody valve. Panels A–H show the fluoroscopic images in both frontal (*upper case*) and lateral (*lower case*) imaging planes from prestenting all the way through to valve deployment and postdeployment angiography. Panels I–V show the corresponding intracardiac echocardiography (ICE) images evaluating the RVOT before valve deployment and after prestenting and subsequent valve deployment.

regarding symptoms, thus providing an objective assessment of exercise capacity. However, it is less clear cut whether CPET should be widely used after tPVR to prove benefit. Published data to date have been mixed in determining whether CPET is useful in demonstrating changes in measured variables, and this may be a consequence of the mixed pathologies encountered (**Table 2**).

Cardiac MRI produces accurate assessment of right ventricular volumes and function and also provides an estimate of regurgitant fraction.

However, cardiac MRI is time consuming and uncomfortable for patients, and transthoracic echocardiography alone may suffice. Recent data from the US Melody clinical trial looking at the reliability and accuracy of echocardiographic right heart evaluation suggested that Doppler echocardiographic assessment of RVOT obstruction shows excellent correlation with gradient at catheterization.[31] Assessment of pulmonary regurgitation using a 3-point severity scale showed good agreement with cardiac MRI-derived pulmonary regurgitant fraction. Moreover, apical diastolic

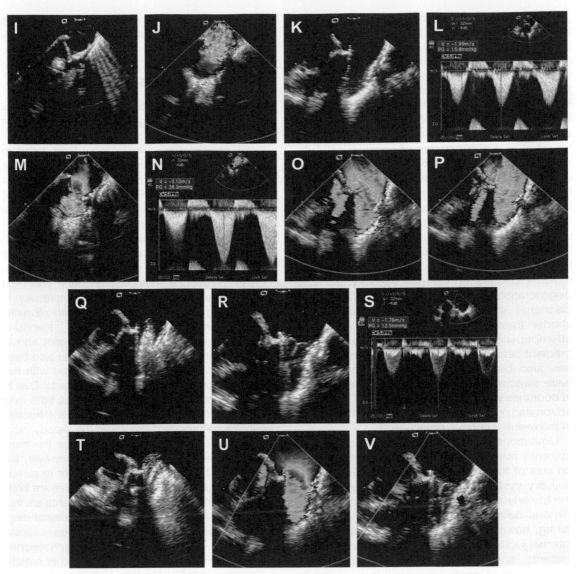

Fig. 4. (continued)

area was highly reproducible and had an excellent correlation with cardiac MRI RV end-diastolic volume with all patients with indexed RV apical diastolic areas ≥30 cm²/m² having cardiac MRI RV end-diastolic volumes ≥160 mL/m². The authors concluded that transesophageal echocardiogram alone may be a suitable screening test for some tPVR candidates with cardiac MRI indicated for decisions hinging on assessment of RV function. This approach may not provide detailed imaging of the RVOT and surrounding tissues, limiting useful information gleaned on degree of conduit calcification, branch pulmonary artery anatomy, and relationship of the coronary arteries to the conduit. These indices can be measured accurately with cardiac computed tomography, with superior temporal and spatial resolution to MRI, and is a far less cumbersome imaging modality. Whether the degree and extent of calcification of the conduit impacts risk for conduit rupture has yet to be delineated; however, computed tomography is deemed a superior imaging modality for identifying calcification and may prove more advantageous in this regard in the future. Anatomic variances may also have implications for likelihood of stent fracture with severely obstructed conduits or conduits positioned directly behind the sternum associated with increased risk of Melody Valve stent fracture.[32]

Although both the Melody and SAPIEN valves have individual delivery systems, certain basic procedural caveats should be adhered to, including pre-assessment of the coronary artery proximity to the RVOT, establishment of a stable safe wire position, and prestenting before valve implantation. Potential coronary artery compression is not uncommon, with 4.4% of the US cohort having unsuitable anatomy,[13] and deaths have been reported as a consequence of coronary compression in this setting. Attention to wire position is also advised because pulmonary hemorrhage secondary to distal arterial damage has been reported.[16] The benefits of prestenting have predominantly focused on reduction of stent fracture, and a recent report with a high incidence of prestenting (95%) found stent fractures as low as 5%.[21] It is also important to consider the potential deleterious effects of residual stenosis on exercise capacity and valve degeneration with higher RVOT gradients at discharge after Melody insertion associated with shorter freedom from valve dysfunction[12]; thus, attempts should be made to abolish any residual gradient before valve implantation. Conduit rupture has also been reported,[12] and some operators have switched to prestenting with covered stents in countries where these are available. Others have advocated preparation of a covered stent as a bailout in the event of conduit disruption.[33]

Limitations to extended application of the currently available valves have generally centered on size of the patient and of the RVOT. The 22F delivery system used most commonly with both the Melody and SAPIEN valves have limited transfemoral delivery to children weighing more than 20 kg; however, other options are available. The internal jugular vein may be used in these smaller patients, and experience with this approach is evolving. An alternative approach is valve delivery directly through the heart (perventricular) via a sheath placed in the right ventricular free wall.

Extended applications of the valve relate not only as an alternative to elective surgical valve replacement but also in establishing valvar competence in those patients who may not otherwise be surgical candidates. Lurz and colleagues[34] described successful tPVR in 7 patients with significant pulmonary hypertension and severe pulmonary regurgitation. After valve implantation there was improvement in patient symptoms with an increase in RV stroke volumes and oxygen saturations and a decrease in RV volumes. The valve has functioned well at median follow-up of 20 months despite near systemic pulmonary artery pressures in some. Attempts to extend the application of preexisting valves to dilated outflow tracts have also included preplacement of an intravascular reducer

(**Fig. 3**)[35] or telescoping stents from one of the branch pulmonary arteries to anchor a Melody Valve in the RVOT.[3]

CLINICAL OUTCOMES

The relevant clinical outcomes relate to procedural success, that is, placing a well-functioning valve in the desired location, number and extent of procedural complications, and longer-term freedom from valvar dysfunction and reintervention. Data from the largest most recently published studies evaluating attempted tPVR (Melody and SAPIEN) in 500 patients are outlined in **Table 3**. Procedural success is generally high, with mean valve deployment of 95%. Procedural complications (**Box 1**) vary according to definition, but in those studies reporting exclusively major complications, the mean procedural complication rate was just greater than 4%. Coronary artery compression in this setting has been associated with mortality and may present after the procedure[21]; therefore, if there is any doubt, valve deployment should not be attempted. Conduit rupture has also been reported,[33] and risk factors associated with this complication need to be elucidated. Overall mean freedom from reintervention was 86% over a mean follow-up of 26 months. Stent fracture remains an important event with the Melody Valve despite prestenting (5%–16%) and is the most common reason for reintervention; however, the extent of stent fracture is also relevant to clinical outcomes (**Box 2**). Type I stent fractures are likely to occur initially, and only 56% of patients are free from type II fractures at 2 years from initial diagnosis of stent fracture and therefore require careful monitoring.[32] Stent fracture has not been reported to date with the SAPIEN valve. The other notable outcome variable is the risk of infective endocarditis, which has been reported consistently at between 1% and 4% with the Melody Valve. Reported data are not available for the SAPIEN valve in the pulmonary position.

THE FUTURE

Although tPVR is evolving into an acceptable alternative to surgery, much uncertainty exists because longer-term data are lacking. It seems that initial benefits on RV remodeling occur within the first 6 months with limited further changes in RVEDV or ejection fraction as measured by MRI at 1 year.[36] However, this is likely to mirror surgical data, and concerns should be targeted less toward continued RV remodeling than valve and stent durability. There is every reason to believe that valve durability will at least be as good as surgical

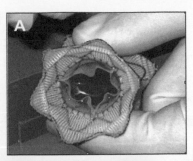

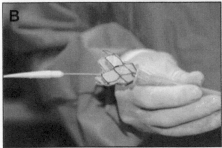

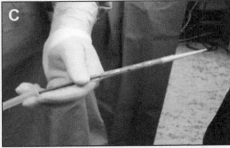

Fig. 5. The new Medtronic self-expanding stent designed for native RVOTs. (*A*) Short axis view of the valve. (*B*) Loading the valve into the delivery system. (*C*) The valve fully loaded and ready for delivery. (*Courtesy of* Medtronic, Mounds View, MN; with permission.)

valve replacement (reports have shown pulmonary regurgitant fractions $\geq$30% at 1 year in 7% of surgical valve replacement patients),[18] although it may be difficult to recruit patients into a randomized clinical trial considering patient preference for tPVR. The most contemporary large dataset evaluating valve dysfunction and reintervention in adolescent patients undergoing surgical PVR revealed mean freedom from valvar dysfunction of 72% and mean freedom from reintervention of 90% at 5 years, and mirroring these figures is a shorter-term goal.[37] Although risk factors for reintervention are being identified,[32] the exact pathologic mechanisms of valve degeneration in a host of different conduits have only been postulated

through case reports.[38] The other attractive option with tPVR is the potential for further valve replacement with the valve-in-valve technique extending the number of repeat percutaneous valve replacements to an as-yet undefined number.[39]

Strategies for the future should be 3-fold. The first strategy should involve consolidating and improving current techniques to minimize procedural risk and simplify follow-up protocols, reducing cost that is not inconsiderable[40,41] and inconvenience to the patient. Intracardiac echocardiography has provided excellent imaging of valve function in the acute phase, confirming valve competency that may be otherwise distorted by catheters required for postdeployment angiography and may provide

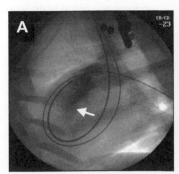

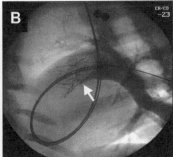

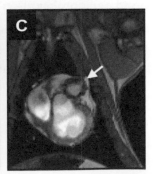

Fig. 6. (*A*) Fluoroscopic image from an animal model shows significant pulmonary regurgitation (*white arrow*). (*B*) Pulmonary competence is restored after valve implantation (*white arrow*). (*C*) MR image shows the valve in the RVOT with the distal end outlined (*white arrow*).

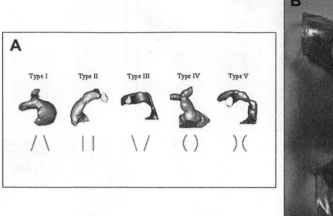

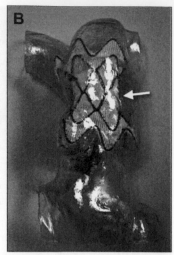

Fig. 7. (*A*) The variety of RVOT morphologies that may be encountered. (*B*) The self-expanding valve in a plastic model of a native RVOT (*white arrow*).

more accurate postdeployment assessment of valve function (**Fig. 4**).

The second endeavor should be aimed at further valve development to extend technology to those with native RVOTs. Although deployment of balloon-expandable stents in native outflow tracts has been described,[4,6] size restriction on the currently available valves (Melody, 22 mm [has been stretched up to 24 mm] and SAPIEN, 26 mm [29-mm SAPIEN valve may be available in the near future for pulmonic position]) prevents deployment in most patients with significant pulmonary regurgitation. Clinical reports exist of a new valve sewn into a self-expanding nitinol frame (**Figs. 5** and **6**)[5]; however, applicability of this technology over the anatomic and dynamic variability that exists within the RVOT[42] remains

questionable (**Fig. 7**) and further modifications may be necessary. Other self-expanding valve systems are in development (**Fig. 8**); however, clinical data are required before longer-term applicability is assessed.

The third endeavor should be to miniaturize the delivery system so that smaller children with dysfunctional conduits/bioprosthetic valves may be treated percutaneously. The newer generation of the SAPIEN valve (the SAPIEN XT) requires a smaller delivery system of 18–19F (NovaFlex, Edwards Lifesciences). However, this system has not been tested yet for deployment in the pulmonary position. Also, newer lower profile pulmonary valves are being evaluated in animal models. One such a new valve is the Colibri Heart Valve (Colibri Heart Valve, LLC, Broomfield, CO) (**Fig. 9**). This

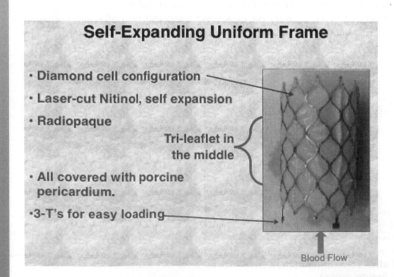

Fig. 8. The Lifetech Scientific valve (Shenzhen, China) is a porcine peri-cardial valve mounted on a self-expanding nitinol frame and is currently undergoing clinical trials. (*Courtesy of Nguyen Lan Hieu, MD, PhD, Hanoi, Vietnam; with permission.*)

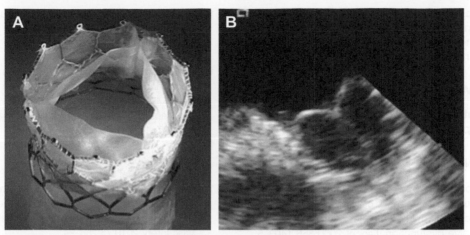

Fig. 9. (*A*) The Colibri valve in seen with an (*B*) ICE image of the valve in the RVOT in a canine model. (*Courtesy of Colibri Heart Valve, LLC, Broomfield, CO; with permission.*)

valve has been tested in a swine model (**Fig. 10**), and it requires 12–16F delivery system for valves ranging in size from 20–30 mm.

The last endeavor should be to merge these approaches with tissue engineering technologies to provide living autologous valve replacements with regenerative and growth potential. This approach has been described in an animal model,[43] and although representing the longer-term goal of valve replacement, this may be some way off.

Although established, tPVR is in its infancy compared with surgical PVR. Extended clinical experience and follow-up have identified new challenges; however, careful evaluation of data through clinical trials has facilitated effective evolution of responses to these challenges. The limited patient population has resulted in less interest in new valve design, but having been the older sibling to transcatheter aortic valve replacement, tPVR is likely to benefit in the future from design modifications to the more popular and

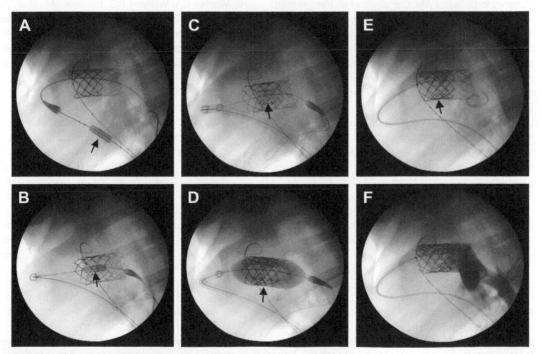

Fig. 10. Series of fluoroscopic images outlining implantation of the Colibri in a swine model (Valve indicated by *black arrow*). (*A, B*) Advancement of the premounted valve across the prestented main pulmonary artery. (*C, D*) Inflation of the inner and outer balloons, with final stent-valve position and angiogram showing valvar competence (*E, F*).

commercially viable transcatheter aortic valve revolution. Improving valve longevity and applying the technology to native outflow tracts remain the short-to-medium goals.

ACKNOWLEDGMENTS

The authors thank Dr Qi-Ling Cao for his assistance in preparing the images used in this report.

REFERENCES

1. Bonhoeffer P, Boudjemline Y, Saliba Z, et al. Percutaneous replacement of pulmonary valve in a right-ventricle to pulmonary-artery prosthetic conduit with valve dysfunction. Lancet 2000;356:1403–5.

2. Momenah TS, El Oakley R, Al Najashi K, et al. Extended application of percutaneous pulmonary valve implantation. J Am Coll Cardiol 2009;53:1859–63.

3. Boudjemline Y, Legendre A, Ladouceur M, et al. Branch pulmonary artery jailing with a bare metal stent to anchor a transcatheter pulmonary valve in patients with patched large right ventricular outflow tract. Circ Cardiovasc Interv 2012;5:e22–5.

4. Guccione P, Milanesi O, Hijazi ZM, et al. Transcatheter pulmonary valve implantation in native pulmonary outflow tract using the Edwards SAPIEN™ transcatheter heart valve. Eur J Cardiothorac Surg 2012;41:1192–4.

5. Schievano S, Taylor AM, Capelli C, et al. First-in-man implantation of a novel percutaneous valve: a new approach to medical device development. EuroIntervention 2010;5:745–50.

6. Khambadkone S, Coats L, Taylor A, et al. Percutaneous pulmonary valve implantation in humans: results in 59 consecutive patients. Circulation 2005;112:1189–97.

7. Lurz P, Puranik R, Nordmeyer J, et al. Improvement in left ventricular filling properties after relief of right ventricle to pulmonary artery conduit obstruction: contribution of septal motion and interventricular mechanical delay. Eur Heart J 2009;30:2266–74.

8. Batra AS, McElhinney DB, Wang W, et al. Cardiopulmonary exercise function among patients undergoing transcatheter pulmonary valve implantation in the US Melody valve investigational trial. Am Heart J 2012;163:280–7.

9. Plymen CM, Bolger AP, Lurz P, et al. Electrical remodeling following percutaneous pulmonary valve implantation. Am J Cardiol 2011;107:309–14.

10. Bonhoeffer P, Boudjemline Y, Saliba Z, et al. Transcathotor implantation of a bovine valve in pulmonary position: a lamb study. Circulation 2000;102:813–6.

11. Bonhoeffer P, Boudjemline Y, Qureshi SA, et al. Percutaneous insertion of the pulmonary valve. J Am Coll Cardiol 2002;39:1664–9.

12. Lurz P, Coats L, Khambadkone S, et al. Percutaneous pulmonary valve implantation: impact of evolving technology and learning curve on clinical outcome. Circulation 2008;117:1964–72.

13. McElhinney DB, Hellenbrand WE, Zahn EM, et al. Short- and medium-term outcomes after transcatheter pulmonary valve placement in the expanded multicenter US melody valve trial. Circulation 2010;122:507–16.

14. Webb JG, Chandavimol M, Thompson CR, et al. Percutaneous aortic valve implantation retrograde from the femoral artery. Circulation 2006;113:842–50.

15. Boone RH, Webb JG, Horlick E, et al. Transcatheter pulmonary valve implantation using the Edwards SAPIEN transcatheter heart valve. Catheter Cardiovasc Interv 2010;75:286–94.

16. Kenny D, Hijazi ZM, Kar S, et al. Percutaneous implantation of the Edwards SAPIEN transcatheter heart valve for conduit failure in the pulmonary position: early phase 1 results from an international multicenter clinical trial. J Am Coll Cardiol 2011;58:594–8.

17. Oosterhof T, van Straten A, Vliegen HW, et al. Preoperative thresholds for pulmonary valve replacement in patients with corrected tetralogy of Fallot using cardiovascular magnetic resonance. Circulation 2007;116:545–51.

18. Frigiola A, Tsang V, Bull C, et al. Biventricular response after pulmonary valve replacement for right ventricular outflow tract dysfunction: is age a predictor of outcome? Circulation 2008;118(Suppl):S182–90.

19. Warnes CA, Williams RG, Bashore TM, et al. ACC/AHA 2008 guidelines for the management of adults with congenital heart disease: a report of the American College of Cardiology/American Heart Association Task Force on Practice Guidelines. Circulation 2008;118:714–833.

20. Feltes TF, Bacha E, Beekman RH 3rd, et al, on behalf of the American Heart Association Congenital Cardiac Defects Committee of the Council on Cardiovascular Disease in the Young, Council on Clinical Cardiology, Council on Cardiovascular Radiology and Intervention. Indications for cardiac catheterization and intervention in pediatric cardiac disease: a scientific statement from the American Heart Association. Circulation 2011;123:2607–52.

21. Eicken A, Ewert P, Hager A, et al. Percutaneous pulmonary valve implantation: two-centre experience with more than 100 patients. Eur Heart J 2011;32:1260–5.

22. Vezmar M, Chaturvedi R, Lee KJ, et al. Percutaneous pulmonary valve implantation in the young 2-year follow-up. JACC Cardiovasc Interv 2010;3:439–48.

23. Lurz P, Giardini A, Taylor AM, et al. Effect of altering pathologic right ventricular loading conditions by percutaneous pulmonary valve implantation on exercise capacity. Am J Cardiol 2010;105:721–6.

24. Gatzoulis MA, Balaji S, Webber SA, et al. Risk factors for arrhythmia and sudden cardiac death late after repair of tetralogy of Fallot: a multicentre study. Lancet 2000;356:975–81.

25. Oosterhof T, Vliegen HW, Meijboom FJ, et al. Long-term effect of pulmonary valve replacement on QRS duration in patients with corrected tetralogy of Fallot. Heart 2007;93:506–9.

26. Khairy P, Harris L, Landzberg MJ, et al. Implantable cardioverter-defibrillators in tetralogy of Fallot. Circulation 2008;117:363–70.

27. Broberg CS, Aboulhosn J, Mongeon FP, et al, Alliance for Adult Research in Congenital Cardiology (AARCC). Prevalence of left ventricular systolic dysfunction in adults with repaired tetralogy of Fallot. Am J Cardiol 2011;107:1215–20.

28. Tobler D, Crean AM, Redington AN, et al. The left heart after pulmonary valve replacement in adults late after tetralogy of Fallot repair. Int J Cardiol 2012;160(3):165–70.

29. Coats L, Khambadkone S, Derrick G, et al. Physiological and clinical consequences of relief of right ventricular outflow tract obstruction late after repair of congenital heart defects. Circulation 2006;113: 2037–44.

30. Giardini A, Specchia S, Tacy TA, et al. Usefulness of cardiopulmonary exercise to predict long-term prognosis in adults with repaired tetralogy of Fallot. Am J Cardiol 2007;99:1462–7.

31. Brown DW, McElhinney DB, Araoz PA, et al. Reliability and accuracy of echocardiographic right heart evaluation in the U.S. Melody valve investigational trial. J Am Soc Echocardiogr 2012;25: 383–92.

32. McElhinney DB, Cheatham JP, Jones TK, et al. Stent fracture, valve dysfunction, and right ventricular outflow tract reintervention after transcatheter pulmonary valve implantation: patient-related and procedural risk factors in the US Melody Valve Trial. Circ Cardiovasc Interv 2011;4:602–14.

33. Sosnowski C, Kenny D, Hijazi ZM. Bailout use of the Gore Excluder following pulmonary conduit rupture during transcatheter valve replacement. Catheter Cardiovasc Interv, in print.

34. Lurz P, Nordmeyer J, Coats L, et al. Immediate clinical and haemodynamic benefits of restoration of pulmonary valvar competence in patients with pulmonary hypertension. Heart 2009;95:646–50.

35. Mollet A, Basquin A, Stos B, et al. Off-pump replacement of the pulmonary valve in large right ventricular outflow tracts: a transcatheter approach using an intravascular infundibulum reducer. Pediatr Res 2007;62:428–33.

36. Lurz P, Nordmeyer J, Giardini A, et al. Early versus late functional outcome after successful percutaneous pulmonary valve implantation: are the acute effects of altered right ventricular loading all we can expect? J Am Coll Cardiol 2011;57:724–31.

37. Batlivala SP, Emani S, Mayer JE, et al. Pulmonary valve replacement function in adolescents: a comparison of bioprosthetic valves and homograft conduits. Ann Thorac Surg 2012;93:2007–16.

38. Law KB, Phillips KR, Butany J. Pulmonary valve-in-valve implants: how long do they prolong reintervention and what causes them to fail? Cardiovasc Pathol 2012. [Epub ahead of print].

39. Nordmeyer J, Coats L, Lurz P, et al. Percutaneous pulmonary valve-in-valve implantation: a successful treatment concept for early device failure. Eur Heart J 2008;29:810–5.

40. Raikou M, McGuire A, Lurz P, et al. An assessment of the cost of percutaneous pulmonary valve implantation (PPVI) versus surgical pulmonary valve replacement (PVR) in patients with right ventricular outflow tract dysfunction. J Med Econ 2011;14:47–52.

41. Gatlin SW, Kim DW, Mahle WT. Cost analysis of percutaneous pulmonary valve replacement. Am J Cardiol 2011;108:572–4.

42. Nordmeyer J, Tsang V, Gaudin R, et al. Quantitative assessment of homograft function 1 year after insertion into the pulmonary position: impact of in situ homograft geometry on valve competence. Eur Heart J 2009;30:2147–54.

43. Butera G, Milanesi O, Spadoni I, et al. Melody transcatheter pulmonary valve implantation. Results from the registry of the Italian Society of Pediatric Cardiology (SICP). Catheter Cardiovasc Interv 2012. [Epub ahead of print].

Pulmonary Vein Stenting for Atrial Fibrillation Ablation–Induced Pulmonary Vein Stenosis

Ameya Kulkarni, MD, Ignacio Inglessis, MD*

KEYWORDS

• Atrial fibrillation • Pulmonary vein stenosis • Stenting

KEY POINTS

• Pulmonary vein stenosis (PVS) is a known complication of pulmonary vein isolation in the treatment of atrial fibrillation.
• Patients with PVS can present with a great variety of symptoms. Clinicians should have a low threshold to evaluate for this potentially morbid and treatable condition.
• PVS can be treated by stenting affected pulmonary veins via transseptal access to the left atrium and use of bare metal biliary stents.

INTRODUCTION

The use of catheter-based ablative therapy in the treatment of atrial fibrillation (AF) has been largely successful in reducing the burden of this exceedingly common condition.[1,2] The technique of electrically isolating the pulmonary veins is well tolerated in most patients. However, for a small subset of patients, pulmonary vein isolation can result in stenosis of the pulmonary veins.[1] When severe, this process can cause pulmonary hypertension, heart failure, and hemoptysis, potentially resulting in significant morbidity for the patient.[3] Transcatheter therapy provides a safe, minimally invasive option to relieve obstructive lesions and shows significant promise as a modality in the treatment of this potentially devastating condition.

Incidence

The rate of significant pulmonary vein stenosis (PVS) after ablative therapy for AF was initially reported as between 2% and 8%,[1,3] although some studies suggested the true prevalence was as high as 42%.[2] Some of this variance explained by changes in ablative technique over time and whether routine follow-up diagnostic imaging studies are performed following the procedure. For example, 20% of patients treated with circular mapping and distal isolation had a severe stenosis of the pulmonary veins (>70%); the electroanatomic approach was associated with an incidence of 15%; 2.9% was the rate with circular mapping and ostial isolation based on PV angiography; 1.4% with circular mapping guided by intracardiac echocardiography; and 0% with circular mapping with energy delivery based on visualization of microbubbles.[4] Continued evolution of ablation technology coupled with increased comfort with established methods have decreased rates of iatrogenic PVS. Current epidemiologic studies suggest a rate closer to 0% to 5%.[5,6]

Clinical Presentation

Clinical manifestations of severe PVS typically require reduction of the luminal area greater than 70% in the pulmonary vein.[3] Many patients with

Interventional Cardiology, Massachusetts General Hospital, Harvard Medical School, Boston, MA, USA
* Corresponding author. Cardiology Division, Massachusetts General Hospital, 55 Fruit Street, GRB 820, Boston, MA 02114.
E-mail address: inglessis.ignacio@mgh.harvard.edu

Intervent Cardiol Clin 2 (2013) 195–202
http://dx.doi.org/10.1016/j.iccl.2012.09.006

interventional.theclinics.com

single pulmonary vein compromise are asymptomatic; however, the likelihood of developing symptoms increases when more than one vein is involved. Median time to symptom onset is 7 to 8 weeks after the procedure, although some patients become symptomatic immediately after the procedure. Respiratory complaints are the typical presenting symptoms.[7] A dry cough or the persistence of a pulmonary infection despite adequate therapy is frequently noted early in the patient's clinical course. If PVS involves multiple pulmonary veins, the obstructive lesions can result in postcapillary pulmonary hypertension, resulting in dyspnea on exertion, pulmonary edema, or clinical findings consistent with right heart failure.[8] Rarely, hemoptysis is seen as the presenting complaint. The relative heterogeneity of symptoms and infrequency of PVS mean that the diagnosis is frequently missed.[7] Because of the great variation in clinical presentations, the diagnosis of PVS should be considered in *any* patient with respiratory complaints or new signs of heart failure after AF ablation.

Asymptomatic Patients

The concern about poor recognition of nonspecific symptoms has prompted some to advocate for routine noninvasive screening after AF ablation.[6] Although there is no clear evidence to support screening in completely asymptomatic patients, the potential morbidity associated with the clinical manifestations of PVS may empirically justify periodic surveillance with a noninvasive imaging modality.

PULMONARY VEIN ANATOMY

In most patients, pulmonary venous drainage follows a standard pattern. Four pulmonary veins drain in to the posterior part of the left atrium. On the left, the left superior pulmonary vein typically enters at an angle 30° superior to the coronal plane and drains the left upper lobe. Similarly, the left inferior pulmonary vein connects to the atrium 30° inferior to the coronal plane and drains the left lower lobe. There is significantly greater variation in the right-sided pulmonary veins; although on average, the right superior pulmonary vein is 50° superior and drains the right upper and middle lobe, the right inferior pulmonary vein is 20° inferior to the coronal plane and drains the right lower lobe **(Fig. 1)**.[9]

A large minority of patients may have significant anatomic variations. In patients imaged before AF ablation, almost one-third were noted to have a right middle pulmonary vein that provided drainage for the right middle lobe and 17% of

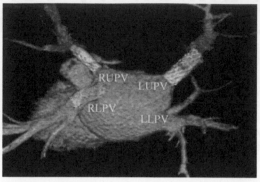

Fig. 1. Routine follow-up computed tomography scan after completion of a staged intervention on 3 stenotic pulmonary veins. The anatomic relationship between the posterior left atrium and the 4 pulmonary veins (right upper pulmonary vein [RUPV], right lower pulmonary vein [RLPV], left upper pulmonary vein [LUPV], and left lower pulmonary vein [LLPV]) is clearly seen. There are widely patent stents in the RUPV, RLPV, and LUPV.

patients had a common ostia for the left pulmonary veins. In addition, even among patients with only 4 pulmonary veins, there was significant variation in the angles of entry to the atrium, especially for the veins draining the right lung.[9]

These variances emphasize the importance of developing an anatomic road map using either computed tomography (CT) or magnetic resonance imaging in anticipation of pulmonary vein transcatheter therapy. Anatomic factors to consider preprocedurally include:

- Anatomic position of the pulmonary veins: The number of ostia, presence of additional veins, anomalous pulmonary venous return, and the angle of entry into the atrium are all important in considering appropriate selection of guiding catheters.
- Venous ostial diameter: On average, the pulmonary venous ostium is 7.8 mm in diameter. However, there is significant variation within and among patients. Preprocedural imaging, as well as review of preablation imaging studies when available, are helpful in determining pulmonary vein size and orientation for guide catheter and stent selection.
- Presence of early side branches: Although the interatrial septum is typically crossed slightly anterior to the posterior wall of the left atrium at the level of the right lower pulmonary vein, once crossed, the right lower pulmonary vein is immediately posterior and the right-sided pulmonary vein is typically immediately superior and posterior.

PREPROCEDURE PLANNING
Clinical Evaluation

A thorough history focusing on respiratory complaints and clinical signs of heart failure is the key part of the initial clinical evaluation. As symptom improvement is the primary determinant of success in pulmonary vein stenting, a detailed understanding of presenting symptoms to establish a baseline is important. Physical examination findings specific to PVS are rare and are usually limited to physical findings associated with pulmonary hypertension and right heart failure.

Femoral venous access and transseptal puncture are required for PV stenting. As such, confirming femoral venous patency and ensuring that there are no obstructions in the inferior vena cava (ie, inferior vena cava filter) is reasonable in the appropriate clinical scenario. An assessment of fitness for dual antiplatelet therapy is critical as all patients receiving pulmonary stents should be placed on Aspirin and Plavix for a minimum of 3 months.

Diagnostic Imaging

Ventilation-perfusion scan
Ventilation-perfusion (V/Q) scanning is the primary modality used to assess the physiologic consequences of PVS. Lobar perfusion defects have been associated with stenosis greater than 80% in the veins providing drainage for that region as well as gradients across the pulmonary veins of less than 5 mm Hg.[10,11] In addition, relief of the stenosis has correlated with an improvement in lobar perfusion (Fig. 2).[12] As such, V/Q scanning is recommended during the initial evaluation. Follow-up V/Q scanning can also be done 6 months after PV stenting to evaluate for improvement and also for the diagnosis of stent restenosis in patients who develop recurrent symptoms.

Spiral CT chest with contrast
Dedicated CT scan of the chest with venous contrast is the preferred noninvasive test to identify the anatomy and stenoses in the pulmonary veins. Lesions occupying more than 70% of the lumen of pulmonary veins are considered significant (Fig. 3). Imaging protocols should be carefully coordinated with radiologists to focus on the left atrial inflow, and contrast infusion should be timed to fill pulmonary veins during image capture. Despite adequate protocoling in experienced centers, there is a significant rate of false-positive diagnoses in the evaluation of PVS. Conversely, total pulmonary vein occlusions can also be overestimated by CT angiography. As such, it is imperative that confirmatory invasive angiography is performed before any intervention.

Cardiac magnetic resonance angiography
Cardiac magnetic resonance angiography (MRA) is also frequently used to evaluate pulmonary veins after AF ablation.[6] The spatial resolution and quantitative analysis of flows can provide detailed information about the relative anatomy of the pulmonary veins and flow limitation.[9] However, the frequency of motion artifact in the left atrium and the inability to use this modality in patients with pacemakers or implantable cardioverter defibrillators limit its utility in this population.

Echocardiogram
The transthoracic echocardiogram has little utility in defining pulmonary venous anatomy or diagnosing stenosis though it can be helpful in defining the anatomy of the atrial septum (presence of atrial septal aneurysm, atrial sepal defect, patent foramen ovale) and the dimensions of the left atrium. Transesophageal echocardiography (TEE) or intracardiac echocardiography (ICE), on the other hand, can provide significant information on the anatomic relationship between the interatrial septum and the individual pulmonary veins. In addition, flow acceleration at the ostium of the pulmonary veins could suggest significant stenosis. Although neither necessary nor sufficient

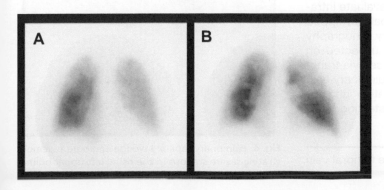

A   B

Fig. 2. Perfusion scans in a patient with severe stenosis of the right upper, left upper, and left lower pulmonary veins before (A) and after (B) stenting. Defects in both the right and left lung fields improve with stenting.

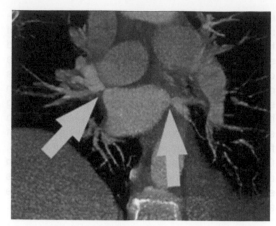

Fig. 3. CT angiogram demonstrating severe stenosis of the right and left upper pulmonary veins (*arrows*).

for the diagnosis of PVS, TEE and/or ICE can be a helpful adjunct to other diagnostic modalities.

PROCEDURAL PREPARATION

Procedures should be done in cardiac catheterization laboratories, preferably with biplane capability, as simultaneous orthogonal planes are extremely helpful in engaging pulmonary veins. Patients are placed in the traditional supine position and placed under general anesthesia. Selective bilateral lung intubation should be considered in patients at high risk for hemoptysis (ie, severe congestive heart failure with multiple pulmonary veins involved). TEE immediately before and during the procedure may be helpful to engage the guiding catheter into affected pulmonary veins, although its use is not critical, especially if biplane fluoroscopy is available.

PROCEDURAL APPROACH
Overview

After the patient is under general anesthesia, a 7F sheath is placed in a femoral vein. Right heart catheterization using a balloon tipped Swan-Ganz catheter is then performed to evaluate intracardiac hemodynamics. Next, a balloon-tipped wedge catheter is used for pulmonary venography via wedge angiography. If PVS is suspected on angiography, the left atrium is accessed via transseptal puncture, and the affected pulmonary vein is selectively engaged for confirmatory angiography, followed by angioplasty and stenting.

Vascular Access

A standard 7F sheath is placed in the femoral vein for initial access.

Hemodynamic Assessment and Wedge Angiography

Using a standard balloon-tipped Swan-Ganz pulmonary artery catheter, right-sided intracardiac and pulmonary hemodynamics are measured. The balloon-tipped catheter is then used to selectively engage the right upper lobe, right lower lobe, left upper lobe, and left lower lobe. In each lobe, a pulmonary capillary wedge pressure is obtained and while the balloon is inflated, contrast is injected distal to the balloon. Pulmonary venous runoff during levophase is assessed.

The resulting pulmonary wedge angiograms are used as screening for significant PVS and as a "road map" to engage the veins directly via transseptal approach (**Fig. 4**). Angiographically evident stenosis greater than 70% is considered severe and should be considered for luminal modification.

Transseptal Puncture

To enter the left atrium, a transseptal puncture needle is advanced over a Mullins sheath through the fossa ovalis (slightly superior to the tricuspid valve and posterior when seen in the lateral projection). Once access to the left atrium has been obtained, the Mullins sheath should be exchanged for a deflectable tip sheath, such as the Agilis sheath (St Jude Medical, St Paul, MN, USA), over a stiff wire. The Agilis sheath has an 8.5F internal lumen, accommodating most currently available stent platforms.

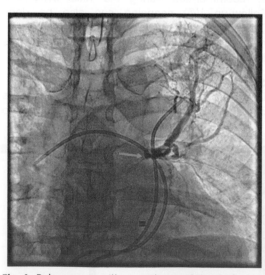

Fig. 4. Pulmonary capillary wedge angiogram demonstrating severe stenosis in the ostial left upper pulmonary vein (*arrow*).

Engagement of Pulmonary Veins

A deflectable tip sheath will provide enough directability to engage the pulmonary veins in most cases. If necessary, especially for lesions in the right middle or right lower pulmonary veins (typically more difficult to access via the transseptal approach), an additional catheter, such as the Judkins Right or the multipurpose catheter, could be used inside the tip deflectable sheath. Pulmonary wedge angiography outlining the stenotic pulmonary vein is often used as a road map to facilitate direct pulmonary vein engagement.

Diagnostic Assessment Before Stenting

Once the stenotic pulmonary vein has been engaged, retrograde selective pulmonary vein angiography is used to evaluate the length and severity of the stenosis as well as to outline the surrounding anatomic landmarks (**Fig. 5**A). Careful attention should be paid to understand the relationship between the stenotic zone and the venoatrial junction. Pulmonary venous branches close to the stenosis should also be identified and avoided, as jailing of side branches could result in less than expected improvement in patient symptoms. Pressure gradients across the stenotic lesion should also be interrogated either using a coronary pressure wire or a small double lumen catheter (**Fig. 6**A).

For lesions that are difficult to evaluate using simple angiography, intravascular ultrasound can be helpful to understand lesion characteristics and complicated anatomy (**Fig. 7**).

Intervention

Wiring the lesion
Both 0.035" and 0.018" platforms can be used for pulmonary vein angioplasty. In our experience, however, a 0.035" platform provides significantly more stability and support.

Angioplasty
Large balloons are frequently required because of the large luminal diameter (typically >5 cm) of the pulmonary veins. Cautious predilation with a slightly undersized balloon is recommended to improve luminal diameter and to help facilitate stent delivery. In those cases where a significant waist is observed during balloon predilation, which indicates a severe and highly resistant stenosis, over dilation should be avoided to prevent pulmonary vein rupture. Smaller and less complaint balloons should be used in this situation.

Stenting
Because of the large caliber of pulmonary veins, drug-eluting stents are frequently too small for pulmonary vein stenting with limited experience to date with these devices.[13] As such, bare metal biliary stents are most often used. We favor balloon-delivered stents over self-expandable stents as the former allows for increased deployment accuracy. The stents should be sized to match the reference diameter of the affected pulmonary vein.

Criteria for Successful Result

Complete angiographic resolution of stenosis is rare as tissue noncompliance and recoil are commonplace in the muscular pulmonary veins. As such, a successful procedure is one that results in less than 25% residual stenosis with less than 5 mm Hg residual gradient across the stent (see **Figs. 5**B and **6**B). If there is uncertainty about deployment, intravascular ultrasound is used to evaluate the reference vessel as well as the stented region.

Procedural Complications

Stent migration or encroachment
Deployed stents occasionally migrate into the left atrium, where they can be a nidus for thrombus or the focus of atrial ectopy. Similarly, stent encroachment on proximal pulmonary vein branches could result in obstructed flow or branch occlusion, resulting in reduced pulmonary outflow and pulmonary hypertension.

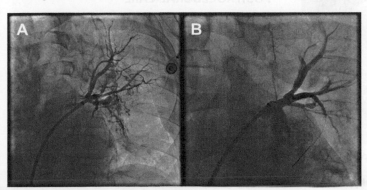

Fig. 5. Left upper pulmonary vein with severe stenosis before (*A*) and after (*B*) stent placement.

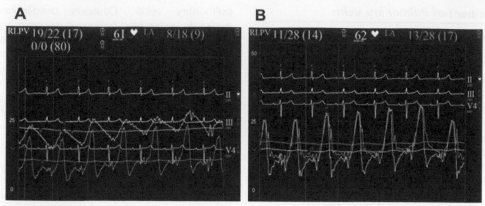

Fig. 6. Pressure measured in the left atrium and in the pulmonary vein proximal to a severe stenosis. Before stenting, there is a significant gradient across the stenotic lesion (*A*). After stenting, there is no residual gradient (*B*).

Pulmonary vein rupture

Overstretching of the pulmonary vein could result in rupture, manifesting as a pericardial effusion or hemoptysis. Covered stents should be readily available to treat this complication.

Pulmonary hemorrhage

Pulmonary vein hemorrhage is a potentially serious procedural complication and is typically the result of perforation of the pulmonary veins or pulmonary capillary leaking in patients with severe pulmonary venous hypertension. Careful assessment of patients who have hemoptysis during the procedure is crucial to prevent significant morbidity.

Stroke

As with any instrumentation of the left atrium, there is a small but significant risk of stroke during and immediately after the procedure. The use of a stable, consistently active anticoagulant such as bivalirudin during the procedure can significantly reduce this risk. In shorter procedures, heparin can also be safely used for procedural anticoagulation, although bivalirudin is still preferred when possible.

Other Considerations

Staged procedures

In patients with stenoses of multiple pulmonary veins, a staged approach with multiple procedures may be necessary to reduce the risks associated with contrast and prolonged radiation exposure.

Selective bilateral lung intubation

In patients presenting with preexisting hemoptysis, severe pulmonary hypertension, history of radiation to the chest, or any other clinical syndrome that suggests a higher risk of hemorrhage, selective bilateral lung intubation can significantly reduce morbidity from pulmonary hemorrhage as the lung not reliant on drainage from the stenotic pulmonary vein can be protected.

POSTPROCEDURAL CARE

After the procedure, patients should be closely monitored with close observation of noninvasive hemodynamics and telemetry. Although rare, significant pericardial effusions, pulmonary hemorrhage, or interruption of pulmonary veins can occur and are potentially devastating. Intensive care unit monitoring, therefore, is strongly recommended for the night after PVS is performed. On average, patients who tolerate the procedure well can be discharged on postoperative day 2.

Apart from routine care of vascular access sites, no designated rehabilitation program is required.

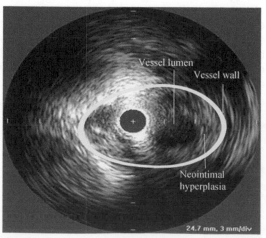

Fig. 7. Intravascular ultrasound image of pulmonary vein lumen with severe stenosis. There is significant luminal encroachment from neointimal hyperplasia.

Clinical Recovery

Most symptoms, including dyspnea and chest pain, will improve immediately after PVS. In a case series of symptomatic patients undergoing stenting for iatrogenic PVS, 9 of 10 patients had complete improvement of their symptoms within 24 hours after PVS; this effect persisted during almost 4 years of clinical follow-up.[12] Although other case series have suggested that the treatment effect is not so profound,[14] most reports in the literature do show some improvement in clinical symptoms (dyspnea, exercise intolerance) after luminal modification of the pulmonary veins.[12,15]

Anticoagulation Strategy

The duration and selection of anticoagulants after stenting of the pulmonary veins vary greatly among practitioners. Some have called for the use of long-term warfarin to prevent pulmonary artery thrombi in the territory of the stented veins.[16] Our experience however, suggests that 3 months of aspirin (Aspirin) and clopidogrel (Plavix) therapy may be sufficient to reduce the risk of stent thrombosis and that the risk benefit analysis of long-term therapy may favor its use only in select cases.

FOLLOW-UP

Clinical evaluation of symptoms should occur on a regular basis, as there is a moderate risk of recurrence even 2 to 4 years after stenting,[12] primarily associated with in-stent restenosis (ISR). If clinical suspicion of stent failure arises, CT angiography (see **Fig. 1**), V/Q scanning (see **Fig. 2**),[17] or transesophageal echocardiography[13] can be used to identify recurrent lesions.

Restenosis

Balloon angioplasty alone has a higher rate of restenosis when compared with stenting (72% vs 33%, respectively, in one series[6]). Therefore, stenting is the favored approach by most operators as the initial mode of therapy. Nevertheless, ISR remains a significant problem, with reports of significant ISR of greater than 50% at one year in other series.[14,15] Late restenosis at more than 24 months has also been reported.[12] Larger stents (>6 mm) are less likely to experience ISR. The relative frequency of ISR and the great variance in clinical presentation have prompted some to advocate for annual screening CT angiography or transesophageal echocardiography in patients undergoing PVS. At least, any symptoms that could be suggestive of ISR should be evaluated immediately with an imaging modality that can define the anatomy. Anatomic resolution is better with CT angiography and is the preferred modality to diagnose ISR.

If ISR is found, the therapeutic options are somewhat limited. Drug eluting stents are rarely available in the size required for pulmonary vein stenting, and even when available, their efficacy is not clear. Covered stents have been used in the past to treat ISR with some success, although further study is required to understand its true efficacy. A novel therapy, enteric sirolimus therapy after pulmonary vein stenting, has met with some success in reducing recurrent restenosis in a small case series.[18] Finally, the use of drug eluting balloons has been suggested in the treatment of congenital PVS.[19] To our knowledge, drug eluting balloons have not been used in adults with iatrogenic PVS, but this therapy may hold promise for the treatment of ISR in this population.

SUMMARY

Pulmonary vein isolation is emerging as a successful treatment strategy for patients suffering from AF. Still PVS remains the most troublesome long-term complication from this procedure. The diagnosis of PVS is not always straightforward, and a high index of clinical suspicion is required to make the diagnosis via CTA angiography/MRA, V/Q scanning, or echocardiography. Endovascular stenting offers the possibility of restoring pulmonary venous blood flow with symptom relief. However, the procedure is technically challenging and associated with ISR rates in excess of 50%.

REFERENCES

1. Haissaguerre M, Jais P, Shah DC, et al. Electrophysiological end point for catheter ablation of atrial fibrillation initiated from multiple pulmonary venous foci. Circulation 2000;101:1409–17.

2. Chen SA, Hsieh MH, Tai CT, et al. Initiation of atrial fibrillation by ectopic beats originating from the pulmonary veins: electrophysiological characteristics, pharmacological responses, and effects of radiofrequency ablation. Circulation 1999;100:1879–86.

3. Purerfellner H, Aichinger J, Martinek M, et al. Incidence, management, and outcome in significant pulmonary vein stenosis complicating ablation for atrial fibrillation. Am J Cardiol 2004;93:1428–31 A1410.

4. Saad EB, Rossillo A, Saad CP, et al. Pulmonary vein stenosis after radiofrequency ablation of atrial fibrillation: Functional characterization, evolution, and

influence of the ablation strategy. Circulation 2003; 108:3102–7.

5. Cappato R, Calkins H, Chen SA, et al. Updated worldwide survey on the methods, efficacy, and safety of catheter ablation for human atrial fibrillation. Circ Arrhythm Electrophysiol 2010;3:32–8.

6. Prieto LR, Schoenhagen P, Arruda MJ, et al. Comparison of stent versus balloon angioplasty for pulmonary vein stenosis complicating pulmonary vein isolation. J Cardiovasc Electrophysiol 2008;19: 673–8.

7. Qureshi AM, Prieto LR, Latson LA, et al. Transcatheter angioplasty for acquired pulmonary vein stenosis after radiofrequency ablation. Circulation 2003;108:1336–42.

8. Packer DL, Keelan P, Munger TM, et al. Clinical presentation, investigation, and management of pulmonary vein stenosis complicating ablation for atrial fibrillation. Circulation 2005;111:546–54.

9. Mansour M, Refaat M, Heist EK, et al. Three-dimensional anatomy of the left atrium by magnetic resonance angiography: implications for catheter ablation for atrial fibrillation. J Cardiovasc Electrophysiol 2006;17:719–23.

10. Nanthakumar K, Mountz JM, Plumb VJ, et al. Functional assessment of pulmonary vein stenosis using radionuclide ventilation/perfusion imaging. Chest 2004;126:645–51.

11. Robbins IM, Colvin EV, Doyle TP, et al. Pulmonary vein stenosis after catheter ablation of atrial fibrillation. Circulation 1998;98:1769–75.

12. Neumann T, Kuniss M, Conradi G, et al. Pulmonary vein stenting for the treatment of acquired severe pulmonary vein stenosis after pulmonary vein isolation: clinical implications after long-term follow-up of 4 years. J Cardiovasc Electrophysiol 2009;20:251–7.

13. De Potter TJ, Schmidt B, Chun KR, et al. Drug-eluting stents for the treatment of pulmonary vein stenosis after atrial fibrillation ablation. Europace 2011;13:57–61.

14. Di Biase L, Fahmy TS, Wazni OM, et al. Pulmonary vein total occlusion following catheter ablation for atrial fibrillation: clinical implications after long-term follow-up. J Am Coll Cardiol 2006;48:2493–9.

15. Latson LA, Prieto LR. Congenital and acquired pulmonary vein stenosis. Circulation 2007;115:103–8.

16. Holmes DR Jr, Monahan KH, Packer D. Pulmonary vein stenosis complicating ablation for atrial fibrillation: clinical spectrum and interventional considerations. JACC Cardiovasc Interv 2009;2:267–76.

17. Wong KK, Gruenewald SM, Larcos G. Ventilation-perfusion mismatch resulting from iatrogenic pulmonary vein stenosis after radiofrequency ablation: a case report. Clin Cardiol 2009;32:E67–70.

18. Bromberg-Marin G, Tsimikas S, Mahmud E. Treatment of recurrent pulmonary vein stenoses with endovascular stenting and adjuvant oral sirolimus. Catheter Cardiovasc Interv 2007;69:362–8.

19. Mueller GC, Dodge-Khatami A, Weil J. First experience with a new drug-eluting balloon for the treatment of congenital pulmonary vein stenosis in a neonate. Cardiol Young 2010;20:455–8.

Percutaneous Mitral Valve Interventions

Alice Perlowski, MD[a], Ted Feldman, MD, FESC, FSCAI[b,c],*

KEYWORDS

- Balloon mitral valvuloplasty • Mitral valve interventions • Mitral regurgitation
- Percutaneous interventions

KEY POINTS

- Balloon mitral valvuloplasty (BMV) was the first effective catheter therapy for mitral valvular heart disease. The technique and device approach was initially reported by Inoue in 1982 and, remarkably, is virtually unchanged between then and now.
- Rheumatic mitral stenosis is historically one of the most common heart diseases worldwide, and BMV is the therapy of choice in most patients with symptomatic rheumatic mitral stenosis.
- Medical therapy is basically ineffectual for mitral regurgitation, one of the most common types of heart valve disease.
- Surgical intervention is the standard of care for patients with symptoms and severe mitral regurgitation, particularly for degenerative mitral regurgitation.
- Several percutaneous approaches based on surgical repair techniques are in development and early clinical use.

PERCUTANEOUS INTERVENTIONS FOR MITRAL VALVE DISEASE

Percutaneous interventions for mitral valve disease represent both the oldest and the newest of catheter interventions. Balloon mitral valvuloplasty (BMV) was the first effective catheter therapy for valvular heart disease. The technique and device approach was initially reported by Inoue in 1982 and, remarkably, has been virtually unchanged between then and now.[1] Conversely, novel catheter therapies to repair mitral regurgitation (MR) are now in their infancy, with only the earliest human experience. This article details both of these therapies.

BALLOON VALVULOPLASTY FOR MITRAL STENOSIS

Rheumatic Mitral Stenosis

Rheumatic mitral stenosis is historically one of the most common heart diseases worldwide. This disease remains an important diagnostic entity globally but is increasingly infrequent in the United States. Most of the rheumatic heart disease in the United States is seen in immigrants importing the entity from Mexico, Central and South America, and Asia. Some strains of streptococci associated with skin or kidney infections have been implicated as causing rheumatic fever and rheumatic heart disease in outbreaks in the United States.[1]

Because the problem of rheumatic fever is so infrequent in the United States, we often forget that the initial disease requires specific therapy.[2] The disease process of rheumatic fever attacks not only the valves but also produces a pancarditis. Pancarditis may affect both atrial and ventricular tissues. Atrial fibrillation in association with rheumatic mitral stenosis is, thus, probably caused by both left atrial distention and primary involvement of the atria in the rheumatic process.

[a] University of Chicago Hospital, Chicago, Illinois, USA; [b] NorthShore University HealthSystem, Evanston, Illinois, USA; [c] Division of Cardiology, Evanston Hospital, Walgreen Building 3rd Floor, 2650 Ridge Avenue, Evanston, IL 60201, USA
* Corresponding author. Division of Cardiology, Evanston Hospital, Walgreen Building 3rd Floor, 2650 Ridge Avenue, Evanston, IL 60201.
E-mail address: tfeldman@northshore.org

Intervent Cardiol Clin 2 (2013) 203–224
http://dx.doi.org/10.1016/j.iccl.2012.09.002
2211-7458/13/$ – see front matter © 2013 Elsevier Inc. All rights reserved.

interventional.theclinics.com

Mitral stenosis is synonymous with rheumatic disease. When rheumatic disease is excluded, there are several infrequent causes of mitral stenosis, which should be considered. Congenital, carcinoid disease, and eosinophilic endomyocardial fibroelastosis are rare causes of this problem. An entity seen with increasing frequency is calcific mitral stenosis. This entity is associated with severe mitral annular calcification. Although several years ago it was seen mostly among patients undergoing chronic hemodialysis, as the population ages and calcific valvular disease becomes more common, mitral stenosis caused by leaflet calcification rather than commissural fusion is becoming more common.

The critical feature that distinguishes rheumatic mitral stenosis from calcific disease is commissural fusion. Rheumatic commissural fusion occurs almost exclusively in association with thickening of the subvalvular apparatus and with associated involvement of other valves. In contrast, patients with non-rheumatic calcification of the leaflets as the cause of mitral stenosis demonstrate calcifications that involve the annulus that extend toward the body of the leaflets, with freedom of movement of the leaflet tips and little or no involvement of the chordae tendineae. In the setting of calcific disease, there is no commissural fusion.

The clinical presentation of mitral stenosis is dyspnea on exertion, which is the hallmark of the disease. Patients present with shortness of breath and are frequently misdiagnosed with other chronic lung diseases, including asthma or pulmonary fibrosis. Exercise intolerance and dyspnea are uniformly present unless patients are sedentary.

The history is confounded by most patients with mitral stenosis downregulating their activity to minimize symptoms. With exercise, the cardiac output increases and there is a disproportionate increase in both left atrial and pulmonary artery pressures. Many patients deny limitations in exercise tolerance, and exercise testing can be helpful when the symptomatic status of patients is ambiguous. Among patients with borderline indications for intervention, serial exercise testing over a period of years can be very helpful (**Fig. 1**).[3]

Echocardiographic Evaluation

Transthoracic echocardiography is critical for defining the cause and severity of mitral stenosis and assessing patients for BMV. A scoring system that uses 4 morphologic characteristics of the valve and valve apparatus has been described to characterize the severity of mitral deformity.[4] Descriptions of leaflet mobility, leaflet thickening, calcification, and subvalvular involvement on a 4-point scale are used. A score of 1 represents minimal deformity and a score of 4 represents severe deformity. This system is subjective and there is significant interobserver variability. Nonetheless, this represents a useful common language for the description of valve deformity in mitral stenosis. Scores of 8 or less have been associated with excellent long-term results from BMV, whereas scores greater than 12 have been

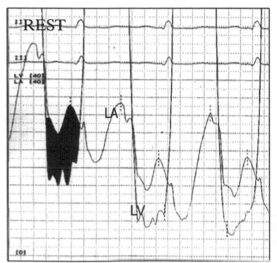 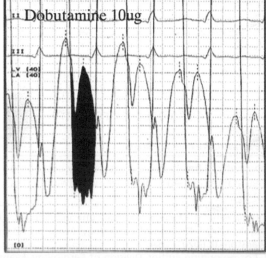

Fig. 1. Dobutamine stress is used to demonstrate a dramatic increase in the transmitral pressure gradient. Simultaneous left atrial (LA) and left ventricular (LV) pressure are shown. The transmitral gradient has been filled in with solid black. There is a dramatic increase in the transmitral gradient with dobutamine infusion, mimicking the increase in LA and pulmonary pressure typically seen with exertion in these patients.

associated with poorer long-term outcomes and, importantly, a higher incidence of MR complicating BMV.[5] Patients with scores between 9 and 12 have intermediate outcomes. The eventual survival rate for low-score patients over 5 years exceeds 80% and declines to about 60% among those with intermediate scores. The score cannot be used to arbitrarily decide which patients are candidates for BMV. Older patients with high scores are often poor candidates for any form of therapy and are treated with BMV rather than surgery because surgical risks are prohibitive. In this setting, BMV is palliative.

Commissural fusion is assessed using a short-axis transthoracic echocardiographic view. Symmetric fusion in the absence of leaflet calcification is associated with the best balloon dilatation outcomes.[6] Asymmetry of the fusion or calcification of the commissures gives poorer results from BMV. Symmetric fusion lends itself to splitting of both commissures in a more predictable fashion, whereas asymmetry with one heavily calcified and one noncalcified but fused commissures may lead to splitting of only the more pliable commissure.

In the assessment of patients for BMV, coronary angiography is indicated for those with symptoms suggestive of ischemia, poor left ventricular function, and history of coronary artery disease. It is also recommended for men and postmenopausal women older than 35 years and for postmenopausal women when risk factors for coronary artery disease are present.

Patient Selection

BMV is the therapy of choice in most patients with symptomatic rheumatic mitral stenosis (**Box 1**).[7] Balloon therapy is recommended for symptomatic patients with a valve area of less than 1.5 cm^2 who have favorable valve morphology, no left atrial

---

Box 1
Indications for balloon mitral commissurotomy

CLASS I

1. Balloon mitral commissurotomy (BMC) is effective for symptomatic patients (NYHA functional class II, III, or IV) with moderate or severe mitral stenosis (MS) and valve morphology favorable for BMC in the absence of left atrial thrombus or moderate to severe MR. (Level of evidence: A)

2. BMC is effective for asymptomatic patients with moderate or severe MS and valve morphology that is favorable for BMC who have pulmonary hypertension (pulmonary artery systolic pressure greater than 50 mm Hg at rest or greater than 60 mm Hg with exercise) in the absence of left atrial thrombus or moderate to severe MR. (Level of evidence: C)

CLASS IIa

1. BMC is reasonable for patients with moderate or severe MS who have a nonpliable calcified valve, are in NYHA functional class III to IV, and are either not candidates for surgery or are at a high risk for surgery. (Level of evidence: C)

CLASS IIb

1. BMC may be considered for asymptomatic patients with moderate or severe MS and valve morphology favorable for percutaneous BMC who have a new onset of atrial fibrillation in the absence of left atrial thrombus or moderate to severe MR. (Level of evidence: C)

2. BMC may be considered for symptomatic patients (NYHA functional class II, III, or IV) with a mitral valve (MV) area greater than 1.5 cm^2 if there is evidence of hemodynamically significant MS based on pulmonary artery systolic pressure greater than 60 mm Hg, pulmonary artery wedge pressure of 25 mm Hg or more, or mean MV gradient greater than 15 mm Hg during exercise. (Level of evidence: C)

3. BMC may be considered as an alternative to surgery for patients with moderate or severe MS who have a non pliable calcified valve and are in NYHA functional class III to IV. (Level of evidence: C)

CLASS III

1. BMC is not indicated for patients with mild MS. (Level of evidence: C)

2. BMC should not be performed in patients with moderate to severe MR or left atrial thrombus. (Level of evidence: C)

Data from Feldman T. Hemodynamic results, clinical outcome and complications of Inoue balloon mitral valvotomy. Cathet Cardiovasc Diagn 1994;2(Suppl):2–7.

thrombus, and with less than severe MR. Treatment of asymptomatic patients is challenging. Asymptomatic patients with a valve area of less than 1.5 cm^2 may be considered for BMV when the pulmonary artery peak pressure is greater than 50 mm at rest or 60 mm with exercise. New onset of atrial fibrillation is also an indication for valvuloplasty in asymptomatic patients. Patients with moderate to severe mitral stenosis and New York Heart Association (NYHA) class III or IV symptoms with restricted and calcified leaflets and who are at a high risk for conventional surgery are also acceptable candidates for BMV.

Acute Outcomes from BMV

There are several methods to accomplish commissurotomy, which will be discussed later. The clinical and hemodynamic results have been similar regardless of the method used to accomplish commissurotomy. The hemodynamic results are immediate and dramatic.[8] The left atrial pressure and transmitral pressure gradient decline within seconds after a balloon inflation, and the cardiac output increases (**Fig. 2**).[9] The mitral valve area increases. A common confounding condition in older patients is associated left ventricular diastolic pressure elevations from ischemic or hypertensive heart disease. These elevations may diminish the transmitral gradient. The decrease in gradient associated with commissurotomy may be blunted by a higher residual left ventricular diastolic pressure.

In most cases, the mitral valve area increases from 1 cm^2 to almost 2 cm^2. Peak pulmonary artery pressure decreases between 10% and 25%. The decrease in pulmonary hypertension is striking and occurs as soon as the valve has been opened. The decreases in left atrial and pulmonary artery pressure are sometimes associated with spontaneous comments from patients on the catheterization table who note an improved sensation of relief of dyspnea. The pulmonary artery pressure often decreases further over several weeks or months after the procedure. Severe pulmonary hypertension at baseline virtually always improves but does not completely resolve. Atrial fibrillation reverts to sinus rhythm in no more than a quarter of patients, likely because of the rheumatic involvement of atrial tissue and the persistent fibrosis caused by chronic left atrial chamber distention and thickening.

Complications of BMV

An increase in MR occurs in about one-third of patients (**Figs. 3** and **4**).[9] Most of these are by a single grade or less and still associated with a clear favorable clinical benefit. About 2% or 3% of patients require mitral valve replacement during their hospitalizations for BMV because of the precipitation of severe MR. Hospital death occurs in less than 1% of patients, although the availability of surgery for those infrequent cases with severe MR or cardiac perforation from catheter devices is a necessary backup.[10]

Stroke or transient ischemic attack occurring in association with BMV has been minimized by the routine use of transesophageal echocardiographic examinations as a screening tool before BMV. The occurrences of cerebral embolic

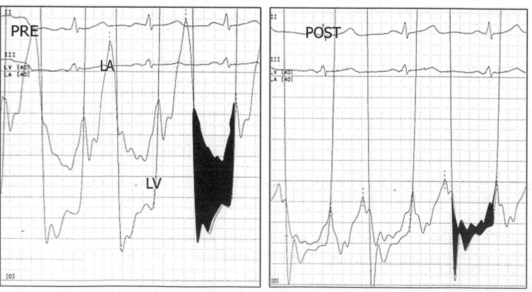

Fig. 2. Results of percutaneous transvenous mitral commissurotomy. The left atrial (LA) and left ventricular (LV) pressures have both decreased with a dramatic decrease in the transmitral pressure gradients.

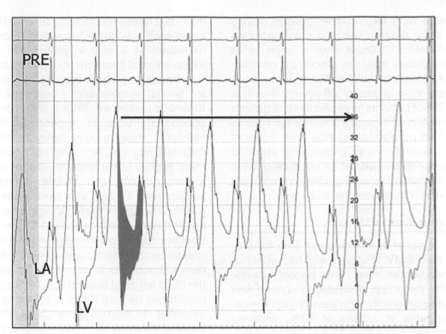

Fig. 3. MR may increase dramatically after percutaneous mitral commissurotomy if the commissures are torn or especially if a leaflet is damaged. The image shows a large persistent transmitral gradient after balloon dilatation with a V wave of 36 mm Hg, which, by itself, is not diagnostic of MR. This image shows the baseline value in a patient with mitral stenosis and only trivial MR by echocardiographic examination. The arrow demonstrates that the peak of the V wave is 36 mm Hg.

complications are, thus, similar to other catheterization procedures. Transseptal puncture may be associated with cardiac perforation in about 1% of cases. Perforations of the ventricle by the

balloon are rare with the Inoue device (Toray Inc, Tokyo, Japan) and are probably more frequent with longer, sharper-tipped balloons used for the double-balloon technique.

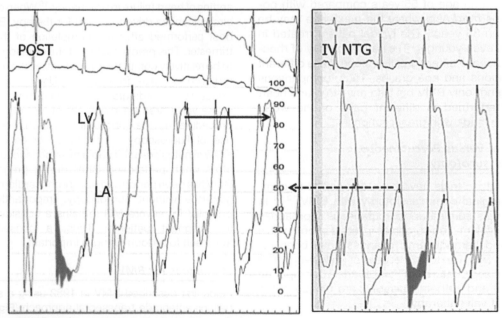

Fig. 4. The *left panel* shows reduction of the transmitral gradient; but the black arrow shows a V wave approaching 90 mm Hg, which represents acute severe MR as a consequence of leaflet damage after balloon inflation. On the *right panel*, intravenous nitroglycerin infusion has been started and the V wave has been decreased to about 50 mm as shown by the dotted line.

The passage of a large-caliber balloon device across the atrial septum requires creation of an atrial septal defect.[11] Shunt flow is seen in all patients immediately after the procedure on color Doppler, but almost all atrial septal defects close spontaneously over a period of several months. Fewer than 2% of patients have shunt ratios greater than 1.5, which might require therapy for volume overload. When persistent shunting does occur, it is typically associated with persistently elevated left atrial pressures because of an insufficient initial BMV result, so that a pressure gradient from the left to the right atrium maintains the shunt flow.

Late Outcomes from BMV

About 70% of patients remain event free for 5 or more years after BMV.[9] Patients with higher echocardiographic scores may have poorer results. Patients with the most desirable anatomy and very little valve deformity may have 5-year event-free survival rates in excess of 80%, whereas those with scores more than 12 and heavily calcified subvalvular apparatus and leaflets may have a 5-year event-free survival of only 50%. In this latter group, palliation is often the goal of therapy.

It is critical to consider the patients individually when defining expectations for BMV outcomes. Similarly, interpreting the results of published reports on BMV requires understanding the patient population that is included in the report. Patients from the United States undergoing BMV are typically a mean age of 55 years compared with populations from Asia where the mean age may be less than 35 years. The typical patient treated in India is even younger. The natural history of rheumatic disease differs greatly among these different populations and age groups. Thus, comparisons among not only BMV but also any structural heart trials performed in different parts of the world must be made with great caution.

Surgical versus Percutaneous Commissurotomy

Randomized trials have been conducted to compare surgical commissurotomy with BMV.[12,13] In these trials, surgical and percutaneous approaches are equivalent. The outcomes in terms of both valve area and hemodynamic changes have been reported with up to a decade of follow-up. The randomized nature of these trials comparing surgical and catheter therapies are unique in the arena of valve therapy.

Special Populations for BMV

The occurrence of left atrial thrombus is frequent in rheumatic mitral stenosis and represents an important relative contraindication for BMV. Transesophageal echocardiographic screening is necessary as a step in preparation for BMV.[14] When left atrial thrombus is detected, anticoagulation therapy may be either initiated or intensified for several months and a reassessment of the thrombus performed. After 2 or 3 months of anticoagulation, 80% of appendage thrombi will resolve.[15] Patients who have a large, mobile thrombus might be best referred for valve replacement surgery to minimize the risk of stroke. Even among patients with mobile thrombus, when surgical risks are also very high, a trial of anticoagulation therapy is useful. In some cases, a laminated thrombus may be seen at the baseline in postanticoagulation transesophageal echocardiographic examinations, usually with a highly echodense shadow as a smooth concave surface in the distal left atrial appendage. Although it is never possible to be sure if this is an organized or soft thrombus, in most of these cases, BMV may be pursued safely. A common misconception is that left atrial smoke on echocardiographic examination is problematic, but this is not a contraindication to BMV.

BMV During Pregnancy

Mitral stenosis will often present during pregnancy as the hemodynamic burden increases and provokes dyspnea or sometimes congestive heart failure. BMV is the procedure of choice in the setting of heart failure in pregnancy.[16] When clinical circumstances drive the need for therapy, BMV is best performed after the completion of the first trimester. This practice allows fetal organogenesis to be relatively complete and minimizes the risks for radiation exposure for the fetus. Use of transesophageal echocardiogram to evaluate improvement in the valve area development of MR during the procedure may be important to help minimize the use of fluoroscopy. Fluoroscopy times of only a few minutes are achievable by experienced operators when performing BMV during pregnancy. BMV has been performed using echocardiographic guidance without fluoroscopy. Importantly, the potential for severe MR remains a consideration for pregnant patients. Thus, a conservative approach to balloon sizing is important.

Techniques for BMV

Inoue first described BMV in 1982 using a single-balloon antegrade transseptal approach (**Fig. 5**).[17] Several techniques have been described to accomplish BMV. The uses of conventional large balloons either as a single- or double-balloon approach have also been used (**Fig. 6**).[18,19] Dilatation is, for

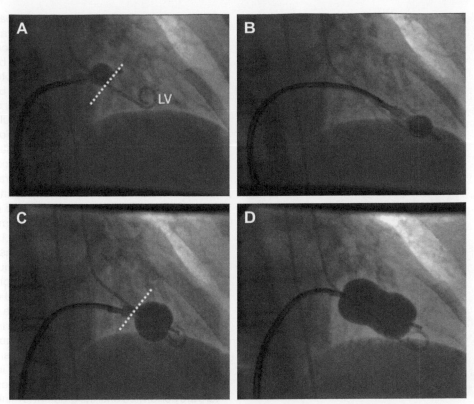

Fig. 5. Inoue balloon commissurotomy. (*A*) The partially inflated balloon on the left atrial side of the plane of the mitral valve, denoted by the dashed line. A pigtail catheter is in the left ventricle (LV). (*B*) The partially inflated balloon has been passed across the mitral orifice into the LV apex. (*C*) The balloon is pulled back to engage the mitral valve and finally inflated in (*D*) to split the mitral commissures.

all practical purposes, always performed using an antegrade approach with a transseptal puncture for left atrial access. Retrograde access to the valve via the aorta is only rarely used.[20] A metal commissurotome that replicated a folder device used in surgical procedures has also been described, but this device is no longer available (**Fig. 7**).[21,22]

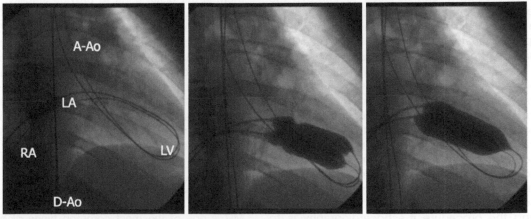

Fig. 6. Double-balloon mitral valvotomy. On the *left panel*, 2 wires are seen looped through the circulation. They traverse from the right atrium (RA) to the left atrium (LA) to left ventricle (LV) to ascending aorta (A-AO) and finally to descending aorta (D-AO). An 8-mm peripheral balloon can be seen on the superior wire dilating the interatrial septum to enable passage of the 2 conventional balloons. The *middle panel* shows the 2 balloons across the mitral valve with a waist caused by the stenotic commissures. In the *right panel*, after full inflation of the balloons, the waist has been eliminated with commissural splitting.

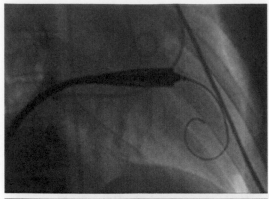

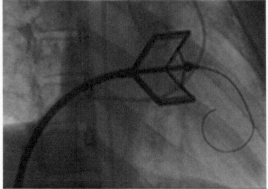

Fig. 7. Metal commissurotome. A rigid commissurotome is passed across the mitral valve over an extra stiff guidewire as seen in the *upper panel*. Squeezing a handle outside of the patient opens the blades of the commissurotome with resultant commissural splitting, with the open blades shown in the lower panel.

Transseptal puncture for access of the left atrium is a ubiquitous part of this procedure. Imaging with transesophageal or intracardiac echocardiography can be used to improve the safety and accuracy of the transseptal puncture. The fossa ovalis is easily seen using echocardiographic imaging; when a transseptal needle is engaged in the fossa, an indentation or tenting of the fossa is seen. One common challenge faced during transseptal pucture in these patients is the bowing of the intraatrial septum caused by left atrial pressure overload. The concave shape often makes it difficult to engage the fossa ovalis because of the inadequate reach of the transseptal needle. Placing a larger curve on the transseptal needle may help with this problem.

Intracardiac echocardiography eliminates the need for general anesthesia or heavy sedation during the procedure if echocardiography is to be used for guidance. The only liability for intracardiac echocardiography is the need for an additional femoral venous puncture.

The most commonly used balloon for BMV is the Inoue balloon catheter (see **Fig. 5**). This catheter is introduced into the left atrium and the partially inflated balloon is used to traverse the mitral annulus and pass into the left ventricle. The balloon inflates in 3 stages.[23] Use of the partially inflated balloon to cross the mitral valve minimizes the potential for entanglement in the chordae. After the balloon is passed into the left ventricular chamber, the distal end is inflated fully and the balloon is pulled back to engage the mitral orifice. As the balloon is inflated further, the proximal portion inflates and creates a dog bone configuration. This configuration self-centers and engages the mitral orifice. When the balloon is completely inflated, the middle section opens and expands the commissures ideally, with splitting of the commissural fusion.

The balloon can be inflated with increasing inflation volumes of dilute contrast. The sequential or stepwise approach is the most common technique for attempting to achieve a maximal diameter while still having the chance to assess the pressure gradient and potential for MR in between inflations. Assessments with hemodynamics, echocardiography, and repeat ventriculography, as needed, are performed in between balloon inflations. Successive inflations at increasing balloon diameters are performed until the gradient is minimized or MR begins to increase. The judgment about when to stop performing additional inflations is one of the most challenging parts of the procedure.

BMV can also be performed using the double-balloon technique (see **Fig. 6**). Two conventional balloons of between a 15 and 20 mm diameter are used together. The most common approach is to place 2 wires into the left ventricle or to route them into the left ventricular apex and anchor them in the distal aorta to provide stability. The conventional balloons are significantly longer than the Inoue balloon and have sharp tip segments. It is more common with conventional balloons to have the balloon catheter tip or guidewire cause left ventricular apical perforation. A double-balloon procedure may also be performed using a single wire across the mitral valve, with a monorail balloon system. This procedure allows 2 balloons to be advanced over a single wire. This technique is called the *multi-track* technique (**Fig. 8**).[24]

PERCUTANEOUS APPROACHES FOR TREATMENT OF MR

MR is one of the most common types of heart valve disease. Medical therapy is basically ineffectual.[25] Surgical intervention is the standard of care for patients with symptoms and severe MR, particularly for degenerative MR. Surgical mitral valve repair uses annuloplasty in almost all cases and

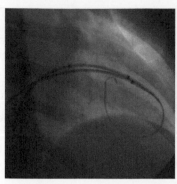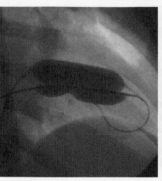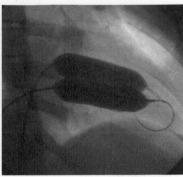

Fig. 8. The Multi-Track system (NuMED, Hopkinton, NY). In the *left panel*, a single wire has been passed through the atrial septum into the left ventricle. Two balloons can then be passed over the wire. In the *middle panel*, a superior balloon can be seen to be riding on a monorail tip while the inferior balloon is over the wire. In the *right panel*, the balloons have been fully expanded.

leaflet and chordal repair for degenerative disease. Less invasive methods for mitral repair are clearly desirable. This point is particularly true for patients with advanced age and other comorbidities. The indications for surgical intervention for MR are for 3 to 4+ MR with symptoms or some indicator of left ventricular dysfunction (**Box 2**).[8]

The earliest suggestions for percutaneous therapy for valvular heart disease involved the use of a wire device for pulmonic valvuloplasty.[26] The idea that MR might be treated nonsurgically was first proposed by Afieri in his description of a surgical method for double orifice mitral valve repair.[27,28] This suggestion preceded the development of viable percutaneous approaches for MR by a decade.

Some of the earliest devices proposed for percutaneous mitral repair attempted to mimic surgical annuloplasty.[29] The simplest approach for percutaneous annuloplasty seemed to be via the coronary sinus. The coronary sinus parallels the mitral annulus and can be accessed easily from the venous system, making it attractive for a catheter therapy. Several methods for direct annuloplasty have also been described using retrograde transventricular delivery. The first percutaneous treatment of MR to be used successfully in large numbers of patients is a leaflet repair technique mimicking the Alfieri edge-to-edge or double-orifice repair.

Technologies for percutaneous mitral valve replacement are in the earliest stages of development. When these catheter devices were first developed in animal models, there were predictions that coronary sinus annuloplasty would be used in thousands of patients within several years because of its simplicity and that percutaneous aortic valve replacement would move more slowly.[30] The opposite has occurred.

Transcatheter aortic valve replacement has now been used in tens of thousands of patients. Percutaneous mitral repair using the MitraClip (Abbott Vascular, Menlo Park, CA) leaflet approach has been used in more than 5000 patients, whereas the aggregate of annuloplasty approaches has been used in only several hundred.

Annuloplasty Approaches

Attempts to mimic surgical annuloplasty with catheter-based methods have used either indirect or direct techniques. Indirect annuloplasty via the coronary sinus has been attempted with several devices. Although the route of delivery is simple, getting devices to work in the coronary sinus has proved remarkably difficult. Among the challenges for coronary sinus annuloplasty are the fact that the coronary sinus is usually superior to the true annulus, there is variability in the crossing over of circumflex coronary artery branches by the coronary sinus, and torsional forces resulting from coronary sinus movement that have led to wire fracture in many of the devices attempted in this location. Device fracture in the coronary sinus and the occurrence of myocardial infarction from circumflex compression have led to several entrants in this field failing altogether and withdrawing from the marketplace.

Indirect Annuloplasty

Among the indirect angioplasty devices, only the Carrillon Mitral Contour System (Cardiac Dimensions, Kirkland, Washington) device remains under development. An initial trial of this device showed some efficacy in reducing MR but suffered wire frame fracture in several cases after a few months following implantation. Importantly, wire fractures were not associated with clinical complications

Box 2
Indications for mitral valve operation for MR

CLASS I

1. Mitral valve (MV) surgery is recommended for symptomatic patients with acute severe MR. (Level of evidence: B)

2. MV surgery is beneficial for patients with chronic severe MR and NYHA functional class II, III, or IV symptoms in the absence of severe left ventricular (LV) dysfunction (severe LV dysfunction is defined as ejection fraction <0.30) and/or an end-systolic dimension greater than 55 mm. (Level of evidence: B)

3. MV surgery is beneficial for asymptomatic patients with chronic severe MR and mild to moderate LV dysfunction, ejection fraction 0.30 to 0.60, and/or end-systolic dimension 40 mm or more. (Level of evidence: B)

4. MV repair is recommended over MV replacement in most patients with severe chronic MR who require surgery, and patients should be referred to surgical centers experienced in MV repair. (Level of evidence: C)

CLASS IIa

1. MV repair is reasonable in experienced surgical centers for asymptomatic patients with chronic severe MR with a preserved LV ejection fraction greater than 0.60 and an end-systolic dimension less than 40 mm in whom the likelihood of successful repair without residual MR is greater than 90%. (Level of evidence: B)

2. MV surgery is reasonable for asymptomatic patients with chronic severe MR, preserved LV function, and a new onset of atrial fibrillation. (Level of evidence: C)

3. MV surgery is reasonable for asymptomatic patients with chronic severe MR, preserved LV function, and pulmonary artery systolic pressure greater than 50 mm Hg at rest or greater than 60 mm Hg with exercise. (Level of evidence: C) MV surgery is reasonable for patients with chronic severe MR caused by a primary abnormality of the mitral apparatus, NYHA class III to IV symptoms, severe LVEF less than 0.30, and/or an end-systolic dimension greater than 55 mm in whom MV repair is highly likely. (Level of evidence: C)

CLASS IIb

1. MV repair may be considered for patients with chronic severe secondary MR caused by severe LV dysfunction (ejection fraction <0.30) who have persistent NYHA functional class III to IV symptoms despite optimal therapy for heart failure, including biventricular pacing. (Level of evidence: C)

CLASS III

1. MV surgery is not indicated for asymptomatic patients with MR and preserved LV function (ejection fraction >0.60 and end-systolic dimension <40 mm) in whom significant doubt about the feasibility of repair exists. (Level of evidence: C)

2. Isolated MV surgery is not indicated for patients with mild or moderate MR. (Level of evidence: C)

Data from Feldman T. Hemodynamic results, clinical outcome and complications of Inoue balloon mitral valvotomy. Cathet Cardiovasc Diagn 1994;2(Suppl):2–7.

and, surprisingly, were also associated with maintained efficacy of reduction of MR in some cases.[31] Further improvements in this device seem to have eliminated the issue of wire fracture. Bench testing is now able to reproduce the wire fracture problem in older-generation devices, and the newest renditions of the device do not commonly have this problem. A recent report documented the outcomes in 50 patients treated with this device.[32] The implant success rate was two-thirds. The remainder of the patients either had coronary sinus anatomy not suitable for the device or transient circumflex compression that precluded leaving the device in place. Among the remainder of the patients, there were improvements in MR severity; left ventricular volumes; and clinical parameters, such as quality of life after 1 year. This device has approval in Europe, and larger trials will be needed to demonstrate the efficacy of the device and reducing MR compared with medical therapy in patients with severe MR and heart failure.

Direct Annuloplasty

Attempts to create direct percutaneous annuloplasty have been divided into transventricular approaches and a transatrial approach. Two companies have transventricular methods. A guide catheter is placed across the aortic valve and into the left ventricle to provide access to the mitral annulus from below the posterior leaflet. The Guided Delivery Systems Accucinch device (Guided Delivery Systems, Santa Clara, CA) places a delivery system below the posterior mitral leaflet on the ventricular side, through which between 10 and 20 nitinol anchors are delivered. These anchors are tethered by a drawstring, which is tensioned to reduce the mitral annulus. Several patients have been treated, but the device is still under development. Mitralign (Mitralign Inc., Tewksbury, MA) is a transventricular device that places 2 pairs of pledgets on either side of the mitral orifice. Each pair is tensioned to reduce the mitral circumference. Similarly, this device is in the early stage of development. A third direct annuloplasty concept is the placement of a mitral band via transseptal catheterization. After access to the left atrium, screwlike anchors are placed in the annulus with a background band that can be tensioned after the anchors have been placed. This device has been used intraoperatively, and a percutaneous technology is under development.

Percutaneous Mitral Leaflet Repair

Afieri described a method for surgical approximation of the mitral leaflets in the early 1990s.[29] Simple sutures were used to create an edge-to-edge repair with a resulting double orifice or figure-of-8 orifice. This method was used primarily in patients with degenerative MR and isolated anterior leaflet prolapse. Stable results for as long as 12 years postoperatively have been reported.[33]

The surgical edge-to-edge technique led to the development of a percutaneous method that recapitulates the double-orifice repair. The MitraClip is delivered percutaneously via transvenous, transseptal access to the left atrium. The device is navigated through the left atrium and across the mitral orifice where it is aligned to grasp the leaflets. It is then closed to approximate the leaflet edges.[34,35]

Animal model studies demonstrated the healing response after application of the MitraClip.[36] A tissue bridge forms over the device, connecting the 2 leaflets,[37] which leads to long-term anatomic durability. The healing response in patients seems to be similar. The first MitraClip implant in a human patient was performed in Caracas, Venezuela in June 2003. The patient was a 49-year-old woman who suffered from bileaflet flail and severe symptomatic MR. The clip was successfully deployed reducing her MR to less than 2+. The patient's symptoms resolved completely, and follow-up echocardiograms demonstrated stable MR grade and normalization of left ventricular dimensions and ejection fraction at the 2-year follow-up. The first case in the United States was performed several days later at Evanston Hospital as part of the initial EVEREST (Endovascular Valve Edge-to-Edge Repair Study) phase I registry.

MitraClip Procedural Steps

The basic steps of the MitraClip procedure are illustrated using a case example in **Figs. 9–22**. The baseline MR is shown in **Fig. 9**. Transseptal puncture is performed to create a favorable trajectory from the atrial septum to the mitral valve orifice (see **Fig. 10**). After the MitraClip is navigated to the mitral orifice at the source of the MR jet, the clip arms are opened and the device oriented so that the arms are perpendicular to the line of mitral coaptation (see **Figs. 11** and **12**). The open clip arms are then passed across the mitral orifice into the left ventricle (see **Figs. 13** and **14**) and then pulled back to grasp the mitral leaflets (see **Fig. 15**). At that point, a careful assessment of leaflet insertion into the clip is made before attention is turned to evaluating a reduction in MR (see **Fig. 14**). Finally, the MR reduction is assessed (see **Fig. 16**). If the reduction in MR is not adequate, a decision must be made regarding the placement of a second clip. Part of this determination requires the measurement of the residual mitral valve area at that point to be sure that mitral stenosis will not be created by the placement of an additional clip (see **Fig. 17**). If a second clip is thought to be necessary, it is passed adjacent to the first clip to the point of origin of the residual MR jet (see **Figs. 18–21**). Follow-up echocardiography is essential to determine the durability of the reduction and MR (see **Fig. 22**).

EVEREST I

The EVEREST I registry was the initial human experience with the device and included 107 patients.[38] Almost 80% had degenerative MR, whereas the remainder had functional MR. A clip device was placed successfully in 90% of patients. Two clips were used in one-third. Acute procedural success, defined as placement of 1 or more clips resulting in 2+ or less MR, was 74%. At the 3-year follow-up, 70% of patients remained free of surgical intervention. Eighty-four percent of the surgical procedures performed after the clip

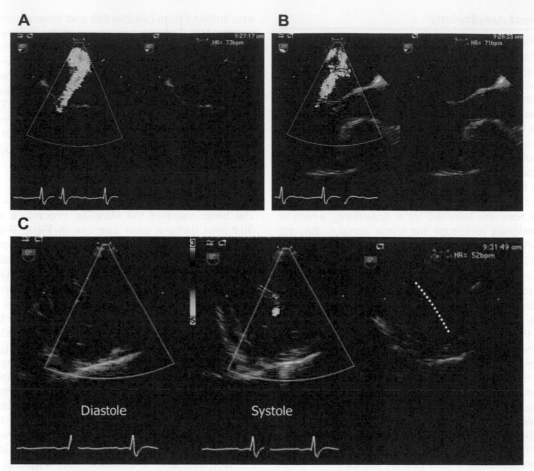

Fig. 9. Preprocedure echocardiographic images of MR in an 81-year-old woman with a history of tuberculosis and resultant chronic obstructive pulmonary disease. She has a history of hypertension with chronic kidney disease and a creatinine level of 2.2. She had coronary artery bypass graft surgery in 1999 and percutaneous coronary intervention several years ago. The left ventricular ejection fraction is 45%. She lived independently and was able to perform light housework and shopping until recent progressive dyspnea on exertion occurred, and she was hospitalized with congestive heart failure. (*A, B*) The preprocedure echocardiogram showed a regurgitant volume of 49 mL, regurgitant fraction of 56%, and an effective regurgitant orifice (ERO) of 30 mm². The echocardiogram findings were consistent with severe diastolic dysfunction, high filling pressures, dilated left ventricle, and ischemic cardiomyopathy with old transmural inferoposterior infarction. There was moderately severe functional mitral insufficiency with a moderately hypokinetic right ventricle and moderate pulmonary hypertension. (*C*) The short-axis echocardiographic examination shows a central jet, most clearly identifiable as originating from the A2 and P2 segments on the short-axis echocardiograms.

placement were successful. The total major adverse event rate was 9%. Blood transfusions represented the most common event. Death, prolonged mechanical ventilation, and periprocedural stroke represented less common adverse events, each affecting less than 1%. Partial clip detachment (detachment of a single leaflet from the clip) occurred in 9%. Most of these were asymptomatic and detected at the scheduled 30-day echocardiography. Most partial clip detachments were successfully treated with mitral valve surgery. There were no clip embolizations. This initial experience with the MitraClip provided evidence of feasibility and safety.

EVEREST II

The randomized EVEREST II trial was an evaluation of both procedural safety and efficacy.[39] The trial compared the use of the mitral clip with conventional mitral valve surgical repair or replacement with a 2:1 randomization.[40] Patients with 3 or 4 + MR and symptoms were included, regardless of the cause of MR. The primary efficacy end point was the composite of freedom

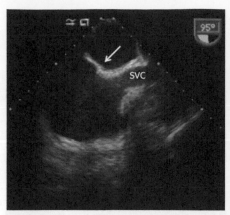
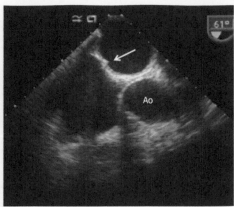

Fig. 10. Transseptal puncture was performed with care to make the puncture posterior and superior. The arrows show tenting of the interatrial septum from the right atrium to the left atrium. The aorta (AO) is anterior, and the superior vena cava (SVC) marks the superior orientation of the puncture.

from surgery for mitral valve dysfunction, 3 or 4 + MR, and death at 12 months. The primary safety end point was defined as a composite of death, myocardial infarction, reoperation for failed mitral valve surgery, nonelective cardiovascular surgery for adverse events, renal failure, stroke, deep wound infection, prolonged mechanical ventilation, gastrointestinal complication requiring surgery, septicemia, new-onset permanent atrial fibrillation, and transfusion of 2 units or more of blood at 30 days.

A total of 279 patients were randomized. Mitra-Clip met the efficacy end point for noninferiority at 12 months. The device group achieved the primary efficacy end point (composite freedom from death, surgery for mitral valve dysfunction, or 3 or 4 + MR) in 55% compared with 73% in the surgical group ($P = .0007$) in an intention-to-treat

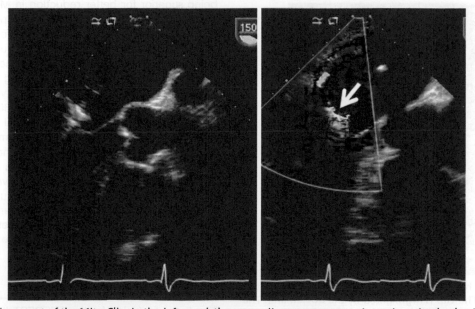

Fig. 11. Placement of the MitraClip. In the *left panel*, the open clip arms are seen above the mitral valve in the left atrium. On the *right panel*, the arrow denotes the MitraClip splitting the regurgitant jet.

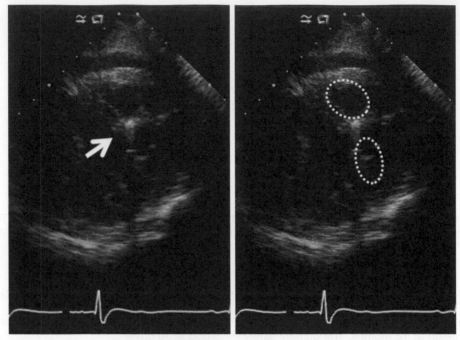

Fig. 12. Short-axis echocardiography demonstrating the MitraClip denoted by the arrow in the center of the *left panel*. On the *right panel*, the double orifice has been marked by the dotted white line.

analysis. The increased rate of surgical referral after MitraClip therapy drove the difference in this composite end point: the need for subsequent surgery was 20.0% in the MitraClip group at 12 months compared with 2.2% for repeat mitral

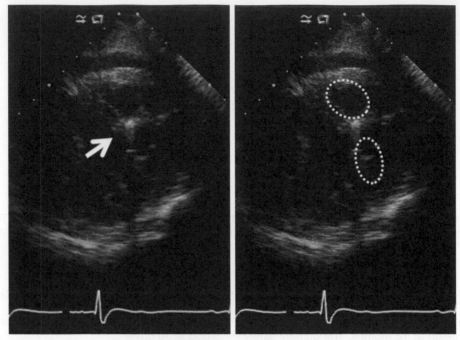

Fig. 13. The open clip arms are seen below the mitral leaflets. The clip is highlighted by the dotted line. The mitral leaflets are seen to be inserted into the closed clip arms.

valve surgery in the surgical group. Importantly, the frequency of death and MR grade 3 to 4 + was not different in the device versus the surgical group, and 80% of the MitraClip recipients avoided surgery in the first 12 months.

The MitraClip continued to meet its efficacy end point for noninferiority at 2 and 3 years, with surgery being superior for better reduction in MR grade. The difference in the composite end point was again weighted by the increased need for surgery for valve dysfunction after the procedure in the percutaneous group (22% vs 4% in the surgical group). The number of patients receiving MitraClip therapy remaining free of surgical intervention at the 2-year follow-up remained close to 80%.

Both percutaneous and surgical groups achieved substantial clinical improvements. At 1 year, 98% of the MitraClip patients and 88% of the surgical patients were NYHA class I/II. Both groups had significant reductions in left ventricular and end diastolic and end systolic volumes and dimensions. Quality-of-life improvements were seen in both groups at 12 months, yet surgery was associated with a transient decrease in quality of life at 30 days.

EVEREST II High Risk Registry

The final conclusion for the EVEREST II randomized trial was that although percutaneous repair

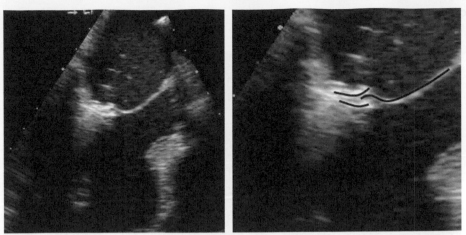

Fig. 14. The leaflet insertion is seen in the *left panel*. The anterior leaflet inserts in between the gripper and clip arm. On the *right panel*, the same image has been enlarged with lines to help identify the gripper, the anterior mitral leaflet, and the clip arm.

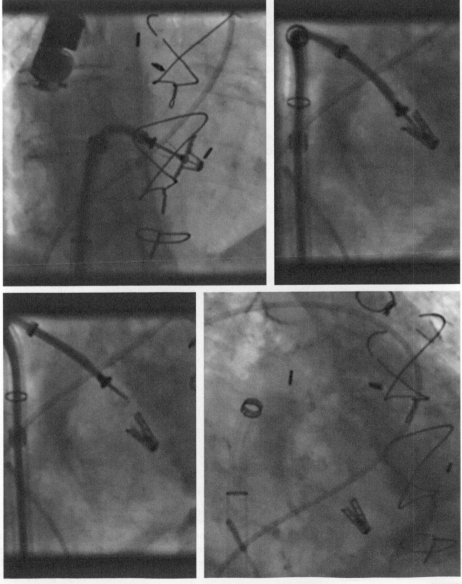

Fig. 15. Fluoroscopic images showing the open clip being passed across the mitral leaflets, the closed clip before release, the closed clip after release, and an image of the first clip implanted on the mitral leaflets.

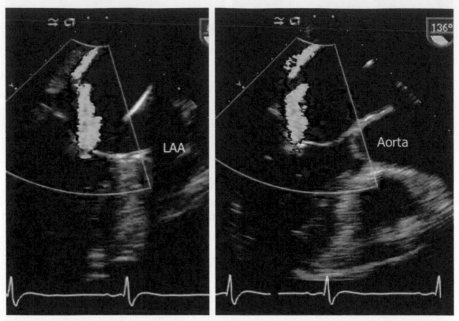

Fig. 16. This transesophageal echocardiographic image shows the degree of residual MR after placement of the first MitraClip. LAA, left atrial appendage.

was less effective at reducing MR than conventional surgery, the procedure was associated with superior safety and similar improvements in clinical outcomes. Subgroup analysis showed that the best results were obtained in older patients with poor LV function and functional rather than degenerative MR.

This finding led to an examination of 211 patients in the high-risk registry.[41] The inclusion criteria included age older than 75 years, left ventricular ejection fraction less than 35%, prior chest surgery, and creatinine levels more than 2.5 mg/dL. Seventy-eight patients with moderate to severe MR and an estimated surgical mortality risk of

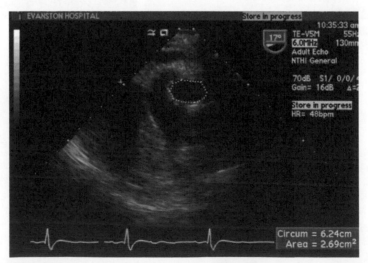

Fig. 17. Planimetry of the short axis shows the superior or medial orifice of the double-orifice valve to have an area of almost 2.7 cm², which verifies that there is enough residual mitral valve area to implant the second clip without causing mitral stenosis. The dotted oval shows tracing of the mitral orifice, from which the area is derived.

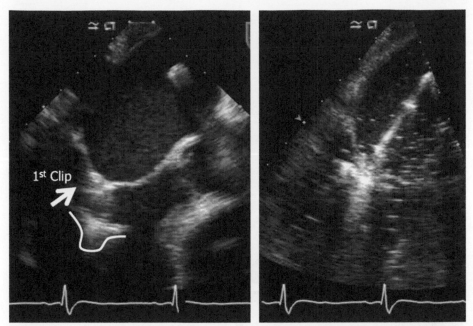

Fig. 18. The first clip is denoted by the arrow on the *left panel*. The white line outlines the MitraClip device. The second clip has been passed across the mitral leaflets into the left ventricle and is seen opened below the mitral leaflets. On the *right panel*, the second clip is pulled back to grasp the leaflets. Bubble contrast is seen in the image, having been released from the delivery system by movement of the clip.

12% or more (measured with the Society of Thoracic Surgery calculator or based on assessment by a surgeon) were enrolled. The prespecified mitral valve anatomic criteria were identical to those used in the randomized trial. The patients were elderly (>75 years of age) with congestive heart failure and coronary artery disease. A substantial number of patients in the high-risk group had previous cardiac surgery (62%), moderate to severe renal disease (23%), chronic obstructive pulmonary disease (35%), and previous myocardial infarction (56%). Most patients in the registry had functional MR (59%), which was substantially higher than the proportion of patients with functional MR in the EVEREST I and EVEREST II randomized trials (approximately 20%). The mean Society for Thoracic Surgery (STS) risk score was more than 12%. Thus, this represented a group of patients who almost never undergo surgery for MR and who present a clinical dilemma for any clinician involved with MR therapy.

Devices were placed successfully in 96% of patients. Most patients had a reduction in MR at discharge (83%), with all but 28.2% achieving a reduction in MR of 2+ or less. At 30 days, 6 months, and 12 months, the patients with MR 2+ or less were 72.9%, 73.3%, and 77.8%, respectively, which represented a statistically significant change from baseline. In the high-risk registry, significant improvements were seen in left ventricular dimensions, NYHA class, and quality-of-life scores at 30 days and 1 year. Annual hospitalizations for heart failure in the high-risk registry were decreased as a result of MitraClip therapy by 45% from baseline. These beneficial effects were present in both the functional MR and degenerative MR groups.

Overall 30-day mortality in the high-risk registry group and control groups were similar (7.7% and 8.3%, respectively), and there was a significantly lower-than-predicted surgical mortality (18.2%) for open-heart MV surgery in this patient cohort (*P* = .006). At 1 year, survival was improved in the high-risk registry group compared with the control group (76.4% vs 55.3%, *P* = .047).

The uniform experience of practitioners treating these very sick patients using this novel device are positive. This group of patients has never had a therapy option in the past, and many respond with excellent clinical outcomes after edge-to-edge repair. The degree of clinical improvement is often discordant with the amount of residual MR. Many patients have persistent 2 + or 3 + MR and, nonetheless, have favorable left ventricular chamber remodeling and symptomatic improvement.

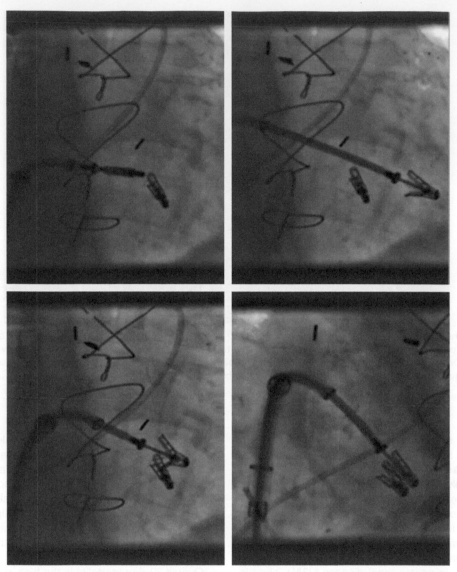

Fig. 19. Fluoroscopic images show implantation of the second clip. On the *upper left panel*, the second clip is closed, positioned in the left atrium before crossing adjacent to the first clip. In the *upper right panel*, the open clip has been passed beyond the mitral leaflets. In the *lower left panel*, the open clip has been pulled back to grasp the leaflets adjacent to the first clip. The *lower right panel* shows the 2 clips in their final position.

Learning Curve

Throughout the course of these trials, substantial experience with a MitraClip device has accrued. These early trials were significantly affected by the learning curve. Even in the randomized pivotal trial, many operators performed only a handful of procedures. Thus, the comparison of MitraClip with conventional surgery represents an embryonic technology in comparison with a decades long established surgical therapy. Between the earliest part of the MitraClip experience, the acute procedure success rate increased from less than 80% to more than 95%. Another important limitation of the device, partial leaflet insertion, was reduced from 90% in the phase I trial to about 1% in the most recent year of international experience. This latter improvement in technique is based on careful attention to the echocardiographic appearance of the leaflets as they drape over the top edge of the MitraClip and insert into the clip. Technique improvements have led to important reductions in procedure duration. The procedure is novel, requiring 3-dimensional navigation through the left atrium and the mitral orifice.

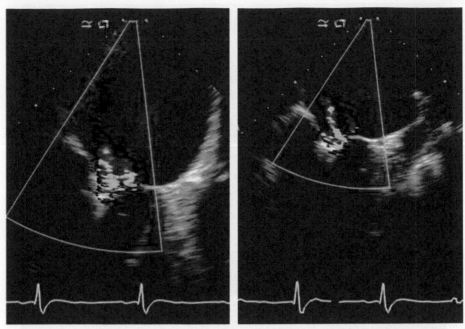

Fig. 20. Transesophageal echocardiographic images show the degree of residual MR after implantation of the second clip.

This procedure often took several hours in the early experience, but improvements in understanding of the steps involved in procedure navigation led to procedure times much closer to 1 hour and often less in the current experience.

Limitations and Anatomic Considerations for MitraClip

The mitral valve morphology requirements for MitraClip therapy are specific. Among patients with

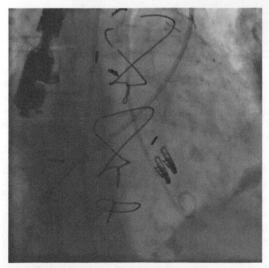

Fig. 21. Fluoroscopic image of the 2 adjacent clips after release. The pigtail catheter is seen in the left ventricular midcavity.

degenerative MR, a coaptation length of at least 1 to 2 mm is needed. A flail gap of less than 1 cm and an MR jet origin less than 15 mm is also recommended. For patients with functional MR, the procedure can be accomplished in the absence of any coaptation length at all; but it is likely that better results for the long-term will occur when there is at least 1 to 2 mm of coaptation initially because when the mitral annulus dilates sufficiently to pull apart the leaflets with no resultant remaining leaflet coaptation, the annular dilatation by itself is a significant problem. These patients may require annuloplasty to ultimately have optimal results. Patients with functional MR and poor left ventricular function have been treated with MitraClip with good 6-month clinical outcomes.[42]

It is not clear what the longer-term response to edge-to-edge repair will be. It is notable that in all of the MitraClip experience, most patients have ejection fractions that are near normal and, thus, do not have sufficient annular dilatation to result in complete separation of the leaflet tips. The concern in the surgical community that annuloplasty is necessary for all patients undergoing repair for MR is counterbalanced by this careful selection for use of the MitraClip, to minimize the proportion of treated patients whereby annular dilatation is a primary part of the etiology of the MR.

A small proportion of patients undergoing MitraClip therapy have significant residual MR requiring surgical repair. A tissue bridge forms over the clip and between the 2 leaflets.[43] Although in

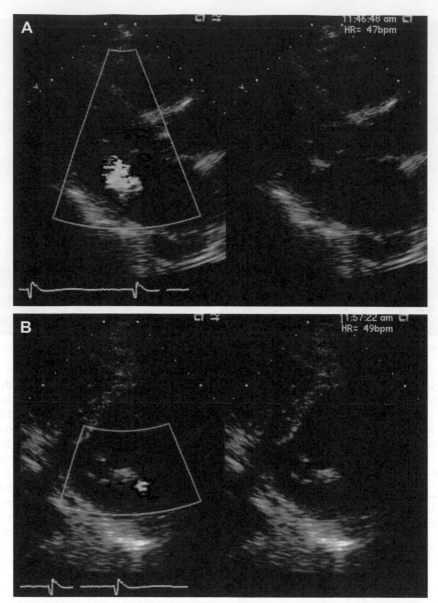

Fig. 22. One-year results in the same patient. In multiple transthoracic echocardiographic views, there is mild residual MR at the conclusion of 1 year. There has been a significant reduction in the quantitative indices of MR severity. The ejection fraction has increased from 45% at baseline to 59% at 1 year. Left ventricular diastolic volume has decreased from 103 mL/m^2 at baseline to 67 mL/m^2 at 1 year. Systolic volume index is decreased from 52 to 31 mL/m^2. The effective regurgitant orifice (ERO) has decreased from 30 mm^2 to 14 mm^2 at 1 year and the regurgitant volume from 46 mL to 22 mL. The regurgitant fraction has decreased from 56% to 35%.

rare cases this may limit the option for subsequent surgical repair, it is clear that, in most cases, surgical repair can be performed. Patients have had successful repair for as long as 5 years after the placement of a MitraClip.[44]

Future Directions for Percuataneous Therapy

The concept of catheter-based mitral valve replacement is a clear logical next step for this field. As a consequence of transcatheter aortic valve replacement, experience with the valve-in-valve therapy for degenerated mitral valve bioprostheses and failed mitral annuloplasty has begun to develop. The placement of a stent mounted bioprosthetic mitral valve in the native mitral annulus is much more complicated. The large size of the orifice and the lack of calcification for anchoring are among the challenges to the development of this therapy. Nonetheless, several

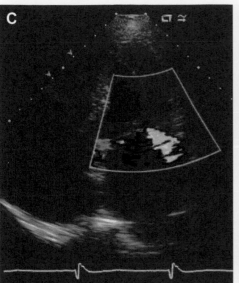 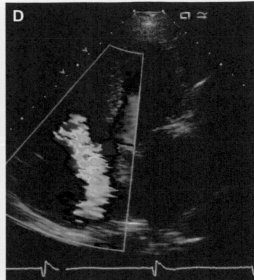

Fig. 22. *(continued)*

efforts are underway to solve this problem. Most of the work in progress is preclinical, but some human experience with percutaneous mitral valve replacement has been done.

Another area for development is chordal replacement. Beating-heart surgical approaches or construction of neo-chordae have been developed. The potential for percutaneous application will require further experience.

REFERENCES

1. Carroll JD, Feldman T. Percutaneous mitral balloon valvotomy and the new demographics of mitral stenosis. JAMA 1993;270:1731–6.
2. Feldman T. Rheumatic heart disease. Curr Opin Cardiol 1996;11:126–30.
3. Hecker SL, Zabalgoitia M, Ashline P, et al. Comparison of exercise and dobutamine stress echocardiography in assessing mitral stenosis. Am J Cardiol 1997;80:1374–7.
4. Wilkins GT, Weyman AE, Abascal VM, et al. Percutaneous balloon dilatation of the mitral valve: an analysis of echocardiographic variables related to outcome and the mecha- nism of dilatation. Br Heart J 1988;60:299–308.
5. Feldman T, Carroll JD, Isner JM, et al. Effect of valve deformity on results and mitral regurgitation after Inoue balloon commissurotomy. Circulation 1992;85:180–7.
6. Levin TN, Feldman T, Bednarz J, et al. Trans-esophageal echocardiographic evaluation of mitral valve morphology to predict outcome after balloon mitral valvotomy. Am J Cardiol 1994;73:707–10.
7. Bonow RO, Carabello BA, Chatterjee K, et al. 2008 focused update incorporated into the ACC/AHA 2006 guidelines for the management of patients with valvular heart disease: a report of the American College of Cardiology/American Heart Association Task Force on Practice Guidelines (Writing Committee to Develop Guidelines for the Management of Patients With Valvular Heart Disease). J Am Coll Cardiol 2008;52:e1–142.
8. Feldman T. Hemodynamic results, clinical outcome and complications of Inoue balloon mitral valvotomy. Cathet Cardiovasc Diagn 1994;2(Suppl):2–7.
9. Ribeiro PA, al Zaibag M, Abdullah M. Pulmonary artery pressure and pulmonary vascular resistance before and after mitral balloon valvotomy in 100 patients with severe mitral valve stenosis. Am Heart J 1993;125:1110–4.
10. Herrmann HC, Lima JA, Feldman T, et al. Mechanisms and outcome of severe mitral regurgitation after Inoue balloon valvuloplasty. J Am Coll Cardiol 1993;22:783–9.
11. Levin TN, Feldman T, Carroll JD. Effect of atrial septal occlusion on mitral area after Inoue balloon valvotomy. Cathet Cardiovasc Diagn 1994;33:308–14.
12. Ben Farhat M, Ayari M, Maatouk F, et al. Percutaneous balloon versus surgical closed and open mitral commissurotomy: seven-year follow-up results of a randomized trial. Circulation 1998;97:245–50.
13. Reyes VP, Raju BS, Wynne J, et al. Percutaneous balloon valvuloplasty compared with open surgical commissurotomy for mitral stenosis. N Engl J Med 1994;331:961–7.
14. Tessler P, Mercier LA, Burelle D, et al. Results of percutaneous mitral commissurotomy in patients

with a left atrial appendage thrombus detected by transesophageal echocardiography. J Am Soc Echocardiogr 1994;7:394–9.

15. Jaber WA, Prior DL, Thamilarasan M, et al. Efficacy of anticoagulation in resolving left atrial and left atrial appendage thrombi: a transesophageal echocardiographic study. Am Heart J 2000;140:150–6.

16. Esteves CA, Munoz JS, Braga S, et al. Immediate and long-term follow-up of percutaneous balloon mitral valvuloplasty in pregnant patients with rheumatic mitral stenosis. Am J Cardiol 2006;98(6): 812–6 [Epub 2006 Aug 2].

17. Feldman T, Herrmann HC, Inoue K. Technique of percutaneous transvenous mitral commissurotomy using the Inoue balloon catheter. Cathet Cardiovasc Diagn 1994;2(Suppl):26–34.

18. Lock JE, Khalilullah M, Shrivastava S, et al. Percutaneous catheter commissurotomy in rheumatic mitral stenosis. N Engl J Med 1985;313:1515–8.

19. Al Zaibag M, Ribeiro PA, Al Kasab S, et al. Percutaneous double-balloon mitral valvotomy for rheumatic mitral valve stenosis. Lancet 1986;1:757–61.

20. Stefanadis CI, Stratos CG, Lambrou SG, et al. Retrograde nontransseptal balloon mitral valvuloplasty: immediate results and intermediate long-term outcome in 441 cases—a multi-center experience. J Am Coll Cardiol 1998;32:1009–16.

21. Cribier A, Rath PC, Letac B. Percutaneous mitral valvotomy with a metal dilatator. Lancet 1997;349:1667.

22. Eltchaninoff H, Koning R, Derumeaux G, et al. Percutaneous mitral commissurotomy by metallic dilator. Multicenter experience with 500 patients. Arch Mal Coeur Vaiss 2000;93:685–92.

23. Feldman T, Carroll JD, Herrmann HC, et al. Effect of balloon size and stepwise inflation technique on the acute results of Inoue mitral commissurotomy: Inoue Balloon Catheter Investigators. Cathet Cardiovasc Diagn 1993;28:199–205.

24. Bonhoeffer P, Piechaud JF, Sidi D, et al. Mitral dilatation with the Multitrack system: an alternative approach. Cathet Cardiovasc Diagn 1995;36:189–93.

25. Fedak P, McCarthy P, Bonow R. Evolving concepts and technologies in mitral valve repair. Circulation 2008;117(7):963–74.

26. Rubio-Alvarez V, Limon R, Soni J. Intracardiac valvulotomy by means of a catheter. Arch Inst Cardiol Mex 1953;23(2):183–92.

27. Maisano F, Torracca L, Oppizzi M, et al. The edge-to-edge technique: a simplified method to correct mitral insufficiency. Eur J Cardiothorac Surg 1998;13(3):240–5.

28. Alfieri O, Maisano F, De Bonis B, et al. The double-orifice technique in mitral valve repair: a simple solution for complex problems. J Thorac Cardiovasc Surg 2001;122:674–81.

29. Feldman T, Cilingiroglu M. Percutaneous leaflet repair and annuloplasty for mitral regurgitation. J Am Coll Cardiol 2011;57:529–37.

30. Stuge O, Liddicoat J. Emerging opportunities for cardiac surgeons within structural heart disease. J Thorac Cardiovasc Surg 2006;132(6):1258–61.

31. Schofer J, Siminiak T, Haude M, et al. Percutaneous mitral annuloplasty for functional mitral regurgitation: results of the AMADEUS trial. Circulation 2009;120: 326–33.

32. Siminiak T, Wu JC, Haude M, et al. Treatment of functional mitral regurgitation by percutaneous annuloplasty-results of the TITAN Trial. Eur J Heart Fail 2012;14(8):931–8.

33. Maisano F, Vigano G, Blasio A, et al. Surgical isolated edge-to-edge mitral repair without annuloplasty: clinical proof of principle for an endovascular approach. EuroIntervention 2006;2:181–6.

34. Cilingiroglu M, Gary G, Salinger MH, et al. Step-by-step guide for percutaneous mitral leaflet repair. Cardiac Interventions Today 2010;4(4):69–76.

35. Gary G, Feldman T. The basic technique for the Evalve MitraClip procedure. In: Feldman T, St Goar F, editors. Percutaneous mitral leaflet repair. London: Informa; 2012. p. 88–101.

36. St Goar FG, Fann JI, Komtebedde J, et al. Endovascular edge-to-edge mitral valve repair: short-term results in a porcine model. Circulation 2003;108(16):1990–3.

37. Fann JI, St Goar FG, Komtebedde J, et al. Beating heart catheter-based edge-to-edge mitral valve procedure in a porcine model: efficacy and healing response. Circulation 2004;110(8):988–93.

38. Feldman T, Wasserman HS, Herrmann HC, et al. Percutaneous mitral valve repair using the edge-to-edge technique: six-month results of the everest phase I clinical trial. J Am Coll Cardiol 2005;46:2134–40.

39. Feldman T, Foster E, Glower DG, et al. Percutaneous repair or surgery for mitral regurgitation. N Engl J Med 2011;364:1395–406.

40. Mauri L, Garg P, Massaro JM, et al. The Everest II Trial: design and rationale for a randomized study of the evalve mitraclip system compared with mitral valve surgery for mitral regurgitation. Am Heart J 2010;160:23–9.

41. Whitlow P, Feldman T, Pedersen W, et al. The EVEREST II High Risk Study: acute and 12 month results with catheter based mitral valve leaflet repair. J Am Coll Cardiol 2012;59:130–9.

42. Franzen O, Baldus S, Rudolph V, et al. Acute outcomes of mitraclip therapy for mitral regurgitation in high-surgical-risk patients: emphasis on adverse valve morphology and severe left ventricular dysfunction. Eur Heart J 2010;31:1373–81.

43. Ladich E, Michaels MB, Jones RM, et al, Virmani R on behalf of the EVEREST investigators. The pathologic healing response of explanted mitraclip devices. Circulation 2011;123:1418–27.

44. Argenziano M, Skipper E, Heimansohn D, et al. Surgical revision after percutaneous mitral repair with the mitraclip device. Ann Thorac Surg 2010;89:72–80.

Transcatheter Occlusion of the Left Atrial Appendage

Mamoo Nakamura, MD[a], Saibal Kar, MD, FSCAI[a,b,*]

KEYWORDS

- Nonvalvular atrial fibrillation • Transcatheter left atrial appendage occlusion
- Ischemic embolic stroke

KEY POINTS

- The left atrial appendage is a major source of thrombi in patients with nonvalvular atrial fibrillation.
- Transcatheter occlusion/exclusion of the left atrial appendage is an important alternative to long-term anticoagulation in patients with nonvalvular atrial fibrillation.
- Morphologic and size evaluation of the left atrial appendage by transesophageal echocardiogram and computerized tomography is crucial for appropriate device selection.
- Transesophageal echocardiogram–guided transseptal puncture is the crucial step of the procedure.
- Most of the clinical experience has been accumulated using the WATCHMAN and the Amplatzer Cardiac Plug devices. Epicardial ligation of the left atrial appendage with the LARIAT device is a novel approach that can be used for selective patients.
- Attention to detail of every procedural step minimizes the complication rate and improves success of the procedure.

INTRODUCTION

Atrial fibrillation (AF) is a major attributable pathology of thromboembolic stroke, particularly in the elderly population.[1] Specifically, in nonvalvular AF, thrombus formation in the left atrial appendage (LAA) is considered to be a main source of major stroke that frequently leads to catastrophic clinical consequence.[2] The current mainstay for the prevention of AF-associated stroke is long-term anticoagulation therapy.[3] However, an incremental risk of bleeding with aging often hampers continuous and long-term use of anticoagulation therapy in the elderly population that generally benefits the most from this treatment.[4] Because the LAA has been shown to be a primary site of thrombus formation in patients with nonvalvular AF,[5] a concept of closure or exclusion of this structure has become an attractive alternative option for oral anticoagulation therapy, specifically in the population with high risk for

anticoagulation-associated bleeding. Accordingly, transcatheter occlusion/exclusion of the LAA has emerged as an innovative procedure that potentially eliminates the necessity for long-term medical anticoagulation therapy to prevent embolic events in patients with nonvalvular AF. This article discusses important key steps that are crucial for successful deployment of these novel devices.

RATIONALE OF TRANSCATHETER LAA OCCLUSION/EXCLUSION FOR STROKE PREVENTION IN NONVALVULAR AF

AF is a powerful predictive factor of ischemic stroke independent of other cardiovascular factors particularly in the elderly population.[1] Moreover, AF-associated ischemic stroke is generally more severe and more likely to be fatal.[2] Most AF-associated stroke is generally considered to occur because of embolism of intracardiac thrombus. This pathology is further supported by the efficacy

[a] Heart Institute, Cedars-Sinai Medical Center, Los Angeles, CA 90048, USA; [b] Interventional Cardiac Research, Heart Institute, Cedars-Sinai Medical Center, UCLA, 8631 West Third Street, Room 415E, Los Angeles, CA 90048, USA
* Corresponding author.
E-mail address: Saibal.Kar2@cshs.org

Intervent Cardiol Clin 2 (2013) 225–234
http://dx.doi.org/10.1016/j.iccl.2012.09.007
2211-7458/13/$ – see front matter © 2013 Published by Elsevier Inc.

of oral anticoagulation in lowering ischemic stroke in this population.[3]

It is well accepted that the LAA is the most common and favorable source of thrombus in patients who develop AF unrelated to rheumatic valvular heart disease. In previously published reviews of multiple studies using transesophageal echocardiography (TEE), autopsy specimens, or direct inspection during surgical intervention, approximately 90% of left atrial thrombi were located in the LAA in patients with nonvalvular AF, whereas only 50% to 60% of thrombi occurred in the LAA in patients with valvular AF.[5,6] Anatomically, the LAA is a pouch-like, discrete trabeculated muscular structure with its orifice located between the left pulmonary vein and the left ventricle. The size of the LAA varies. However, in patients with AF, it tends to be more voluminous and broader, and have larger orifice and fewer branches compared with those with sinus rhythm.[7] AF is also associated with low contractility of the LAA.[8] These anatomic and physiologic changes potentially predispose the LAA to thrombus formation.

Although oral anticoagulation is the gold standard approach for prevention of thromboembolic stroke in patients with AF, this treatment is often underused because of various clinical reasons. Specifically, in elderly patients who are at higher risk of ischemic stroke related to AF and better benefit from this therapy, the oral anticoagulation tends to be suboptimal because this population is more likely to have relative or absolute contraindications or intolerance for this therapy.[4] Furthermore, long-term compliance of oral anticoagulation also progressively declines.[9]

Because most intracardiac thrombus occurs in the LAA in patients with nonvalvular AF, a concept of occlusion/exclusion of the LAA has emerged as an alternative option for stroke prevention. Transcatheter LAA occlusion or exclusion offers several benefits compared with a surgical approach. It is less invasive and therefore carries a safer profile. Furthermore, because of its lesser invasiveness, the postprocedural recovery process is expected to be faster when compared with a surgical approach.

PERCUTANEOUS APPROACHES FOR LAA OCCLUSION/EXCLUSION

There are two major categories of devices available. The first are endovascular devices, which are designed to occlude the ostium of the LAA (**Figs. 1** and **2**). Two main endovascular devices for the LAA occlusion are clinically used worldwide: the WATCHMAN Left Atrial Appendage Closure Device (Boston Scientific, Natick, MA) and the AMPLATZER Cardiac Plug device (ACP device; AGA Medical Corporation, Golden Valley, MN). Both of these devices have CE mark approval in Europe and are available in the United States only as an investigational device. The second approach is an epicardial approach to ligate and exclude the LAA (LARIAT Suture Delivery Device; SentreHEART, Redwood City, CA) (**Fig. 3**). This

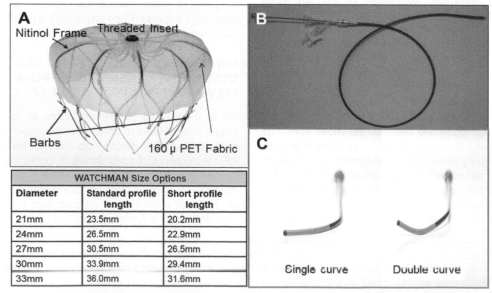

WATCHMAN Size Options		
Diameter	Standard profile length	Short profile length
21mm	23.5mm	20.2mm
24mm	26.5mm	22.9mm
27mm	30.5mm	26.5mm
30mm	33.9mm	29.4mm
33mm	36.0mm	31.6mm

Fig. 1. The WATCHMAN LAA closure technology. The system consists of LAA closure device (A), delivery system (B), and access system (C). Available sizes are listed in **Table 1**.

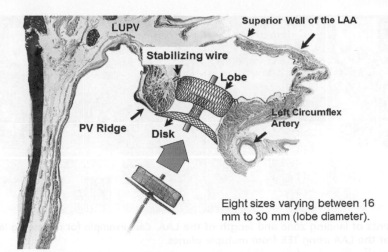

Eight sizes varying between 16 mm to 30 mm (lobe diameter).

Fig. 2. The AMPLATZER Cardiac Plug device. LUPV, left upper pulmonary vein; PV, pulmonary vein. Each arrow indicate anatomic site or a part of device as described.

device has 510 K approval in the United States and is available for clinical use in both markets.

PREPROCEDURAL EVALUATION AND PLANNING
Echocardiography

All candidates for the LAA closure should be evaluated by transthoracic echocardiogram (TTE) for ventricular and valvular function and chamber size. It is important to exclude significant left ventricular dysfunction or severe valve stenosis, which would preclude the patient for an LAA

occlusion procedure. TEE is essential to assess the presence of thrombus and the morphology of the LAA, to help determine the suitability and appropriate size of the device for LAA closure.

The evaluation of orifice (LAA ostium) diameter and length of the LAA is particularly important and should be obtained for multiple angles including 0, 45, 90, and 135 degrees (**Fig. 4**). This can be done by using a three-dimensional TEE probe, which offers X plane function that enables extraction of two orthogonal views concurrently (ie, 0–90 and 45–135 degrees). When assessing the LAA ostial diameter, identification of the LAA

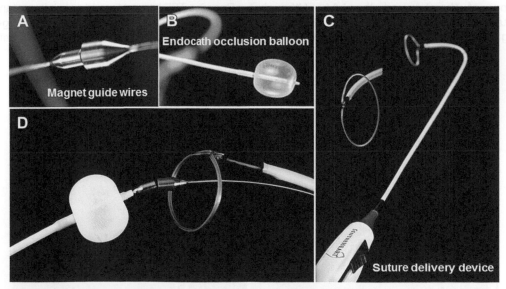

Fig. 3. Components for the percutaneous LAA ligation LARIAT device. (*A*) A 0.025-in endocardial magnet-tipped and an 0.035-in epicardial magnet-tipped guidewire, each with a magnet of opposite polarity enabling an end-to-end alignment. (*B*) A 15-mm compliant occlusion balloon catheter to identify LAA ostium. (*C*) The LARIAT suture delivery device. (*D*) Demonstration of the use of the components as a system to ligate the LAA.

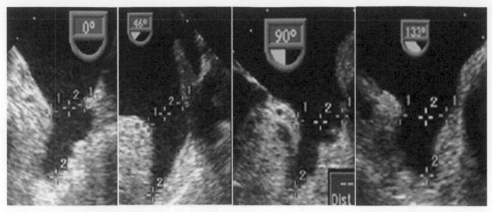

Fig. 4. Measurements of landing zone and length of the LAA. Case example for measuring landing zone (1–1) and length (2–2) of the LAA using TEE from multiple planes.

orifice using certain anatomic landmarks is also an important step. The LAA ostium or landing zone should be measured from the plane of the left coronary trunk to a point approximately 1 to 2 cm from the tip of limbus of the left upper pulmonary vein (see **Fig. 4**). Generally, the measurements are largest in 0- and 135-degree views. Accordingly, it is crucial to obtain measurements in these angles to avoid undersizing of the device. This angle also projects the long axis of the LAA, which is also crucial for positioning of the occluder device (see **Fig. 4**).

Computerized Tomography

Computed tomography of the left atrium (LA) is a very useful noninvasive test to assess the anatomy of the LA and the LAA. Although computed tomography is superior to TEE in determining the morphology of the LAA, TEE is more reliable in measuring the ostium or landing zone for device size selection. There are several morphologic shapes of the LAA, described as chicken wing, broccoli, and so forth. The computed tomography scan is particularly useful when selecting patients for transpericardial ligation of the LAA using the LARIAT device because patients with LAA greater than 40 mm wide in the approach angle or that runs posterior to the pulmonary artery are not suitable candidates for this procedure (**Fig. 5**).

PROCEDURAL APPROACH: COMMON KEY STEPS AND TIPS FOR ENDOVASCULAR APPROACH FOR THE LAA OCCLUSION

Because TEE is used to guide each important step of the procedure, it is performed under general anesthesia, mainly for the safety and comfort of

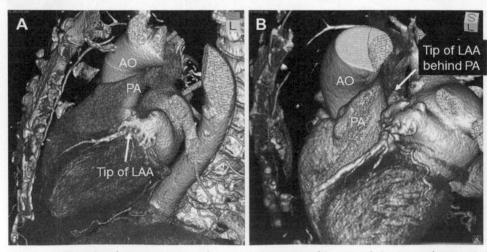

Fig. 5. (A) Three-dimensional reconstruction of computed tomographic scan of the heart shows suitable LAA anatomy for the LARIAT device for ligation. (B) Tip of the LAA (*arrow*) behind the pulmonary artery (PA). This anatomy is not suitable for the LARIAT device. AO, aorta.

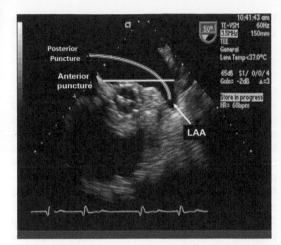

Fig. 6. Transseptal puncture using transeshophageal echocardiogram. The figure shows posterior puncture allows the sheath to be coaxial to the LAA (*arrow*), whereas anterior puncture results in unfavorable sheath position.

the patient. Immediately before obtaining vascular access, preprocedural TEE is performed for repeat assessment of the LAA ostium and to confirm absence of thrombus. Intravenous administration of antibiotics is also given for prophylactic purposes. After venous access is obtained, a transseptal puncture is performed. The location of the transseptal puncture is the most crucial step for the LAA occlusion procedure. Because the LAA arises anterolaterally from the superior aspect of the LA, the puncture site should be at the posterior and inferior aspect of fossa ovalis. This allows the delivery sheath to be coaxial to the long axis of the LAA (**Fig. 6**). For this purpose, fluoroscopic and TEE guidance should be used for site selection of the septal puncture. Bicaval view (90–100 degrees) helps in localizing the puncture site at the inferior aspect, and the short axis view (45–60 degrees) helps in positioning the puncture site at the posterior aspect of the atrial septum (**Fig. 7**). In cases where there is difficulty in crossing the septum, radiofrequency energy can be applied to the hub of the needle to allow easy access into the LA. After successful access is achieved into

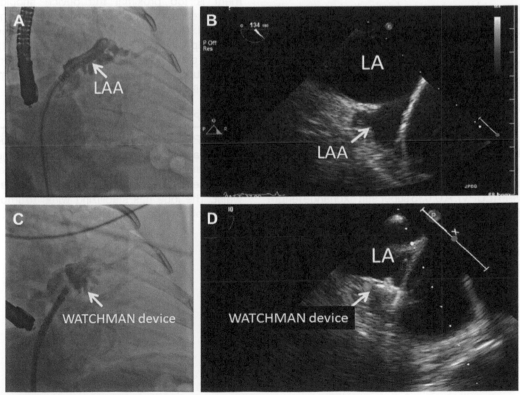

Fig. 7. The WATCHMAN deployment procedure. (*A*) Baseline LAA angiogram from right anterior oblique (RAO) caudal projection. (*B*) Baseline TEE image of the LAA from 135 degrees. (*C*) Final left atrium (LA) angiogram after deployment of the WATCHMAN device shows complete occlusion of the LAA. (*D*) TEE post-WATCHMAN deployment shows successful occlusion of the LAA. (*Arrow* in *A* and *B* indicated the LAA and in *C* and *D* indicated the WATCHMAN device.)

the LA, intravenous heparin is administered and left atrial pressure is measured. If the left atrial pressure is low (<10 mm Hg), additional intravenous fluids are administered, and the LAA dimensions are remeasured.

After successful transseptal puncture, selective access to the LAA is performed using device-specific approaches, discussed later. On successful device deployment, the sheath is then removed from the body. Hemostasis can be achieved through several different approaches. The most common approach is manual compression. However, this requires prolonged bed rest and may not be comfortable for patients. Alternative approaches, such as use of a suture-mediated device or application of figure-of-eight suture on the skin, have been introduced for venous hemostasis of large-caliber sheaths.[10,11]

DEVICE-SPECIFIC PROCEDURAL STEPS AND TIPS
The WATCHMAN Device

The implant is comprised of a self-expanding nitinol frame structure with fixation barbs and a permeable polyester fabric that covers the atrium-facing surface of the device. The implant device is available in five different diameters (21, 24, 27, 30, and 33 mm). The height of the device is equal to the diameter. The device size should be selected based on the LAA ostial/landing zone diameter and it should be 10% to 20% larger.[12,13] The device is preloaded in the delivery system. Delivery of the closure device requires a 12F catheter access sheath that has two different shapes (single and double curves) available.

After successful transseptal puncture, the transseptal sheath is advanced into the left upper pulmonary vein (LUPV). A 0.035 super stiff exchange length wire is then advanced into the LUPV. The sheath is then exchanged for the 12F catheter double or single curve access sheath. The dilator and wire are removed and the large-bore sheath is carefully deaired. A pigtail catheter is then advanced into the large-bore access sheath. Under TEE and fluoro guidance, the pigtail and sheath assembly is gradually withdrawn from the LUPV and gently rotated counterclockwise into the ostium of the LAA. The pigtail is advanced in the LAA and the sheath is then advanced over the pigtail into the LAA. The use of the pigtail catheter minimizes the chance of perforation of the LAA. LAA angiography is then performed by the pigtail catheter in 30-degree right anterior oblique (RAO), 20-degree caudal, and 20-degree cranial projections. The RAO caudal projection is especially useful because it helps in separating the anterosuperior and posterior lobes. It is preferable that the sheath and pigtail be positioned in the anterosuperior lobe.

Then, the device-preloaded delivery catheter is advanced into the tip of the access sheath. The device is deployed by gentle retraction of the sheath (**Fig. 8**). In case of suboptimal distal deployment, the device can be partially recaptured and redeployed again. If the initial deployment is too proximal the device should be recaptured completely and a new device should be used. Before complete release of the device, three important steps must be performed: (1) tug test, (2) compression of the device, and (3) color flow around the device. These three steps confirm the stability of the device.

The ACP Device

The AMPLATZER Cardiac Plug is a transcatheter, self-expanding device constructed from a nitinol mesh and two polyester patches. The device comprises a lobe and a disk connected by a central waist. The lobe has stabilizing wires to improve device placement and retention (see **Fig. 2**). The

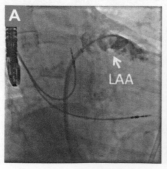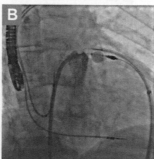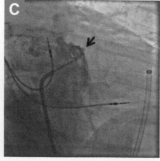

Fig. 8. Fluoroscopic guidance for epicardial LAA ligation using the LARIAT device. All images are in RAO caudal projection. (A) The LAA angiography identifies the ostium and body of the LAA (*arrow*). (B) After verification of the correct position of the snare with the balloon catheter, a left atrial (LA) angiogram is performed before the release of the pretied suture to exclude the existence of a remnant trabeculated LAA lobe. (C) A final LA angiogram is performed to verify LAA exclusion (*arrow*).

device has threaded screw attachments at each end for connection to the delivery and loading cables. The device is available in various sizes from 16 to 30 mm with 2-mm differences. The delivery sheath comes in three different sizes (9F, 10F, and 13F catheter) and three different shapes. The size and shape of the sheath depends on the size and orientation of the LAA.

After successful septal puncture, a 5F or 6F marker pigtail catheter is advanced into the LAA. The LAA angiogram is then performed in RAO cranial and caudal projection. The landing zone of the LAA is measured by angiography and TEE. It is recommended to choose the device size 2 to 4 mm larger than maximum diameter of the landing zone as measured by angiography and TEE. After completion of the angiogram, a 0.035 exchange length extra stiff wire is advanced through the pigtail catheter and the transseptal sheath and pigtail catheter are exchanged for a delivery sheath of suitable shape and size. A tip of the sheath is placed in middle of the body of the LAA. The ACP device is then advanced through the tip of the sheath. The lobe of the ACP is deployed in the LAA at the end of the landing zone by push-pull technique. After the lobe is deployed and anchored, the disk of the device is deployed by retracting the sheath. Ideal device deployment results in tirelike appearance of the device with slight separation of the disk and the lobe. After retraction of the sheath, and before the deployment of the device, adequate size and position of the device is confirmed by TEE and fluoroscopy. The orientation of the device lobe must be consistent with the axis of the intended landing zone in the LAA. Accurate sizing is essential because oversizing and undersizing of the device can cause risk of device embolization.

LAA Suture Ligation Using the LARIAT Device

The LARIAT device comprises three components: (1) a compliant balloon occlusion catheter (Endo-CATH); (2) 0.025- and 0.035-in magnet-tipped guidewires (FindrWRZ); and (3) a 12F catheter suture delivery device (LARIAT) (see **Fig. 3**).

The procedure involves four steps: (1) pericardial followed by a transseptal access, (2) placement of the endocardial magnet-tipped guidewire in the distal aspect of the LAA with the balloon at the ostium of the LAA, (3) connection of the epicardial and endocardial magnet-tipped guidewires for stabilization of the LAA, and (4) snare capture of the LAA with closure confirmation and release of the pretied suture for LAA ligation.

After baseline TEE, anterior pericardial access is achieved using anteroposterior and lateral fluoroscopy using a 17-gauge epicardial needle.[14] After epicardial access is achieved, a 0.035-in guidewire is left in the pericardial space and then the transseptal puncture is performed. The 15-mm occlusion balloon catheter with a magnet-tipped 0.025-in wire is advanced into the apex of the LAA. A 14F catheter epicardial guide cannula is advanced into the epicardial space over the guidewire. A 0.035-in epicardial magnet-tipped guidewire is advanced into the pericardial space through the sheath and the epicardial magnet tip is attached to the endocardial magnet tip. The attached magnet-tipped wire acts as a rail for delivery of the LARIAT snare to the base of the LAA. The endocath balloon helps to position the snare at the ostium of the LAA. After fluoroscopic confirmation the snare is closed. Complete capture of the LAA is confirmed by LA angiography and TEE. The suture is tightened and cut near the LA with a specialized cutter. The pigtail catheter is kept in the pericardial space for 6 to 12 hours.

POSTPROCEDURAL CARE

For the WATHCMAN and the ACP device, the patient is hospitalized in the telemetry floor for overnight monitoring and discharged the following day. All patients are discharged with aspirin and regular dose of warfarin for 45 days. The TEE is performed at 45 days to confirm successful closure and absence of significant thrombus on the device. If the peridevice leak by color flow is less than 5 mm and there is no large thrombus, warfarin is discontinued and clopidogrel is started and continued until 6 months follow-up. At 6 months follow-up, repeat TEE is performed and if this is satisfactory, clopidogrel is discontinued and the patient is treated with aspirin alone indefinitely.

For the LARIAT device, the patient is observed in the intensive care unit overnight. Because the patient has pericardial access, TTE is performed next day. If there is no significant pericardial effusion, the pericardial drainage pigtail catheter is removed. Because there is no device implanted inside the LAA, the patient can be discharged without warfarin and continued on aspirin alone. Similarly, 45-day and 6-month follow-up with TEE is performed. Some patients may require nonsteroidal anti-inflammatory drugs for prolonged chest pain because of reactive pericarditis.

CLINICAL RESULTS: SUMMARY FROM PUBLICATION

Currently, most of the worldwide experience is with the WATCHMAN and the ACP devices.

Between the two devices, the WATCHMAN device has been evaluated more systematically. Both of these devices have CE mark approval in Europe and are available in the United States only as an investigational device. The epicardial LARIAT Suture ligation device has 510 K approval in the United States and CE mark approval in Europe, and is available for clinical use in both markets. A brief summary of trials evaluating each device is presented in **Table 1**.

After demonstration of its feasibility and safety in the pilot study,[12] the WATCHMAN device was studied in a randomized trial (PROTECT AF trial) that enrolled 707 adult patients with nonvalvular AF who had CHAD2 score of one or more in 2:1 ratio (463 for the WATCHMAN and 244 for anticoagulation with warfarin).[13] The patients who received the WATCHMAN device subsequently continued warfarin for 45 days, when it was discontinued if the TEE demonstrated complete occlusion of the LAA or if there was peridevice flow with the jet less than 5 mm in width. These patients then were treated with aspirin (81–325 mg daily) and clopidogrel (75 mg daily) until 6-month follow-up, at which point aspirin alone was continued indefinitely. At 1065 patient-years of follow-up, the trial demonstrated the noninferiority of the WATCHMAN device for primary composite efficacy end point that comprises stroke, cardiovascular death, and systemic embolism compared with oral anticoagulation with warfarin to maintain international normalized ratio between two and three. However, the more frequent primary safety end point that includes major bleeding, pericardial effusion, and device embolization occurred in the patients who underwent the WATCHMAN deployment, raising a concern of the safety profile of this device.

To obtain further efficacy and particularly safety data, the WATCHMAN device was studied in the Continuous Access Protocol registry by experienced operators who participated in PREVENT AF trial. The results of the Continuous Access Protocol registry confirmed a higher procedural success rate (see **Table 1**) and significantly lower complication rate compared with the PROTECT AF trial (3.7% vs 7.7%; P = .007).[15] Importantly, there were no periprocedural strokes, and the pericardial effusion rate was only 2.2% compared with 5.5% in the PROTECT AF trial. The second confirmatory randomized PREVAIL trial has just completed enrolling 400 patients with AF with CHADS2 score greater than two. Patients were randomized 2:1 to the Watchman device or warfarin therapy. It is hoped that if the efficacy data are similar and the complication rate is low, the device will receive Food and Drug Administration approval in the next year.

In contrast to the WATCHMAN device, the clinical published data related to the ACP device have been limited to initial safety and feasibility trials that include small numbers of patients. Two international studies investigated the safety and feasibility of the device.[16,17] In both trials, the successful implantation of the ACP device was performed in 95% or greater than 95% of the enrolled patients. The safety profile of this device from these trials seems to be equivalent to very early experience of the WATCHMAN. A pivotal clinical trial for the ACP device has been initiated and is underway in the United States.[18]

Finally, there has been no randomized study comparing the LARIAT suture device with the other devices or medical therapy. The initial experience of 89 patients has shown that that the procedural success was 96%.[19] Of all the patients who underwent ligation of the LAA, 98% showed complete closure at 1-year follow-up. As expected, there was small number of pericardial access related complications (see **Table 1**).

POTENTIAL COMPLICATIONS AND MANAGEMENT

There are four potential major complications that can be associated with the WATHCMAN and the ACP device: (1) vascular complications, (2) pericardial effusion, (3) periprocedural stroke, and (4) device embolization. The complication rate has dropped significantly with experience. Pericardial effusion seems to be the most common complication, occurring in 1% to 3% of patients. This complication occurs because of faulty transseptal puncture or manipulation of the sheath or the device in the LAA. This complication rate can be minimized by routine use of TEE-guided transseptal puncture and routine use of a pigtail catheter during access into the LAA. The periprocedural stroke rate has dropped dramatically to almost 0%. Careful deairing of the sheath and appropriate anticoagulation can prevent air and thrombus embolization. Device embolization is a rare complication in both devices occurring in less than 2%. Accurate measurement of the LAA size and appropriate placement of the device are essential to avoid this complication. Finally, bleeding from the venous access can occur and cause significant blood loss. Preclosure of the vein with a Proglide suture or application of figure-of-eight subcutaneous suture, and avoidance of low-molecular-weight heparin immediately after the procedure can significantly reduce access site bleeding.

In addition to the previously mentioned complications, pericardial access-related complications

Table 1
Summary of the trials evaluating the WATCHMAN and the AMPLATZER Cardiac Plug device

Study	Device	Study Design	Number of Patients	Summary of Results
Sick et al,[12] 2007	WATCHMAN	Nonrandomized pilot study	66	Implant success; 93% Two device embolization, one air embolism, one delivery wire fracture, two transient ischemic attack, two noncardiac-related deaths
PROTECT AF Holmes et al,[13] 2009	WATCHMAN	Multicenter randomized noninferiority trial	707 (463 for device and 244 for warfarin)	Implant success; 88% No difference in primary efficacy composite end point of stroke, cardiovascular death, and systemic embolism (3% vs 4.9% for device vs control) More frequent primary safety composite end point of major bleeding, pericardial effusion, and device embolization in device arm (7.4 vs 4.4%)
Continuous Access Protocol registry[a] Reddy et al,[15] 2011	WATCHMAN	Nonrandomized continuous access registry	460	Implant success; 95% Procedure- or device-related safety adverse event including bleeding and procedure-related events (pericardial effusion, stroke, device embolization) within 7 d; 3.7% (17 of 460)
ASAP Sievert H TCT 2011	WATCHMAN	Nonrandomized single arm registry (warfarin contraindicated patient)	150	Implant success; 94.7% 1.7% ischemic stroke rate (per 100 patient-years); 77% reduction in expected event rate
Park et al,[16] 2011	ACP	Single-center retrospective preregistry study	143	Implant success; 96% Ten serious complications including three strokes, two device embolizations, five serious pericardial effusions
Lam et al,[17] 2012	ACP	Open-label nonrandomized pilot study	20	Implant success; 95% One catheter-related thrombus, one coronary air embolism, and one TEE-related esophageal injury
Bartus et al,[19] 2012	LARIAT	Open-label single arm	89	Implant success; 96% 98% complete closure at 1 y Three pericardial effusions, two pericarditis, and two late strokes

[a] Results were presented as part of the study comparing complication rate between the device arm of the PROTECT AF trial and the continuous access registry trial.

are uncommon but unique to the LARIAT device. The patient can have pericarditis, accidental right ventricular puncture, or transseptal complications. In addition, reactive pericarditis can occur in a small number of patients (2%–3%) that usually responds to anti-inflammatory medication. Attention to detail at every step of the procedure is critical to minimize the complication rate.

SUMMARY

LAA thrombus is the most important cause of stroke in patients with nonvalvular AF. Transcatheter occlusion/exclusion of the LAA has emerged as an important alternative to long-term anticoagulation in the prevention of stroke associated with AF. Studies using different devices and approaches have been completed or are ongoing that support this hypothesis. Careful preprocedural imaging and attention to detail in the procedure are key factors in ensuring the efficacy and safety of the procedure.

REFERENCES

1. Wolf PA, Abbott RD, Kannel WB. Atrial fibrillation as an independent risk factor for stroke: the Framingham Study. Stroke 1991;22(8):983–8.

2. Lin HJ, Wolf PA, Kelly-Hayes M, et al. Stroke severity in atrial fibrillation. The Framingham study. Stroke 1996;27(10):1760–4.

3. Hart RG, Pearce LA, Aguilar MI. Meta-analysis: antithrombotic therapy to prevent stroke in patients who have nonvalvular atrial fibrillation. Ann Intern Med 2007;146(12):857–67.

4. Hylek EM, D'Antonio J, Evans-Molina C, et al. Translating the results of randomized trials into clinical practice: the challenge of warfarin candidacy among hospitalized elderly patients with atrial fibrillation. Stroke 2006;37(4):1075–80.

5. Blackshear JL, Odell JA. Appendage obliteration to reduce stroke in cardiac surgical patients with atrial fibrillation. Ann Thorac Surg 1996;61(2):755–9.

6. Onalan O, Crystal E. Left atrial appendage exclusion for stroke prevention in patients with nonrheumatic atrial fibrillation. Stroke 2007;38(Suppl 2):624–30.

7. Al-Saady NM, Obel OA, Camm AJ. Left atrial appendage: structure, function, and role in thromboembolism. Heart 1999;82(5):547–54.

8. Pollick C, Taylor D. Assessment of left atrial appendage function by transesophageal echocardiography. Implications for the development of thrombus. Circulation 1991;84(1):223–31.

9. Glader EL, Sjolander M, Eriksson M, et al. Persistent use of secondary preventive drugs declines rapidly during the first 2 years after stroke. Stroke 2010;41(2):397–401.

10. Cilingiroglu M, Salinger M, Zhao D, et al. Technique of temporary subcutaneous "figure-of-eight" sutures to achieve hemostasis after removal of large-caliber femoral venous sheaths. Catheter Cardiovasc Interv 2011;78(1):155–60.

11. Mahadevan VS, Jimeno S, Benson LN, et al. Preclosure of femoral venous access sites used for large-sized sheath insertion with the perclose device in adults undergoing cardiac intervention. Heart 2008;94(5):571–2.

12. Sick PB, Schuler G, Hauptmann KE, et al. Initial worldwide experience with the WATCHMAN left atrial appendage system for stroke prevention in atrial fibrillation. J Am Coll Cardiol 2007;49(13): 1490–5.

13. Holmes DR, Reddy VY, Turi ZG, et al. Percutaneous closure of the left atrial appendage versus warfarin therapy for prevention of stroke in patients with atrial fibrillation: a randomised non-inferiority trial. Lancet 2009;374(9689):534–42.

14. Sosa E, Scanavacca M, d'Avila A, et al. A new technique to perform epicardial mapping in the electrophysiology laboratory. J Cardiovasc Electrophysiol 1996;7(6):531–6.

15. Reddy VY, Holmes D, Doshi SK, et al. Safety of percutaneous left atrial appendage closure: results from the Watchman left atrial appendage system for embolic protection in patients with AF (PROTECT AF) clinical trial and the continued access registry. Circulation 2011;123(4):417–24.

16. Park JW, Bethencourt A, Sievert H, et al. Left atrial appendage closure with Amplatzer cardiac plug in atrial fibrillation: initial European experience. Catheter Cardiovasc Interv 2011;77(5):700–6.

17. Lam YY, Yip GW, Yu CM, et al. Left atrial appendage closure with AMPLATZER cardiac plug for stroke prevention in atrial fibrillation: initial Asia-Pacific experience. Catheter Cardiovasc Interv 2012;79(5): 794–800.

18. Landmesser U, Holmes DR Jr. Left atrial appendage closure: a percutaneous transcatheter approach for stroke prevention in atrial fibrillation. Eur Heart J 2012;33(6):698–704.

19. Bartus K, Han FK, Bednarek J, et al. Percutaneous left atrial appendage suture ligation using the LARIAT in patients with atrial fibrillation: initial clinical experience. J Am Coll Cardiol 2012. [Epub ahead of print].

Index

Note: Page numbers of article titles are in **boldface** type.

A

Alagille syndrome, pulmonary artery stenosis in, 143–145, 148–149

Amplatz devices
    for atrial septal defect closure, 42–46
    for coronary artery fistula closure, 162
    for left atrial appendage occlusion, 226, 230–232
    for membranous ventricular septal defect closure, 90
    for patent foramen ovale closure, 60, 63–64, 68, 70, 73–79
    for sinus of Valsalva rupture repair, 168
    for venous baffle closure, after transposition of the great arteries correction, 156, 160
    for ventricular septal defect repair, after myocardial infarction, 175–177, 179

AndraStents, for aortic coarctation, 117–121, 124

Aneurysm(s)
    atrial septal, patent foramen ovale with, 53, 56, 65–66, 68, 70
    Sinus of Valsalva, 164–169
    ventricular septal, 88

Angel-wings Occluder, for patent foramen ovale closure, 73–79

Angioplasty
    for pulmonary artery stenosis, 132
        in single-ventricle physiology, 148
        lobar branch, 142–143
        proximal main branch, 138–139
        segmental and subsegmental, 143–145
        unifocalized aortopulmonary collaterals, 145–147
    for venous baffle closure, after transposition of the great arteries correction, 157

Annuloplasty approaches, for mitral regurgitation, 211–213

Anticoagulants
    after left atrial appendage occlusion, 231
    after pulmonary vein stenting, 201

Aorta, patent ductus arteriosus origin in, 94

Aortic coarctation, **115–129**
    description of, 115
    diagnosis of, 116
    neonatal, 17, 19–20
    repair of, history of, 115–116
    stenting of
        balloons for, 122
        devices for, 117–122
        indications for, 116–117

outcomes of, 125–127
        technique for, 122–125

Aortic root, enlargement of, patent foramen ovale with, 56–57

Aortic stenosis
    fetal interventions for, 1–2, 6
    neonatal, 11–18

Aortic valvuloplasty
    for aortic stenosis, 11–18
    in fetus, 2, 4–5, 7

Aortopulmonary collaterals, stenosis of, 145–147

Arrhythmias, in atrial septal defect closure, 45

Atrial fibrillation
    ablation of, pulmonary vein stenosis after, stenting for, **195–202**
    left atrial appendage thrombi in, **225–234**

Atrial septal defect
    closure of, **39–49**
        complications of, 44–46
        outcomes of, 42–44
        percutaneous, 39–46
        surgical, 41–42
        techniques for, 39–42
    small, patent foramen ovale with, 56, 68, 70
    with coronary artery fistula, 161

Atrial septoplasty, in fetus, 2, 4–5

Atrial septum, patent foramen ovale in. *See also* Patent foramen ovale.
    aneurysm of, 53, 56, 65–66, 68, 70
    lipomatous hypertrophy of, 54–55, 66–68
    rims of, deficiency in, 57–58

Atrial switch, for transposition of the great arteries, venous baffle stenosis after, 154–157, 160

Avanta stents, for aortic coarctation, 126–127

B

Baffles, in transposition of the great arteries, stenosis or leaks of, 154–157, 160

Balloon(s)
    cutting, for pulmonary artery stenosis, 132–133
    for patent ductus arteriosus stenting, 103, 105

Balloon detunnelization technique, for patent ovale foramen closure, 64

Balloon dilation
    for aortic coarctation, 19
    for aortic stenosis, 11–18

Balloon valvuloplasty, for mitral stenosis, 203–210
    complications of, 206–208
    echocardiography for, 204–205

Intervent Cardiol Clin 2 (2013) 235–239
http://dx.doi.org/10.1016/S2211-7458(12)00152-6

interventional.theclinics.com

Moving?

Make sure your subscription moves with you!

To notify us of your new address, find your **Clinics Account Number** (located on your mailing label above your name), and contact customer service at:

Email: journalscustomerservice-usa@elsevier.com

800-654-2452 (subscribers in the U.S. & Canada)
314-447-8871 (subscribers outside of the U.S. & Canada)

Fax number: 314-447-8029

Elsevier Health Sciences Division
Subscription Customer Service
3251 Riverport Lane
Maryland Heights, MO 63043

*To ensure uninterrupted delivery of your subscription, please notify us at least 4 weeks in advance of move.

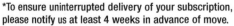

Printed and bound by CPI Group (UK) Ltd, Croydon, CR0 4YY

03/10/2024

01040348-0005